Basic Surgical Skills & Techniques

Basic Surgical Skills & Techniques

FOURTH EDITION

Editors

Sudhir Kumar Jain
MBBS MS FRCS (Edinburgh) FICS FACS MBA (HCA)
Dean/Principal
Hamdard Institute of Medical Sciences and Research
Jamia Hamdard University
New Delhi, India

Mrunal Bharat Kshirsagar
MBBS FCPS (General Surgery) FAMS
Dip MAS (Laparoscopic and General Surgery)
Faculty
Rama Medical College Hospital and Research Centre
Hapur, Uttar Pradesh, India

JAYPEE

JAYPEE BROTHERS MEDICAL PUBLISHERS

The Health Sciences Publisher

New Delhi | London

JAYPEE **Jaypee Brothers Medical Publishers (P) Ltd**

Headquarters
EMCA House
23/23-B, Ansari Road, Daryaganj
New Delhi 110 002, India
Landline: +91-11-23272143, +91-11-23272703,
+91-11-23282021, +91-11-23245672
E-mail: jaypee@jaypeebrothers.com

Corporate Office
4838/24, Ansari Road, Daryaganj
New Delhi 110 002, India
Phone: +91-11-43574357
Fax: +91-11-43574314
E-mail: jaypee@jaypeebrothers.com

Overseas Office
J.P. Medical Ltd
83 Victoria Street, London
SW1H 0HW (UK)
Phone: +44 20 3170 8910
E-mail: info@jpmedpub.com

EU GPSR Authorised Representative
Logos Europe, 9 rue Nicolas Poussin
17000, La Rochelle, France
Phone: +33 (0) 6 67 93 73 78
E-mail: contact@logoseurope.eu

Website: www.jaypeebrothers.com
Website: www.jaypeedigital.com

Inquiries for bulk sales may be solicited at: jaypee@jaypeebrothers.com

Basic Surgical Skills & Techniques
First Edition: 2008
Second Edition: 2013
Third Edition: 2018
Fourth Edition: 2025
Reprint: 2026
ISBN: 978-93-6616-720-6
Printed in India

Dedicated to

Our families,
for their support in spite of their neglection
by us during the process of this work
Our parents, for their blessings
Our teachers, for their wisdom
Our students who inspire us
Our patients, from whom we continue to learn daily

Contributors

David L Stoker BSc MS FRCS
Consultant Upper Gastrointestinal Surgeon
Department of Surgery
North Middlesex University Hospital
London, UK

MD Raihan MD (Dermatology)
Professor and Head
Department of Dermatology
Rama Medical College Hospital and Research Centre
Hapur, Uttar Pradesh, India

Mrunal Bharat Kshirsagar
MBBS FCPS (General Surgery) FAMS
Dip MAS (Laparoscopic and General Surgery)
Faculty
Department of Surgery
Rama Medical College Hospital and Research Centre
Hapur, Uttar Pradesh, India

Raman Tanwar MBBS MS MCh (Urology)
Consultant Urologist
Department of Urology
Jyoti Urocentre
Gurugram, Haryana, India

Sudhir Kumar Jain
MBBS MS FRCS (Edinburgh) FICS FACS MBA (HCA)
Dean/Principal
Hamdard Institute of Medical Sciences and Research
Jamia Hamdard University
New Delhi, India

Preface to the Fourth Edition

The art and science of surgery is rapidly advancing year by year. Newer techniques and instruments are being added every year, and emphasis is on zero-error surgery. We are bringing the fourth edition of this book. The present edition is an attempt to provide far insight of recent advances.

Many chapters such as "Informed Consent, Enhanced Recovery After Surgery, WHO Safety Checklist, Wrong-site Surgery, and Duty of Candor" have been added for the first time. It is a humble effort to cultivate culture of surgical safety. Many chapters, such as General Surgical Instruments, Principles of Robotic Surgery, Basic Surgical Procedures, and Basics of Staplers have been thoroughly revised and updated. All the diagrams have been redrawn to make them more simplified.

With the fourth edition, which has taken an altogether different shape, we hope to enrich the readers with knowledge. We thank the readers for the feedback and support and look forward to constructive criticism.

Sudhir Kumar Jain
Mrunal Bharat Kshirsagar

Preface to the First Edition

Apprentices in surgery need a basic set of practical skills in order to care for their patients well. Although many of these skills are same as those used by their 20th century predecessors, today's trainees need to keep abreast of rapidly changing and advancing technologies that were not available even 10 years ago.

At the same time, basic surgical training for medical students and junior doctors is being compressed into a shorter time frame, as other medical specialties evolve and need to be taught in growing curricula. There is an increasing emphasis on communication skills, and self-directed learning in many undergraduate programs, and the student of surgery today has, therefore, to learn more in less time. He/she will have less "Hands-on" experience in theater, ward, or clinic, and inevitably the practical aspects of surgery tend to suffer.

The aim of this book is to facilitate the more rapid learning required in a modern surgical program, with concise chapters on the main techniques that need to be mastered in the early years of training. It is intended to be read mainly by senior medical students and housemen/interns, but may also be a useful revision for those about to take their first surgical postgraduate examinations. It is the book written by working general surgeons to enhance the practical training of their own teams. It is also an international collaboration between London and New Delhi, and will be of use for students studying the art and science of surgery everywhere. It is not an exhaustive reference book, but more of a brief guide, to be used as a learning tool mainly in operating theaters and emergency rooms.

This book contains simple lists and diagrams with no superfluous text. There are clear explanations which should aid the student from scrubbing up to suturing up. This book is designed to enhance practical training, and the student is encouraged to spend as much time as possible putting the basic skills described to good use in a clinical environment. Surgery remains largely an apprenticeship specialty, where only lots of practice will make perfect.

Sudhir Kumar Jain
David L Stoker

Acknowledgments

Our sincere thanks to Shri Jitendar P Vij (Group Chairman) and Mr Ankit Vij (Managing Director) of M/s Jaypee Brothers Medical Publishers (P) Ltd, New Delhi, India, for the encouragement, support and inspiration. We are grateful to Ms Chetna Malhotra (Senior Director—Professional Publishing, Marketing and Business Development), for helping us by valuable suggestions during the process of this work. We express our special thanks to the whole production team of M/s Jaypee Brothers Medical Publishers (P) Ltd, especially Mr Priyansh Saxena (Development Editor) for their hard work professionalism, and helped throughout the process of this publication.

Contents

CHAPTER 1

Enhanced Recovery after Surgery

Sudhir Kumar Jain, Mrunal Bharat Kshirsagar

"ERAS gives positive and joyful experience to patients, reduces hospital stay and is associated with less complications"

HISTORY OF ENHANCED RECOVERY AFTER SURGERY

Enhanced recovery after surgery (ERAS) originated in 1997 when a group of pioneering general surgeons, led by Henrik Kehlet, introduced the concept during colorectal fast-track surgery. Their collaborative research aimed to improve perioperative care by reducing surgical stress, optimizing nutrition, using nonopioid analgesia, and advocating early postoperative nutrition. As ERAS gained traction, it expanded internationally, leading to significant enhancements in postoperative recovery. The establishment of the ERAS Society in 2010 furthered its mission by disseminating guidelines and launching implementation programs globally. ERAS continues to evolve, representing a flexible approach to patient care that transcends geographical boundaries and fosters innovation in surgical practice and research. Since the late 1990s, ERAS protocols have gained prominence. Spearheaded by a multidisciplinary team including dietitians, surgeons, anesthesiologists, and nurses, ERAS emphasizes a collaborative approach to enhance surgical care across preoperative, intraoperative, and postoperative stages. This evolution reflects a departure from conventional practices toward patient-centric, evidence-based methodologies.

DEFINITION OF ENHANCED RECOVERY AFTER SURGERY

"Enhanced recovery after surgery" embodies a systematic and evidence-based approach to perioperative care aimed at optimizing patient's recovery following surgical interventions. This approach encompasses customized interventions and protocols tailored to each patient's needs throughout the preoperative, intraoperative, and postoperative phases.

PRINCIPLES OF ENHANCED RECOVERY AFTER SURGERY

The principles underlying ERAS focus on patient-centered care and evidence-based practices aimed at enhancing surgical outcomes. Key tenets include:

- *Multidisciplinary collaboration:* ERAS emphasizes seamless collaboration among healthcare professionals from various disciplines to optimize patient's care.
- *Patient's education:* Empowering patients with information about their surgical journey fosters active participation and adherence to ERAS protocols.
- *Preoperative optimization:* Comprehensive preoperative assessments and personalized care plans to identify and

mitigate potential risks, setting the stage for improved outcomes.

- *Minimally invasive techniques:* Utilization of minimally invasive surgical approaches reduces surgical stress and accelerates recovery.
- *Personalized anesthesia:* Tailoring anesthesia regimens to individual patient's needs minimizes postoperative complications and enhances recovery.
- *Effective pain management:* Implementing opioid-sparing pain management strategies reduces reliance on opioids, facilitating faster recovery.
- *Early nutrition and mobilization:* Prompt initiation of oral nutrition and early mobilization promote physiological recovery and reduce the risk of complications.
- *Standardized postoperative care:* Consistent postoperative care protocols ensure continuity of care and further contribute to improved surgical outcomes.

HOW ENHANCED RECOVERY AFTER SURGERY DIFFERS FROM PREVIOUS PERIOPERATIVE PROTOCOL?

The ERAS protocol differs from previous perioperative management protocols in several key aspects, including the *exclusion of certain traditional practices.* Here are some examples of previous protocols or practices that are not typically included in ERAS:

Exclusion Criteria

Prolonged Fasting

Traditional perioperative protocols often involved prolonged fasting periods before surgery to reduce the risk of aspiration. However, ERAS protocols advocate for shorter fasting times, typically around 2 hours for liquids and 4 hours for solids, to minimize patient's discomfort and reduce the risk of dehydration and metabolic stress.

Routine Use of Nasogastric Tubes

Previous perioperative management often included the routine placement of nasogastric tubes to decompress the stomach and prevent postoperative ileus. In contrast, ERAS protocols generally discourage the routine use of nasogastric tubes, opting instead for early removal to promote early oral intake and gastrointestinal function.

Extended Bed Rest

Traditional perioperative care often prescribed extended bed rest following surgery to promote wound healing and prevent complications. However, ERAS protocols emphasize early mobilization and ambulation to reduce the risk of complications such as deep vein thrombosis, pneumonia, and muscle atrophy, and to facilitate faster recovery.

Liberal Fluid Administration

Previous perioperative protocols often involved in liberal fluid administration during surgery to maintain blood pressure and organ perfusion. In contrast, ERAS protocols advocate for euvolemic fluid management strategies to prevent fluid overload, minimize postoperative complications such as pulmonary edema and delayed recovery, and improve patient's outcomes.

High Opioid Use for Pain Management

Traditional perioperative pain management often relied heavily on opioids for pain relief, which can lead to adverse effects such as respiratory depression, nausea, constipation, and prolonged recovery. In contrast, ERAS protocols promote multimodal analgesia techniques that minimize opioid use while providing effective pain control, thereby reducing opioid-related side effects and accelerating recovery.

Routine Use of Urinary Catheters

Previous perioperative management often included the routine placement of urinary catheters during surgery to monitor urine output and prevent urinary retention. However, ERAS protocols advocate for the judicious use of urinary catheters and early removal to reduce the risk of catheter-associated urinary tract infections and facilitate early mobility and discharge.

Overall, the ERAS protocol represents a departure from traditional perioperative management practices by excluding certain protocols or practices that have been associated with increased patient's discomfort, prolonged recovery, and higher complication rates. Instead, ERAS focuses on evidence-based and patient-centered strategies that aim to optimize patient's outcomes, enhance recovery, and improve the overall surgical experience **(Fig. 1)**.

Preoperative phase:

- *Preoperative nutritional assessment:* Comprehensive evaluation of nutritional status to identify and address deficiencies.
- *Advice on termination of cigarette use and alcohol consumption:* Counseling patients to cease smoking and limit alcohol intake to optimize perioperative outcomes.
- *Optimization of chronic diseases:* Management of chronic conditions to ensure stability and reduce perioperative risks.
- *Optimization of physical condition and functionality:* Assessment using standardized scales and interventions to improve physical fitness and functionality.

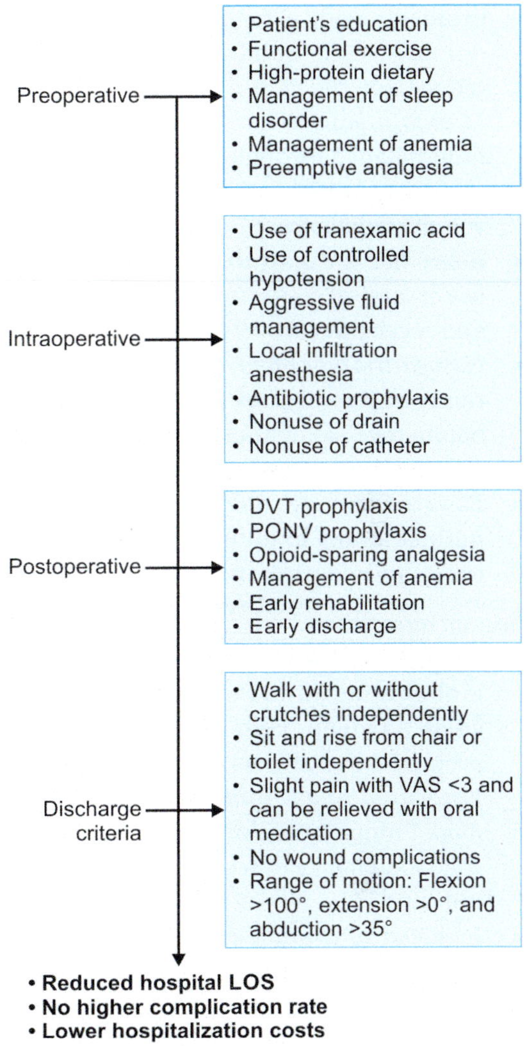

Fig. 1: Enhanced recovery after surgery (ERAS) program protocol. (DVT: deep vein thrombosis; LOS: length of stay; PONV: postoperative nausea and vomiting; VAS: visual analogue scale)

- *Favor minimally invasive surgery:* Preference for minimally invasive surgical approaches to reduce surgical trauma and enhance recovery.

Intraoperative phase:

- *Standardized anesthesia, avoid opioids:* Utilization of standardized anesthesia protocols with a focus on minimizing opioid use to enhance recovery and reduce side effects.

- *Maintain euvolemia:* Ensuring optimal fluid balance throughout the procedure to prevent complications associated with volume imbalances.
- *Restrictive use of drains:* Minimizing the use of surgical drains to reduce discomfort and accelerate recovery.
- *Nasogastric tube removal before anesthetic reversal:* Removal of nasogastric tubes before reversal of anesthesia to facilitate early recovery of gastrointestinal function.
- *Body temperature control:* Maintenance of normothermia to optimize patient's outcomes and reduce the risk of complications.

Postoperative phase:

- *Early mobilization:* Encouraging early mobilization to prevent complications such as deep vein thrombosis and promote faster recovery.
- *Early fluid intake and initiation of solid food:* Prompt initiation of oral fluids and solid food intake to restore hydration and nutrition.
- *Removal of urinary catheter and intravenous fluids:* Early removal of urinary catheters and intravenous fluids to minimize the risk of infections and facilitate mobility.
- *Use of coffee, gum, and laxatives:* Implementation of strategies such as coffee, gum chewing, and laxatives to stimulate bowel function and reduce postoperative ileus.
- *Multimodal strategies for pain control (opioid savers):* Utilization of multimodal analgesia techniques to reduce reliance on opioids and improve pain management.
- *Multimodal approach for control of nausea and antiemetics:* Implementation of multimodal antiemetic strategies to prevent postoperative nausea and vomiting.
- *Early discharge and periodic audit of results:* Facilitation of early discharge and regular audit of outcomes to evaluate the effectiveness of the enhanced recovery program.
- *Preoperative education and patient and family participation:* Provision of preoperative education to patients and their families to enhance understanding and engagement in the recovery process.

KEY POINTS

- *Evidence-based, patient-centered approach:* ERAS replaces traditional practices with evidence-based strategies to enhance recovery and improve patient outcomes.
- *Preoperative optimization:* Focus on nutritional assessment, smoking/alcohol cessation, chronic disease management, physical fitness, and preference for minimally invasive surgery.
- *Standardized anesthesia:* Use of standardized anesthesia protocols, minimizing opioids, and maintaining fluid balance to improve recovery.
- *Minimized surgical trauma:* Restrictive use of drains, early removal of nasogastric tubes, and body temperature control during surgery to reduce complications.
- *Postoperative recovery:* Early mobilization, quick reintroduction of food and fluids, and removal of catheters/IVs to promote faster recovery and reduce infection risks.
- *Pain and Nausea Management:* Multimodal strategies for pain control and antiemetic treatment to reduce opioid use and manage nausea effectively.
- *Early discharge & audit:* Support for early discharge with regular audits to assess ERAS effectiveness and optimize outcomes.
- *Patient and family education:* Preoperative education for patients and families to ensure understanding and active participation in the recovery process.

CHAPTER 2

Informed Consent

Sudhir Kumar Jain, Mrunal Bharat Kshirsagar

"Every surgical trainee should learn to take informed consent to avoid future medicolegal complications"

OBJECTIVE

Objectives of informed consent can be enumerated as follows based on the provided information:

- *Disclosure of adequate information:* The first objective of informed consent is to ensure that patients or research subjects receive comprehensive information about the procedures and treatments they are consenting to. This includes understanding the risks, benefits, and alternatives.
- *Capacity or competency to understand information:* Another objective is to determine whether the patient has the cognitive ability to comprehend the disclosed information. This ensures that consent is given by individuals who are capable of understanding the implications of their decision.
- *Voluntary decision-making:* Informed consent aims to guarantee that the decision to consent is made willingly, without any coercion, force, or deception. This objective emphasizes the importance of autonomy in decision-making.
- *Comprehension of the given information:* It is essential that patients not only receive information but also understand it sufficiently to make an informed decision. This objective ensures that consent is based on a clear understanding of the relevant facts.
- *Consent or agreement to the proposed treatment or procedure:* Ultimately, informed consent seeks to obtain the explicit agreement or consent from the patient or research subject regarding the proposed course of action. This objective formalizes the decision-making process and acknowledges the patient's or subject's acceptance of the outlined risks and benefits.

TYPES OF INFORMED CONSENT

Informed consent is crucial in various aspects of healthcare to ensure patient's autonomy and understanding. Here is a brief explanation of each in **Table 1**.

Treatment

Patients must give informed consent before any medical treatment or intervention, ensuring they understand the nature of the treatment, its potential benefits, risks, and alternatives.

Dissemination of Patient's Information

Patients need to consent to how their personal health information is shared or disclosed,

TABLE 1: Types of consent of healthcare to ensure patient autonomy and understanding.

Standard informed consent	Typical consent used in medical practice and research, where information about treatment or study is disclosed, and the patient/participant decides whether to consent
Implied consent	Consent inferred from actions or circumstances, often used in routine procedures where the patient's presence implies consent
Verbal consent	Consent obtained through spoken communication between the provider/ rsearcher and the patient/participant, suitable when written documentation is not necessary
Written consent	Consent documented by the patient/participant signing a consent form, detailing treatment/study information, risks, benefits, and alternatives
Assent	Agreement from individuals without full legal capacity (e.g., minors or those with cognitive impairments), explaining procedures or studies in understandable terms
Informed consent in emergencies	Waiving or deferring formal consent in emergency situations where immediate intervention is crucial, with information provided as soon as possible
Extended/Detailed Informed consent	Detailed process for complex procedures or experimental treatments, involving thorough information and discussions to ensure understanding and agreement
Broad consent	Agreement for future unspecified research, common in biobanking or genetic studies where specific projects are not yet defined

ensuring privacy and compliance with data protection laws.

Discussion of the Health Insurance Portability and Accountability Act Laws

Healthcare providers must inform patients about their rights under the Health Insurance Portability and Accountability Act (HIPAA), which protects the confidentiality and security of their medical information.

Specific Procedures

Before undergoing any specific medical procedures (such as diagnostic tests or therapies), patients must be informed about the procedure itself, its purpose, and potential risks.

Surgery

Informed consent is particularly critical for surgical procedures, where patients need detailed information about the surgical procedure, potential complications, and postoperative care.

Blood Transfusions

Patients must consent to receive blood transfusions, understanding the purpose, risks (like allergic reactions or infections), and alternatives (if any).

Anesthesia

Before administering anesthesia, patients must be informed about the type of anesthesia planned, its effects, potential side effects, and risks associated with anesthesia administration.

In all these scenarios, informed consent ensures that patients have adequate information to make informed decisions about their healthcare, promoting respect for their autonomy and protecting their rights.

The checklist of informed consent process for surgical procedures:

- *Procedure's name:* Clearly identifies the surgical treatment or procedure proposed.
- *Intended benefits:* Describes expected positive outcomes such as symptom relief, improved function, disease prevention, or life-saving intervention.
- *Alternatives considered:* Discusses alternative treatments, comparing their benefits and drawbacks to the proposed procedure.
- *Risks:*
    - *Frequent:* Common risks include infection, bleeding, organ damage, and anesthesia-related complications.
    - *Serious but rare:* Uncommon risks may include severe bleeding, nerve injury, or adverse reactions to anesthesia.
- *Possible additional procedures:* Addresses supplementary procedures that may be necessary based on the primary procedure's outcome.
- *Sequelae of disease if untreated:* Explains potential disease progression consequences without surgical intervention, such as worsening symptoms or increased health risks.
- *Postoperative complications:* Includes both surgical (infections, bleeding, and organ damage) and anesthetic risks (allergic reactions, respiratory issues, and cardiovascular effects), managed through meticulous preoperative assessment and personalized anesthesia care.
- *Name, signatures, and date:* Documents patient or representative consent, ensuring formal acknowledgment of understanding and agreement with the discussed information.

This structured approach ensures patients to comprehend the full scope of their surgical decision, including potential benefits, alternatives, and associated risks, thereby enabling them to make informed choices about their healthcare.

WHO CAN GIVE INFORMED CONSENT?

Inclusion Criteria

- *Competence:* Individuals must demonstrate the ability to understand the information provided to them.
- *Legal age or emancipation:* They must meet the legal age (India—18 years, United States—16 years) requirement or have legal emancipation status.
- *Voluntariness:* Consent must be given voluntarily without coercion or undue influence.
- *Understanding:* Individuals should comprehend the implications and details of the decision being made.
- *Authorization:* Authorized individuals can provide consent on behalf of someone else, following legal guidelines.

Exclusion Criteria

- *Lack of competence:* Individuals who are unable to understand the information due to cognitive impairment or other factors.
- *Legal incapacity:* Minors who do not meet the legal age requirement or lack emancipation status.
- *Coercion or duress:* Consent obtained under pressure, coercion, or undue influence.
- *Lack of understanding:* Individuals who do not comprehend the information provided.

- *Unauthorized representative:* Individuals lacking legal authorization to provide consent on behalf of another person.

These criteria ensure that informed consent is obtained ethically and legally, respecting the autonomy and rights of individuals while protecting against exploitation or misunderstanding in healthcare decisions.

KEY POINTS

- *Definition of informed consent:* Informed consent is the process by which a patient voluntarily agrees to a medical procedure or treatment after understanding its risks, benefits, alternatives, and potential consequences.
- *Core components:* It includes providing information about the procedure, intended benefits, risks, alternatives, and the consequences of not undergoing treatment.
- *Patient understanding:* The patient must be capable of understanding the information provided, ensuring they can make an informed and voluntary decision.
- *Legal and ethical requirements:* Informed consent is both a legal and ethical obligation to respect patient autonomy and prevent medical malpractice.
- *Competence and voluntariness:* Only competent individuals (of legal age or emancipated minors) can provide consent, and it must be given freely, without coercion or undue pressure.
- *Documentation:* Consent must be documented formally, often through signed consent forms, which include the patient's acknowledgment of understanding.
- *Exclusion criteria:* Individuals who lack competence (due to cognitive impairment), minors not legally allowed to consent, or those under duress cannot give valid informed consent.
- *Role of healthcare providers:* Healthcare providers must ensure patients have received sufficient information, answer questions, and confirm the patient's decision-making capacity before obtaining consent.

CHAPTER 3

Duty of Candor

Mrunal Bharat Kshirsagar, Sudhir Kumar Jain

"Honesty is the best policy"

INTRODUCTION

In light of the duty of candor, transparency means being open and honest, especially when addressing healthcare issues, particularly those that have gone awry.

When mistakes occur, patients rightfully expect:

- A clear and honest explanation of what went wrong.
- Steps that will be taken to address any harm caused.
- Measures to prevent similar incidents from happening again.

To achieve this:

- We must *avoid* fostering a culture of *blame or defensive behavior*.
- Encourage reporting of incidents and conduct objective reviews of these cases.
- Learn from past errors and implement changes to prevent their recurrence.
- Audit changes in practice to ensure lasting improvements.
- Provide necessary support and training to staff for disclosing unforeseen events in patient care and offering apologies when appropriate.

TABLE 1: Principles of candor and their actions.

Principle of candor	***Actions***
Transparency and honesty	• Be open and honest about all aspects of healthcare, especially when things go wrong
Institutional review	• Following the Mid-Staffordshire Public Inquiry, led by Professor Norman Williams and Sir David Dalton, review how to enhance a culture of candor within the NHS
Patient's expectations	• *Patients expect:* – Honest disclosure of what went wrong – Steps to address any harm caused – Actions to prevent future occurrences
Cultural change	Avoid a blame culture and defensive behavior
Incident reporting and review	Encourage structured, objective incident reporting, and review
Learning and improvement	Learn from mistakes and implement changes to prevent recurrence
Auditing and accountability	Audit changes in practice to ensure sustained improvements
Support and training	Provide support and training for staff in disclosing information about unexpected events and offering apologies when appropriate.

(NHS: National Health Service)

SUMMARY

The principle of candor in health care emphasizes transparency and honesty, particularly when addressing errors or adverse events **(Table 1)**. Following the Mid-Staffordshire Public Inquiry, efforts were made to enhance openness within the National Health Service (NHS). Patients rightly expect clear explanations of what went wrong, steps taken to mitigate harm, and measures implemented to prevent future occurrences. Achieving this involves fostering a culture that discourages blame, encourages incident reporting, and conducts objective reviews. Learning from mistakes, implementing changes, and continuously auditing practices are crucial for sustained improvement. Providing support and training for staff to disclose information and apologize when necessary, further strengthens this commitment to patient's safety and accountability.

KEY POINTS

- *Transparency and honesty:* The principle of candor emphasizes openness and honesty in healthcare, especially when addressing errors or adverse events.
- *Post-mid-staffordshire inquiry:* Following the Mid-Staffordshire Public Inquiry, the NHS focused on improving openness and transparency in patient care.
- *Patient expectations:* Patients expect clear, honest explanations regarding what went wrong, what steps were taken to mitigate harm, and measures to prevent future errors.
- *Blame-free culture:* A key aspect of candor is fostering a blame-free culture that encourages reporting incidents and conducting objective reviews to identify issues.
- *Learning and improvement:* Continuous learning from mistakes, implementing changes, and auditing practices are essential for long-term improvement and patient safety.
- *Staff support and training:* Providing staff with training and support to disclose information and apologize when necessary is vital for ensuring accountability and building trust with patients.
- *Commitment to safety:* Candor strengthens the commitment to patient safety by encouraging transparency, improving communication, and holding healthcare providers accountable.

CHAPTER 4

World Health Organization Safety Checklist

Sudhir Kumar Jain, Mrunal Bharat Kshirsagar

"WHO safety check list should be followed in operation theatre to avoid dreaded complications"

INTRODUCTION

The World Health Organization (WHO) estimates that globally, over 7 million individuals will experience complications after undergoing surgery, leading to approximately 1 million deaths. Approximately half of these complications could be prevented. Research by Haynes et al. has shown that there can be reduction of more than one-third in both postoperative morbidity and mortality rates after "WHO Surgery Checklist".

The different components of WHO surgery checklist are following:

1. "Team Brief (Before Anesthesia)"
    - All team members introduce themselves and their roles.
    - Facilitate communication and break down barriers.
    - Empower team members to speak up if they see a departure from routine practice.
    - Discuss each case thoroughly to ensure everyone is informed about patient's history, anesthesia plan, surgical approach, and equipment.
2. "Sign In (Before Induction of Anesthesia)"
    - Confirm patient's identity, surgical site, procedure (make sure that surgical site has been marked), and proper informed consent is taken duly signed by a patient and a surgeon.
    - Mark the surgical site (if applicable).
    - Complete anesthesia checks (machine is properly working and all required drugs are present).
    - Ensure pulse oximeter is attached and functioning.
    - Assess for allergies, difficult airway risk, and blood loss risk.
3. "Time Out (Before Skin Incision)"
    - Confirm each team member introduces himself or herself.
    - Verify patient's identity, surgical site, and procedure with surgeon, anesthetist, and nurse.
    - Confirm prophylactic antibiotic administration and essential imaging.
    - The surgeon reviews critical or unexpected steps, expected blood loss, and operative duration.
    - An anesthetist addresses patient-specific concerns.
4. "Sign Out (Before Patient Leaves Operating Room)"
    - Confirm procedure's name is recorded.
    - Ensure instrument, sponge, and needle counts are correct.
    - Verify specimen labeling.
    - Address any equipment issues.
    - Discuss key concerns for patient's recovery.
    - Document completion of checklist and any issues raised during the procedure.

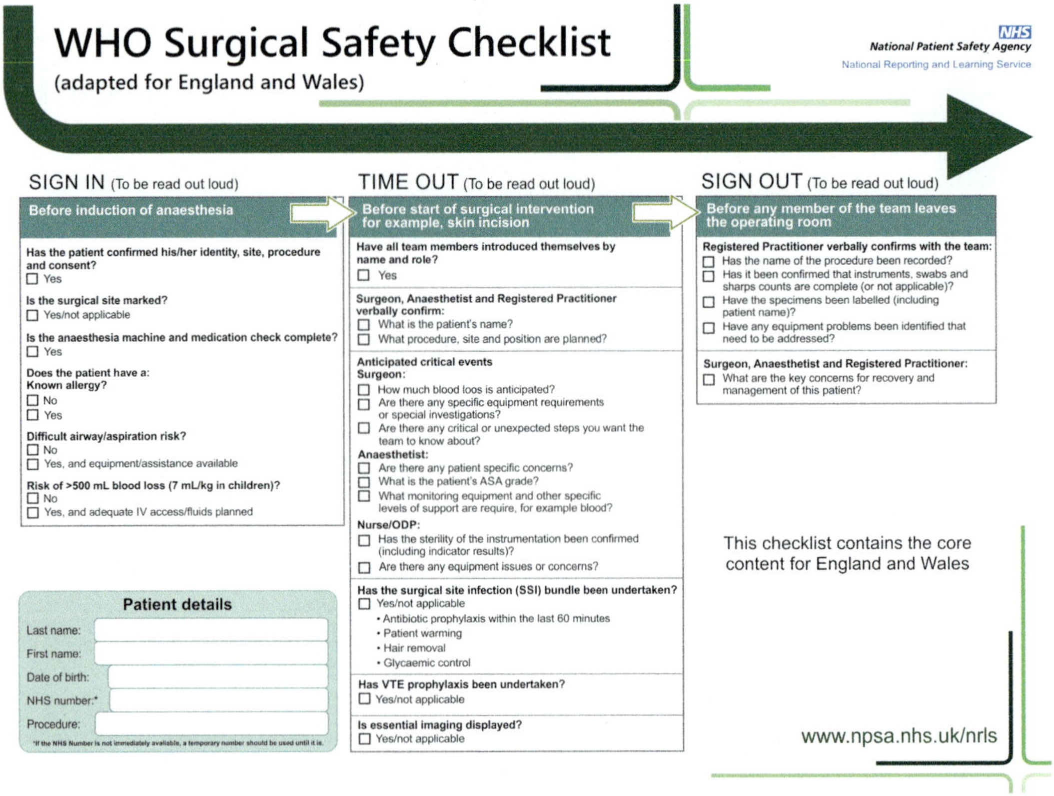

WHO Surgical Safety Checklist
(adapted for England and Wales)

NHS
National Patient Safety Agency
National Reporting and Learning Service

SIGN IN (To be read out loud)

Before induction of anaesthesia

Has the patient confirmed his/her identity, site, procedure and consent?
- ☐ Yes

Is the surgical site marked?
- ☐ Yes/not applicable

Is the anaesthesia machine and medication check complete?
- ☐ Yes

Does the patient have a:
Known allergy?
- ☐ No
- ☐ Yes

Difficult airway/aspiration risk?
- ☐ No
- ☐ Yes, and equipment/assistance available

Risk of >500 mL blood loss (7 mL/kg in children)?
- ☐ No
- ☐ Yes, and adequate IV access/fluids planned

Patient details

Last name:
First name:
Date of birth:
NHS number:*
Procedure:

*If the NHS Number is not immediately available, a temporary number should be used until it is.

TIME OUT (To be read out loud)

Before start of surgical intervention for example, skin incision

Have all team members introduced themselves by name and role?
- ☐ Yes

Surgeon, Anaesthetist and Registered Practitioner verbally confirm:
- ☐ What is the patient's name?
- ☐ What procedure, site and position are planned?

Anticipated critical events
Surgeon:
- ☐ How much blood loos is anticipated?
- ☐ Are there any specific equipment requirements or special investigations?
- ☐ Are there any critical or unexpected steps you want the team to know about?

Anaesthetist:
- ☐ Are there any patient specific concerns?
- ☐ What is the patient's ASA grade?
- ☐ What monitoring equipment and other specific levels of support are require, for example blood?

Nurse/ODP:
- ☐ Has the sterility of the instrumentation been confirmed (including indicator results)?
- ☐ Are there any equipment issues or concerns?

Has the surgical site infection (SSI) bundle been undertaken?
- ☐ Yes/not applicable
  - Antibiotic prophylaxis within the last 60 minutes
  - Patient warming
  - Hair removal
  - Glycaemic control

Has VTE prophylaxis been undertaken?
- ☐ Yes/not applicable

Is essential imaging displayed?
- ☐ Yes/not applicable

SIGN OUT (To be read out loud)

Before any member of the team leaves the operating room

Registered Practitioner verbally confirms with the team:
- ☐ Has the name of the procedure been recorded?
- ☐ Has it been confirmed that instruments, swabs and sharps counts are complete (or not applicable)?
- ☐ Have the specimens been labelled (including patient name)?
- ☐ Have any equipment problems been identified that need to be addressed?

Surgeon, Anaesthetist and Registered Practitioner:
- ☐ What are the key concerns for recovery and management of this patient?

This checklist contains the core content for England and Wales

www.npsa.nhs.uk/nrls

Fig. 1: The World Health Organization (WHO) Surgical Safety Checklist.

5. "Team Debrief (End of Session)"
   - Discuss any issues or complications that occurred.
   - Recognize and reinforce good performance.
   - Provide support for team members, especially after difficult scenarios.

Each phase of the checklist is now clearly enumerated to highlight the sequence of actions and considerations **(Fig. 1)**.

KEY POINTS

- *Team brief (before anesthesia):*
  - All team members introduce themselves and their roles.
  - Discuss patient history, anesthesia plan, surgical approach, and equipment to ensure full team awareness.
  - Encourage open communication and empower team members to speak up about potential issues.
- *Sign In (before induction of anesthesia):*
  - Confirm patient identity, surgical site, and procedure.
  - Mark the surgical site (if applicable) and complete anesthesia checks.
  - Attach and check pulse oximeter, assess allergies, and evaluate risks like difficult airway or blood loss.

- *Time out (before skin incision):*
  - Verify patient identity, surgical site, and procedure with the whole team.
  - Confirm antibiotic administration, review critical steps, blood loss expectations, and operative duration.
  - Anesthetist addresses specific patient concerns.
- *Sign out (before patient leaves operating room):*
  - Ensure the procedure name is recorded and instrument, sponge, and needle counts are correct.
  - Verify specimen labeling, address equipment issues, and discuss recovery concerns.
  - Document any issues raised during the procedure.
- *Team debrief (end of session):*
  - Discuss any complications or issues that arose.
  - Acknowledge good performance and provide support to team members after challenging situations.

CHAPTER 5

Wrong Site Surgery: Consequences, Prevention, and Medicolegal Aspect

Mrunal Bharat Kshirsagar, Sudhir Kumar Jain

"Wrong site surgery is a punishable offense"

INTRODUCTION

Surgery represents a critical domain within healthcare where preventable medical errors and near misses can significantly impact patient's safety. Prior to the groundbreaking 1999 Institute of Medicine report, "To Err Is Human," clinicians lacked a clear understanding of the magnitude of surgery-related injuries, fatalities, and near misses due to the absence of standardized processes for recognizing, reporting, and tracking these incidents.

Among the most concerning types of surgical errors is wrong site surgery (WSS). This term encompasses a range of grave mistakes, including surgeries performed on the incorrect side or site of the body, the wrong surgical procedure being executed, or operations conducted on the wrong patient altogether. Notably, WSS is not limited to traditional operating rooms; it also includes any invasive procedure that subjects patients to more than minimal risk in other settings, such as special procedure units, endoscopy suites, and interventional radiology departments.

The Joint Commission—previously known as the "Joint Commission on Accreditation of Healthcare Organizations"—categorizes WSS as a sentinel event. This designation highlights its serious nature, marking it as one of the top three types of events that can lead to significant patient's harm, including death or severe physical or psychological injuries. The recognition of WSS as a sentinel event emphasizes the urgent need for comprehensive strategies to prevent such occurrences and enhance the overall safety of surgical practices.

CAUSES OF WRONG SITE SURGERY (TABLE 1)

TABLE 1: Factors causing the wrong site surgery.

System factors	*Process factors*
• Lack of institutional controls/formal system to verify the correct site of surgery • Lack of a checklist to make sure every check was performed • Exclusion of certain surgical team members • Reliance solely on the surgeon for determining the correct surgical site • Unusual time pressures (e.g., unplanned emergencies or large volume of procedures)	• Inadequate patient's assessment • Inadequate care planning • Inadequate medical record review • Miscommunication among members of the surgical team and the patient • More than one surgeon involved in the procedure

Contd...

Contd...

System factors	***Process factors***
• Pressures to reduce preoperative preparation time • Procedures requiring unusual equipment or patient's positioning • Team competency and credentialing • Availability of information • Organizational culture • Orientation and training • Staffing • Environmental safety/security • Continuum of care • Patient's characteristics, such as obesity or unusual anatomy, that require alterations in the usual positioning of the patient	• Multiple procedures on multiple parts of a patient performed during a single operation • Failure to include the patient and family or significant others when identifying the correct site • Failure to mark or clearly mark the correct operation site • Incomplete or inaccurate communication among members of the surgical team • Noncompliance with procedures • Failure to recheck patient's information before starting the operation

Universal Protocol for Preventing Wrong Site, Wrong Procedure, and Wrong Person Surgery (Table 2)

TABLE 2: Universal protocol for preventing wrong site, wrong procedure, and wrong person surgery.

Step	***Purpose***	***Process***
Preoperative verification	To ensure all relevant documents and studies are available, reviewed, and consistent with patient's expectations and the team's understanding of the intended procedure, patient, and site. Any missing information or discrepancies must be resolved before the procedure begins	An ongoing process of information gathering and verification that starts with the decision to proceed with the surgery. This continues through all preoperative settings and interventions, culminating in the "time out" just before the procedure
Marking the operative site	To clearly identify the intended site for incision or insertion, eliminating ambiguity	For procedures requiring right/left distinction, multiple structures (e.g., fingers and toes), or various levels (e.g., spinal surgery), the intended site must be marked visibly, even after the patient has been prepared and draped
"Time out" before the procedure	To conduct a final verification of the correct patient, procedure, site, and, where applicable, any implants	All surgical team members engage in active communication, initiated by a designated individual, ensuring a "fail-safe" mode. The procedure will not commence until all questions or concerns are addressed

CONCLUSION

The reported instances of WSS are on the rise as healthcare organizations become increasingly transparent about medical errors. Many of these organizations are leveraging error-prevention theories and lessons from the aviation industry, recognizing that such transparency can lead to systemic changes and improved patient's outcomes. However, complete reporting of WSS remains unlikely due to factors such as industry-wide report cards, concerns about litigation, and varying perspectives among professionals. While the overall numbers of WSS may not be alarming, the consequences for affected patients are severe and often life-altering.

KEY POINTS

- *Increase in reported wrong site surgeries (WSS):* Instances of WSS are on the rise, largely due to greater transparency in healthcare organizations about medical errors.
- *Use of error-prevention theories:* Healthcare organizations are adopting error-prevention strategies and lessons learned from the aviation industry to reduce medical mistakes, including WSS.
- *Impact of transparency:* Greater transparency about errors is seen as a means to drive systemic changes and improve patient's outcomes over time.
- *Challenges in complete reporting:* Full reporting of WSS remains unlikely due to challenges such as:
  - Industry-wide report cards
  - Concerns about litigation
  - Varying perspectives among healthcare professionals on what constitute a reportable incident.
- *Severity of consequences:* While the overall number of WSS cases may not be alarming, the consequences for affected patients are severe and often lead to life-altering outcomes.

CHAPTER 6

Scrubbing, Gowning, and Gloving Techniques

Sudhir Kumar Jain, David L Stoker

"The ritual of scrubbing, gowning, and gloving should be observed religiously"

SURGICAL HAND SCRUB

A surgical hand scrub is performed prior to donning a sterile gown and gloves. Hand scrub does not render the skin sterile, but makes it surgically clean, by reducing the number of organisms, hence reducing the risk to the patient in case a glove is perforated during surgery. In 1846, the Hungarian physician Ignaz Semmelweis recognized the fact that hand cleaning with an antiseptic agent was more effective than simply using plain soap and water. Semmelweis adopted hand disinfection into his practice and immediately mortality rates associated with infections decreased.

The surgical hand scrub continues to be one of the most important procedures in infection prevention and control.

The purpose of surgical hand scrub is threefold:

- To remove transient microorganisms and debris from the skin of hands, forearm, and nails.
- To inhibit the re-growth of microorganisms in between two procedures.
- To reduce the resident microorganism counts to the lowest possible level.

Surgical scrub can be defined as systematic washing and scrubbing of the hands and forearms with an effective antibacterial cleaning solution to render the skin free from bacteria as far as possible.

The following two types of bacterial population are normally present on the skin:

1. *Transient organisms:* These organisms are introduced on to the skin surface by soil, dust, and by various other substances that come in contact with the skin. Surgical scrub will remove most of these organisms.
2. *Resident organisms:* These are mainly gram-negative and gram-positive bacteria with a natural habitat under the fingernails and in the deeper layers of skin, e.g., in hair follicles, sweat glands and in sebaceous glands. Scrubbing removes bacteria from the skin surface and from just beneath the surface. After gloving, resident bacteria from the deeper layers are brought to the skin surface by perspiration and oily secretions, and the bacterial count on the skin again increases. Hand scrub, therefore, needs to be repeated between procedures.

Preparation before Scrubbing

Personal cleanliness is of paramount importance for members of the surgical team. This includes daily showers, frequent shampoos, and attention to hands and fingernails. Staff with rashes, infective lesions, or open wounds of the skin on hands, nails or arms should not scrub for a procedure. Staff with a common cold, sore throats or systemic infections should also not scrub.

Scrubbed personnel should have short nails, such that they are not visible over the tips of the fingers. Short nails are easy to clean and if kept smooth will not puncture the gloves. Fingernails should be free from nail varnish, as chipped fingernail polish can harbor greater numbers of bacteria. Artificial nails should never be worn as fungal growth can occur when moisture becomes trapped between the artificial nail and the natural nail. Watches, bracelets, and rings should be removed and kept in a safe place. Bacteria and dead skin cells accumulate beneath jewelry. Every surgical team member should wear a clean and short-sleeved cotton scrub suit before entering the semi-restricted/restricted areas of the surgical suite. Sleeves of the scrub shirt should be 4 inches above the elbow.

Street clothes or hospital uniforms are not allowed in restricted areas. A scrub shirt should be tucked in to the trousers to avoid contamination by the shirt tail flapping into the sterile field. Trouser legs should not touch the floor as this may transport bacteria from one place to another. Personnel should wear shoes especially assigned for the surgical suite. Shoes should cover the toes completely. This is to prevent injury from sharp or heavy instruments falling from the operating table, and to prevent soiling of toes by the patient's blood or body fluids. Shoes should be cleaned at the end of the day. Street shoes are not allowed in restricted areas unless covered by sterile shoe covers. Shoe covers should be used on a single use basis and must be discarded on leaving the restricted area.

Personnel should wear a disposable surgical cap in such a manner that hair is covered completely to avoid contamination of the sterile field by falling hair or dandruff **(Fig. 1)**.

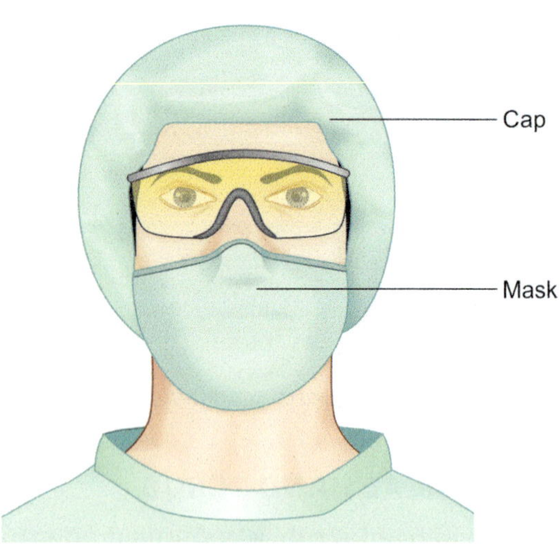

Fig. 1: Proper method of wearing cap and mask.

A surgical mask is worn to protect the patient from bacteria exhaled by operating room personnel and it is mandatory for members of scrub team. The wearing of a mask by other persons present in the operating theater is a matter of local hospital policy. The exception to this rule is when implant or prosthesis surgery is taking place when everyone in theater should wear a mask. A surgical mask should be worn by the surgeon, and assistant to cover the nose and mouth completely **(Fig. 1)**. It may not be necessary to wear a mask for all laparoscopic or endoscopic surgical procedures. The mask should be donned in such a way that it fits snugly to the face and does not allow passage of air around the sides and to prevent fogging of glasses if worn. A fresh mask should be donned immediately before the beginning of the every scrub procedure. If the mask becomes damp or moist it will allow the passage of droplets from the nose and mouth and the mask will no longer serve as a barrier to germs. The mask may need to be changed more often if it becomes damp or moist. Immediately the mask should be placed in a designated receptacle on its removal and the hands should be washed.

The mucous membranes of the eyes, mouth, and nose should be protected in procedures which involve splashing or spraying of blood, body fluids, or bone chips. This can be achieved by donning protective eye wear covering the front and side of the eyes, or by full face visors. These should either be disposable or cleaned according to manufacturer's instructions after use.

Environment and Equipment in Scrub Area

The scrub area should be large enough to allow the scrub personnel to gown and glove safely without hindrance. A wall clock should be strategically placed to time the scrub, and there should be provision to control water temperature. Sink height should be sufficient to minimize splashing, and taps should be elbow or knee operated.

Solutions Used

Three main types of preparations for hand hygiene are used:

1. 4% Chlorhexidine gluconate (clear/pink solution)
2. Iodine-based preparations (Povidone iodine 7.5%) have potential to cause skin irritation.
3. Aqueous alcoholic solutions, e.g., ethyl alcohol and isopropyl alcohol.

Antiseptic soap can be used if the above-mentioned preparations are not available.

These solutions are available in a liquid form. The advantages of liquid preparations over soap are:

- They are nonirritating to most people.
- They leave a minimum number of microorganisms on the skin.
- They have a prolonged antibacterial effect on the skin when used regularly. They leave a film on the skin which keeps the resident bacteria to a minimum and do not interfere with the skin's natural resistance to transient bacteria.
- They lather easily in hot, cold, or hard water.
- The amount of detergent needed is small.

Scrubbing Method

Scrub should be performed before the first case in the morning and then in-between cases. Two methods of scrub technique may be used, the time method or the brush stroke method. Rinsing time is not included in the total scrub time if the time method is used. In the brush-stroke method, a prescribed number of brush strokes are applied lengthwise to each surface of fingers, hands, and arms. An ideal surgical hand scrub should take no longer than 5 minutes.

Unsterile objects should not be touched once the scrub process has begun. If this happens accidentally, the entire scrub process should be repeated.

Scrub Up Technique

Scrubbing procedure must take a minimum of 2 minutes if scrub solutions are used and 5 minutes if antiseptic soap is used. Water temperature should be set at a comfortable level. Wet hands and forearms at the start of scrub up **(Figs. 2A and B)**. Dispense around 5 mL of antibacterial soap solution into the palm. A nail brush should be used only on nails or in web spaces and not on rest of the skin **(Fig. 3)**. Scrubbing should start from fingers to 1 inch below the elbow, not from the elbow to the fingers **(Fig. 4)**. Hands should be held higher than the elbow, so that water flows downward draining off

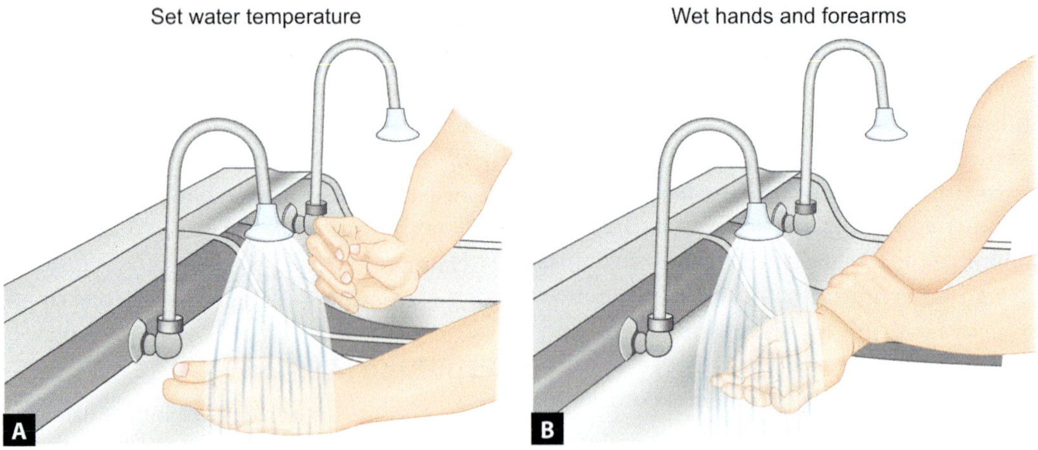

Figs. 2A and B: Wet hands and forearms before starting scrub up.

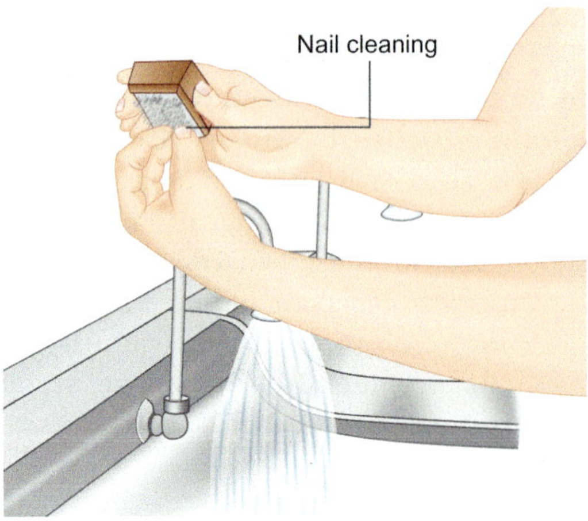

Fig. 3: Scrub fingernails with nail brush.

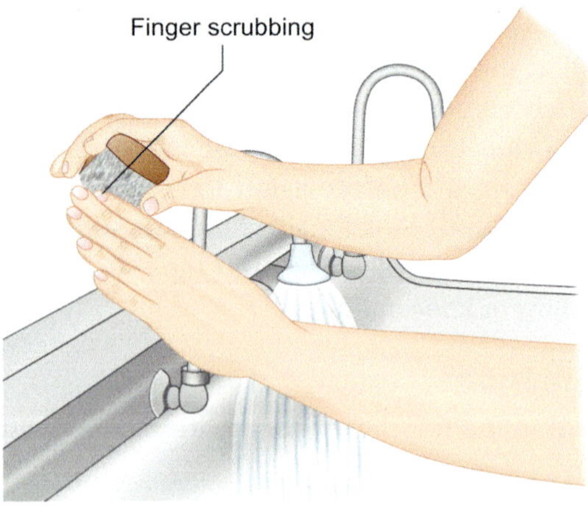

Fig. 4: Scrub anterior, posterior, and lateral sides of fingers.

the elbows **(Fig. 5)**. Scrubbing comprises three washing cycles: (1) hands and arms extending to 1 inch above the elbow; (2) hands and half-way up the forearms; and (3) hands only. The principle of washing from a clean area (the hand) in the direction of the less clean area (the arm) should be followed. The hands should be held above the level of elbows at all times in order to prevent dirty water from dripping from the upper arm in to lower sterile areas. Water splashing on theater clothes should be avoided as wet clothes may cause contamination of the sterile gown. Hands and forearms should be washed and rinsed at least twice after scrubbing **(Figs. 6A and B)**. Following the final rinse, the hands and forearms should be elevated away from the body allowing water to drop from the elbows. Hands and forearms should be dried using a folded disposable hand towel separately for each side. Drying should start from the fingers going toward the elbows.

The towels should be discarded immediately after drying the hands and forearms. Towel should remain folded to double thickness while drying **(Figs. 7 to 10)**.

SURGICAL GOWN TECHNIQUE

Gowns should be properly fitting, permitting adequate freedom of movement. Each sleeve should be provided with a tight-fitting cuff. Gowns should ideally be water repellent.

Standard-of-care for surgical gowns are:

- Gowns must be free of holes, punctures, and tears. They should be resistant to punctures and tears to prevent microbial contamination of the sterile field and prevent surgical site infection (SSI).
- Gowns should be resistant to blood and body fluid penetration. They should have microbial and fluid resistance.
- Intraoperatively patient body fluids and irrigating solutions come into contact with gowns. Gowns should be impervious and fluid-resistant to prevent strike-through contamination from microorganisms. Prevention of strike-through contamination reduces the risk of SSI.
- They should be comfortable and loosely fitting to prevent excess heat build up.
- Gowns, in particular gowns composed of reusable woven material, should be free of toxic substances, such as dyes and laundry detergent residues.
- Flame-resistant gowns should be used especially when using lasers, fiber optics, and electrosurgery within the sterile field.
- The gowns should be lint free as lint is recognized as a vector for causing SSI. Additionally, airborne lint serves as a medium for transport of microbes.

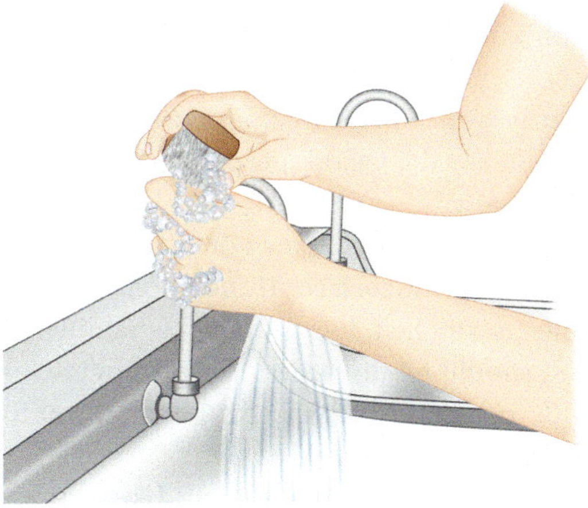

Fig. 5: Continuing scrub process on hands.

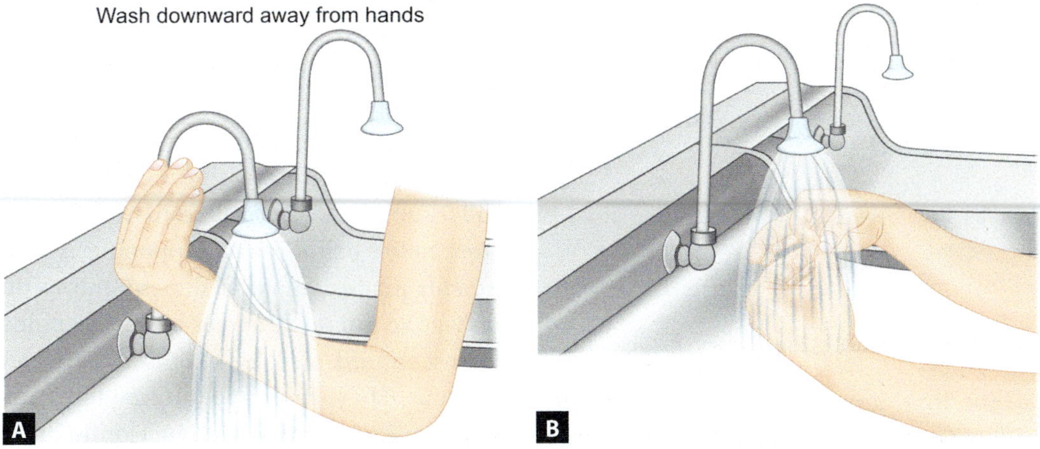

Figs. 6A and B: Rinsing forearms and hands.

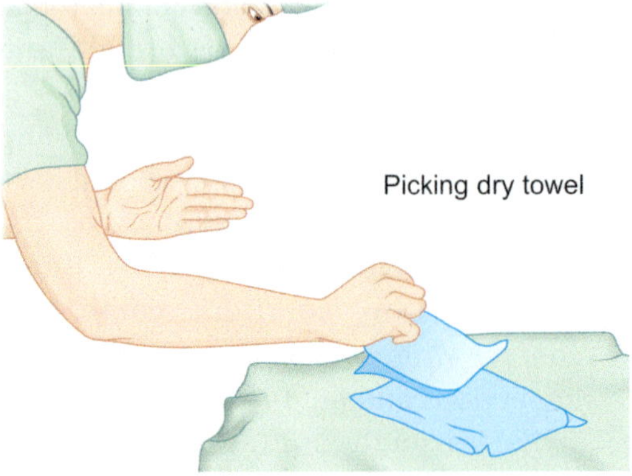

Fig. 7: Picking up folded hand towel.

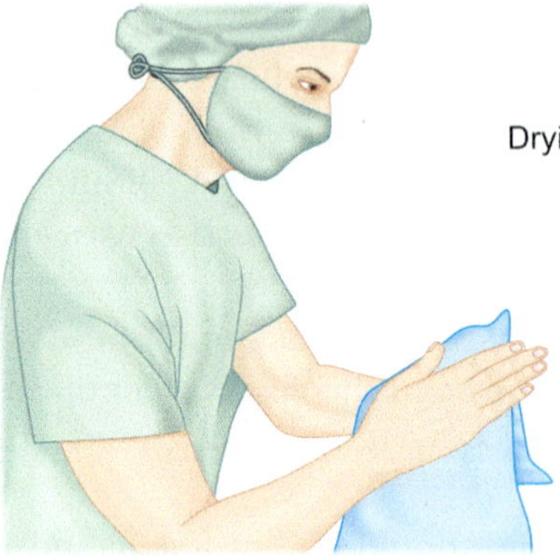

Fig. 8: Drying the elbows.

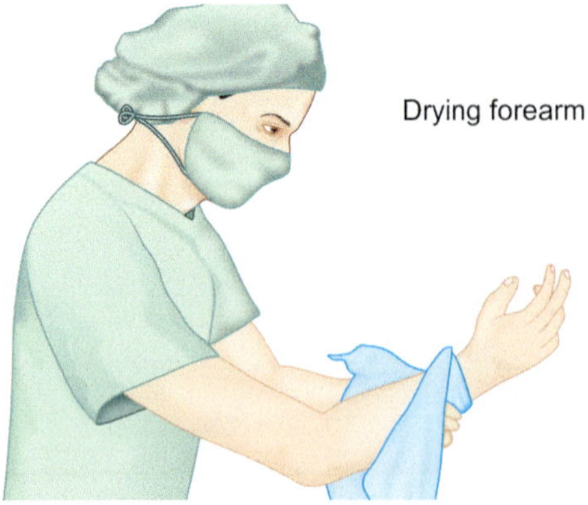

Fig. 9: Drying hands using rotating movements.

Lint-free gowns minimize airborne contamination and spreading of particles into the surgical wound.

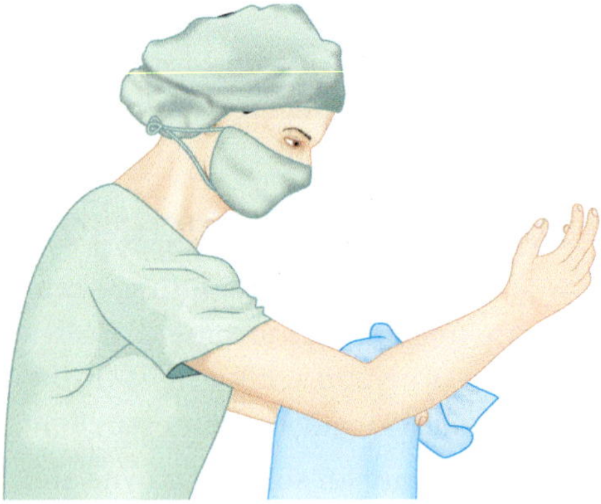

Fig. 10: Drying the forearms.

It is recommended that woven fabrics with a thread count of 270–280 be used as sterile gown material. It is recommended that woven fabrics treated with chemicals to increase the barrier properties be used as sterile gowns.

When donning a gown one should touch only the back surface. If the outside of the gown is touched, it is deemed contaminated and should be discarded. Gowns are folded with the back facing the scrubbed person to facilitate sterile gowning.

Scrubbed personnel should keep their hands and arms above the waist and away from the body at an angle of 20–30° above the elbows. If scrubbed hands and arms fall below waist level, they are considered contaminated.

After donning, the parts which are considered sterile are sleeves (except the axillary area) and the front from waist level to a few inches below the neck opening. As well as being made of material that minimizes the passage of microorganisms and body fluids, gowns should also be tear and puncture resistant. They should be lint free to reduce particle dissemination into the wound or the environment.

PROCEDURE FOR GOWNING

Lift the inner or back side of the neck of the gown upward and away from the table **(Fig. 11)**. While holding at the neckline, the gown is allowed to unfold completely with the inner side facing the wearer **(Fig. 12)**.

Slip both hands into the open armholes keeping the hands at shoulder level and away from the body. Push both hands and forearm into the sleeves of the gown but advance hands up to the proximal edge of the cuff only. Do not allow hands to come out of the cuff **(Figs. 13 and 14)**. An ungloved hand should not touch the front of the gown. The gown is secured at the back by the circulating staff **(Figs. 15 and 16)**.

Rules to observe while wearing sterile gowns and gloves:

- Do not drop your hands below the level of the umbilicus or below the sterile working area.
- Never place hands behind the back.
- Gloved hands must be kept within full view at all times.
- Do not tuck gloved hands under the armpits, as axillary region is considered contaminated.
- Never touch a nonsterile area with gloved hands.

SURGICAL GLOVING TECHNIQUE

There are two types of gloving technique, i.e., (1) open and (2) closed gloving. Closed

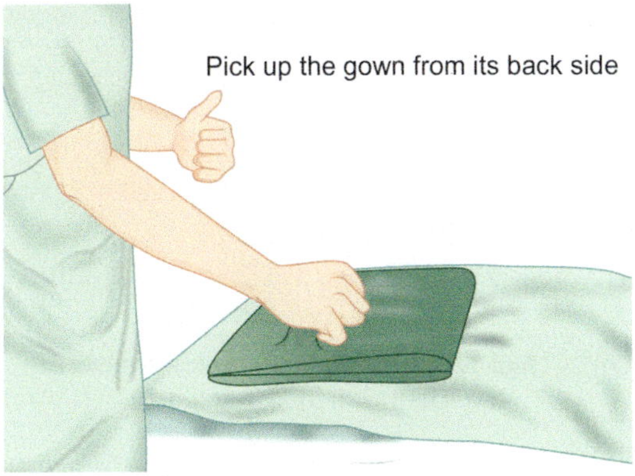

Fig. 11: Pick up the gown from its inner side near the neck.

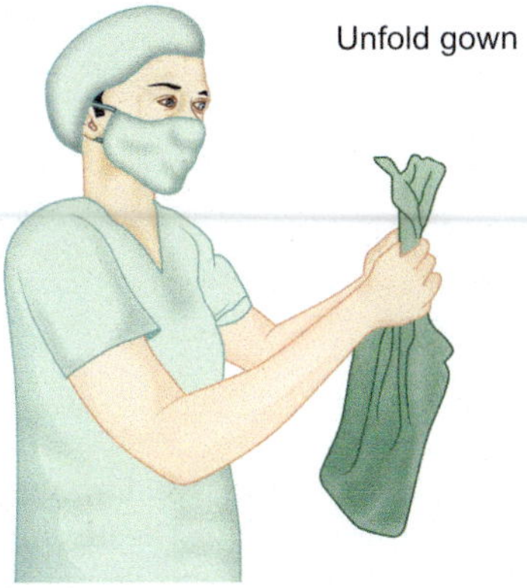

Fig. 12: Unfold the gown.

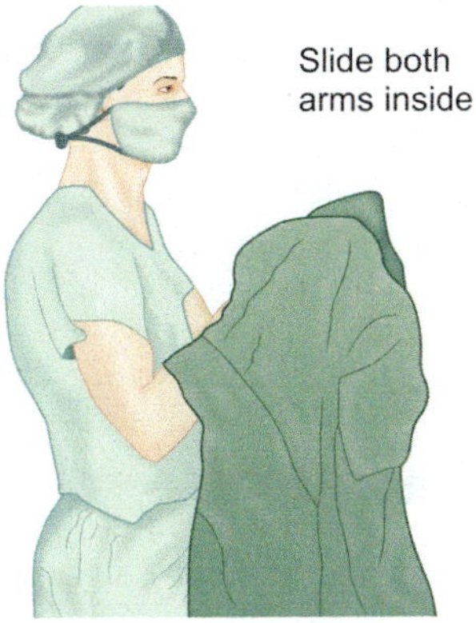

Fig. 13: Slide hands and arms into the sleeves.

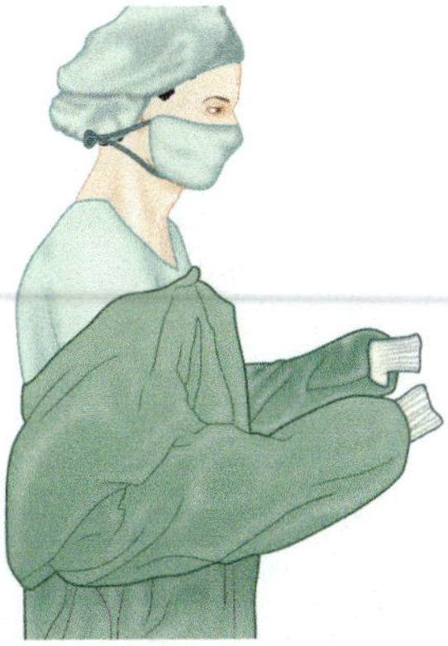

Fig. 14: Slide the arms into the sleeves completely but without protruding fingers out of cuffs.

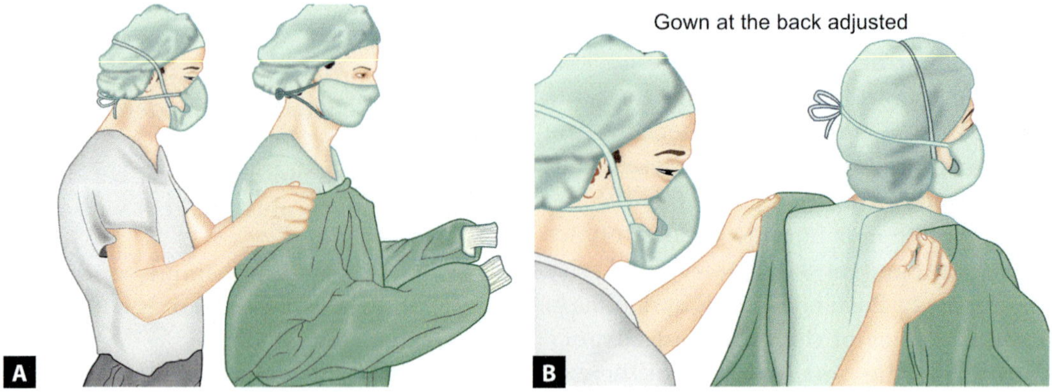

Figs. 15A and B: Adjustment of the (A) Gown over the shoulder and (B) grown at the back.

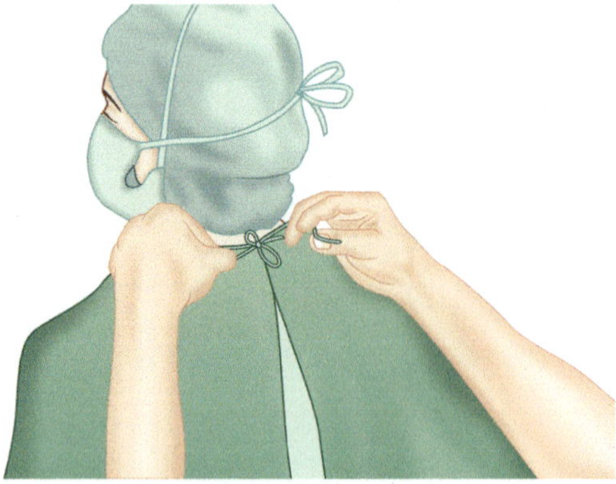

Fig. 16: Circulating staff secures the gown at the neck.

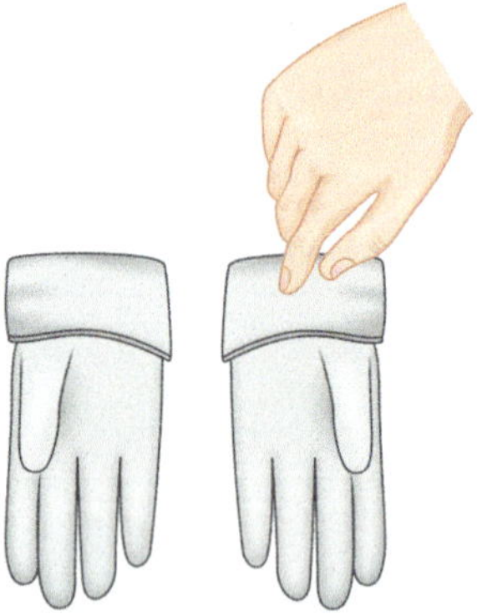

Fig. 17: The cuff of the right glove is picked with the left hand.

gloving is the technique of choice because gloves are handled through the fabric of the gown sleeves, thereby preventing bare hands from coming into contact with the outside of the glove.

Double gloving is recommended for all surgical procedures.

Open Glove Technique (Figs. 17 to 20)

This technique should be used if contamination has occurred at the table. This technique can also be used if a catheterization is performed on table by the circulating nurse.

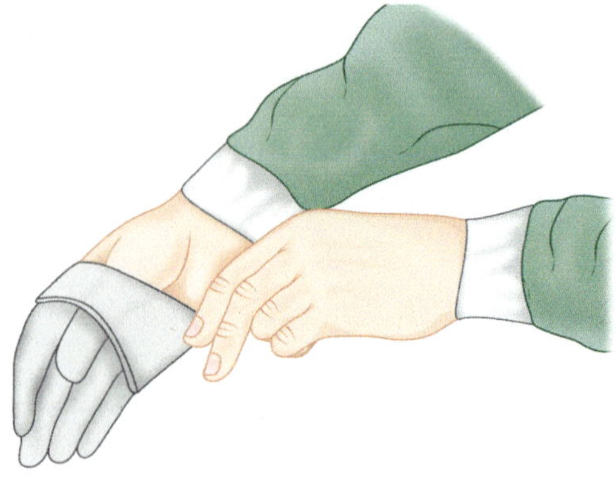

Fig. 18: The right hand is slid into the glove until there is a snug fit over the thumb joints and knuckles. The bare left hand should only touch the folded cuff—the rest of the glove remains sterile.

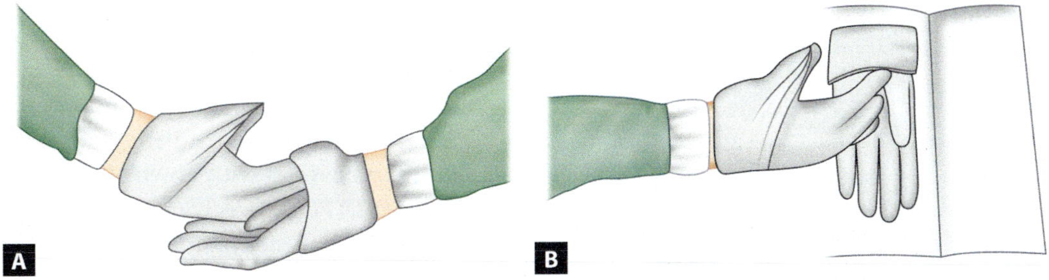

Figs. 19A and B: With the gloved left hand, the folded cuff of right glove is picked and pulled up onto gowned wrist.

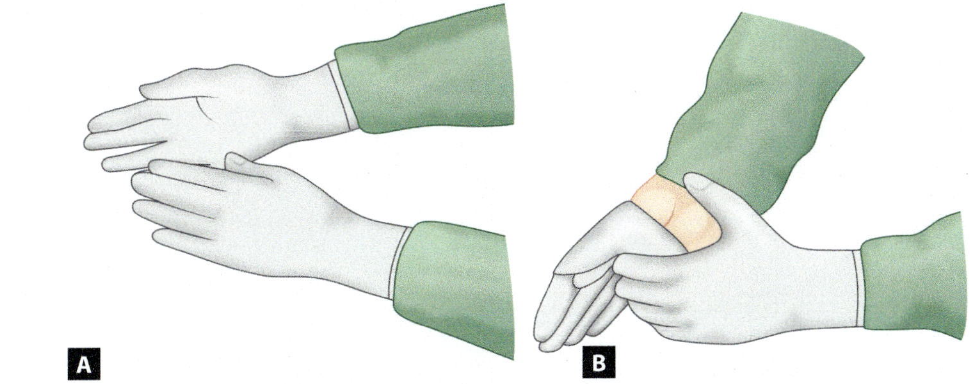

Figs. 20A and B: The fingers of the gloved right hand are placed under the cuff of the partially gloved left hand. The cuff is unfolded down over your gown sleeves. During this process, gloved fingertips should not touch your bare forearms or wrists.

Closed Glove Technique

- Hands are advanced into the sleeves of the gown till the cuff is reached.
- The glove packet is opened in such a way that the right glove faces the right hand.
- Pick up the left glove by its folded cuff edge with a sleeve covered right hand **(Fig. 21)**.
- Place the glove on the opposite gown sleeve, palm down, with the glove fingers pointing toward shoulder **(Figs. 22 to 24)**. The palm of the hand inside the gown sleeve must be facing upward toward the palm of the glove. Hold the bottom rolled

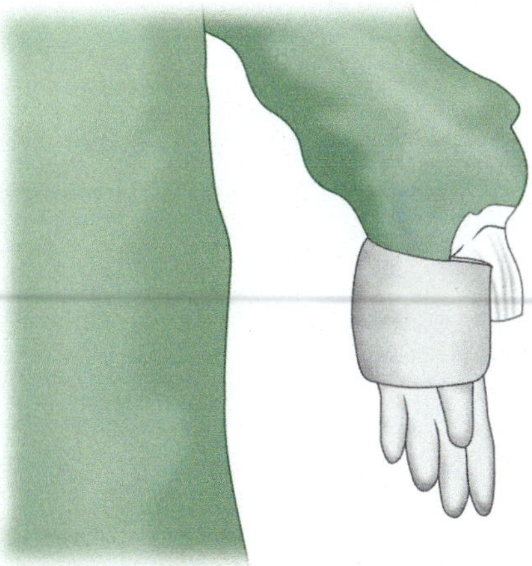

Fig. 21: Picking up a glove by its folded cuff edge with a sleeve-covered hand.

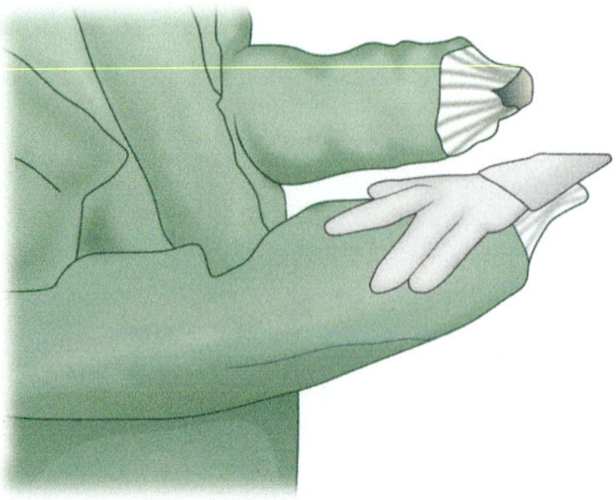

Fig. 22: Place the glove on the opposite sleeve.

edge of the glove with thumb and index finger **(Fig. 25)**.

- Grasp the uppermost edge of the glove's cuff with the opposite hand and stretch the cuff of the glove over the hand. Put left hand covered with gown sleeve into glove's cuff **(Fig. 26)**. Advance your fingers out of the gown sleeve into the cuff of the glove and adjust them into the respective finger stalk. Adjust the glove over the gown sleeve with the right hand covered with gown sleeve **(Fig. 27)**.
- Don the right glove in a similar manner.

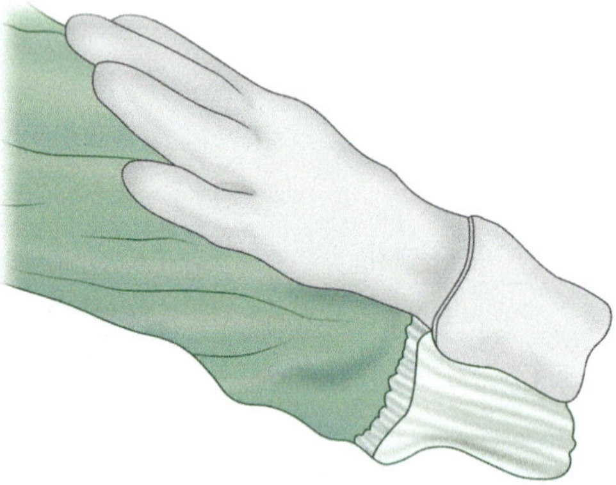

Fig. 23: Place the glove on the opposite sleeve (left glove on right sleeve).

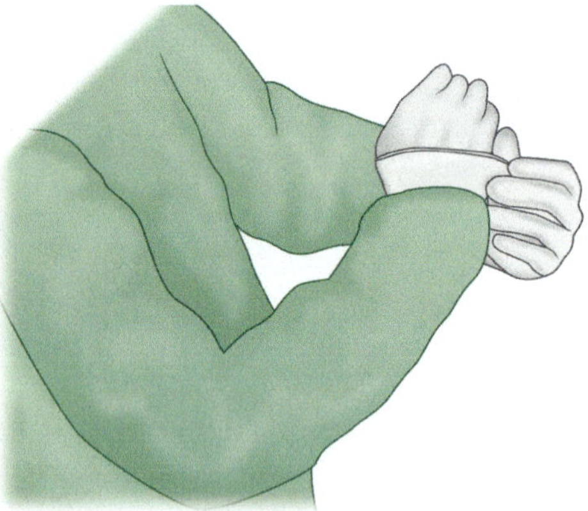

Fig. 25: Hold the bottom rolled edge of the glove with thumb and index finger.

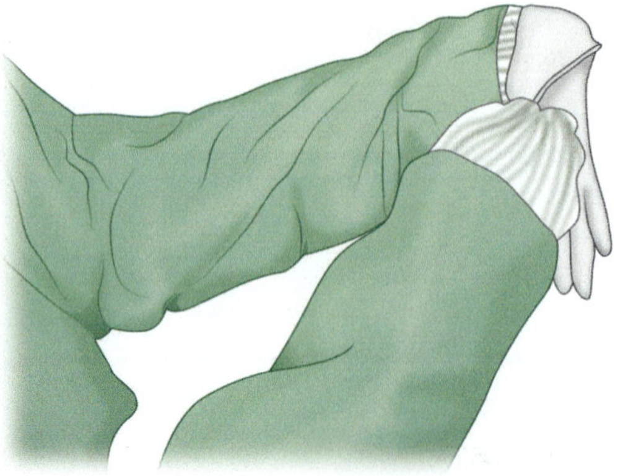

Fig. 24: Glove should be placed in such a way that the rolled edge of the gloved cuff is at the junction of gown cuff and sleeve.

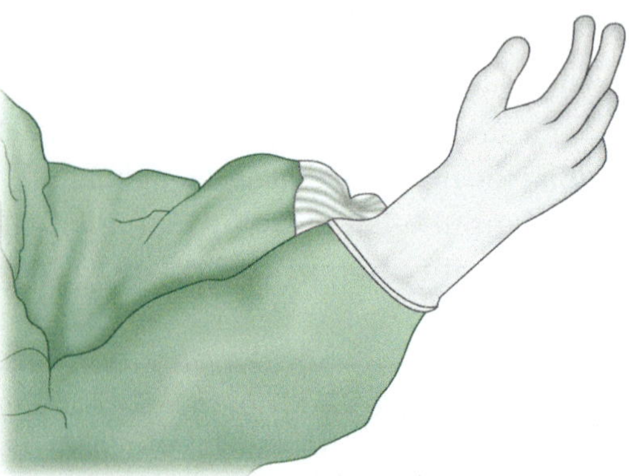

Fig. 26: Stretching the glove cuff over the hand.

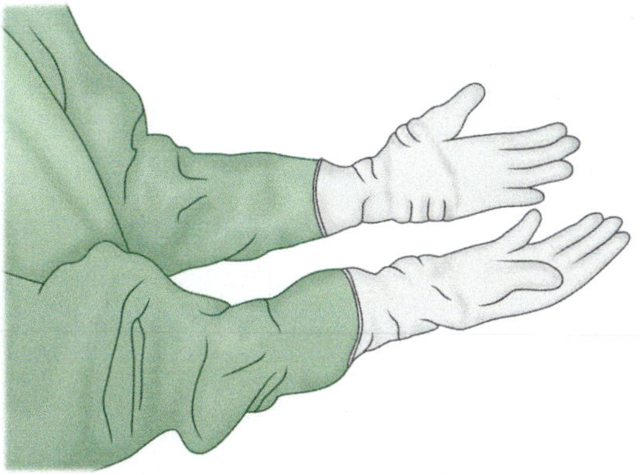

Fig. 27: Pulling the glove on to the hand.

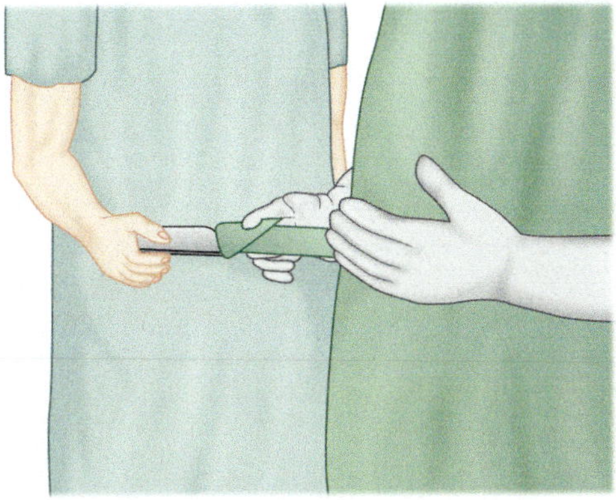

Fig. 29: Paper tab holding belt passed to circulating staff.

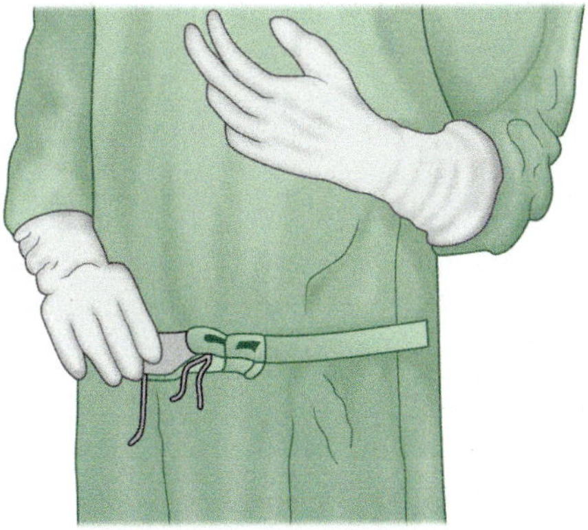

Fig. 28: Scrubbed person holds the paper tab attached to the belt and belt tie.

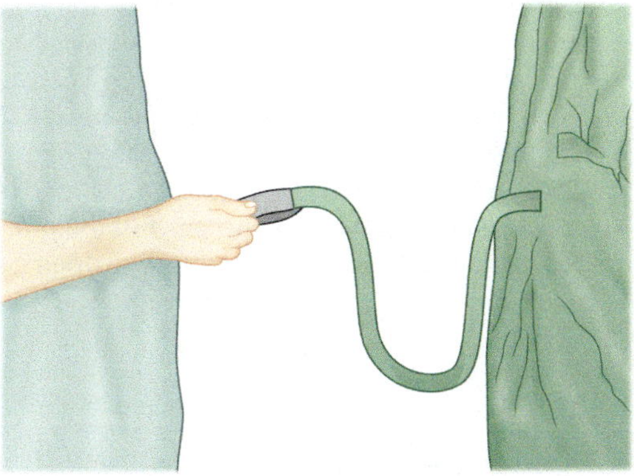

Fig. 30: Circulating staff holding paper tab comes to the other side of the scrubbed person.

Final Tie of the Gown (After Donning Gloves)

If the gown is made of cotton, the waist tie can only be passed around and behind the gowned person by a scrubbed and gowned member of staff to maintain sterility.

If the gown is a paper disposable one, then a disposable tab attached to the waist tie can be handed to a nonscrubbed member of staff to be passed around the waist. The disposable tab is then discarded **(Figs. 28 to 32)**.

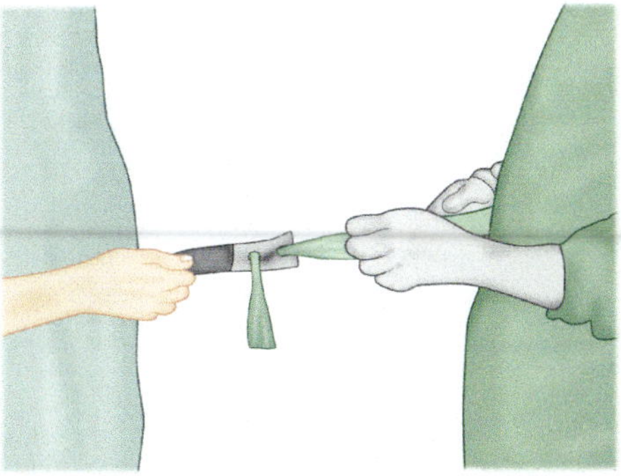

Fig. 31: Scrubbed person should hold the belt without touching the paper tab and pull out the belt.

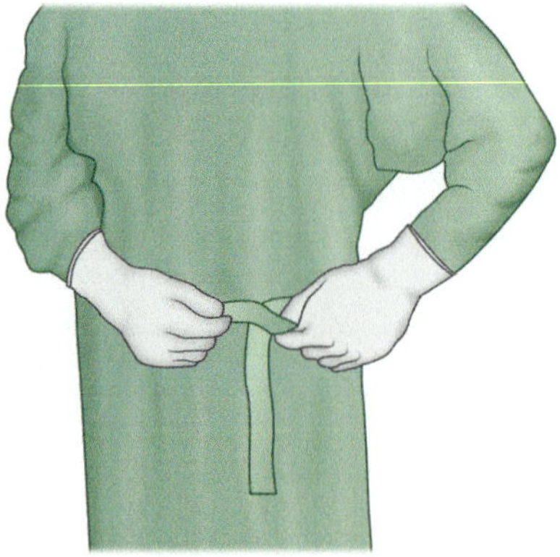

Fig. 32: Scrubbed person will take hold of the belt tie and tie the belt to it.

KEY POINTS

- The purpose of scrubbing is to reduce the number of organisms on the skin so that the risk to the patient is less if gloves are accidentally perforated during surgery.
- One can scrub with an antiseptic solution or soap.
- Recommended scrubbing time is 2 minutes with antiseptic solution and 5 minutes with soap.
- Scrubbing time does not include rinsing time.
- While wearing a gown one should touch only the inside or back of the gown.
- A gown is contaminated if one touches the outside surface.
- Closed gloving technique is better than open gloving technique.

CHAPTER 7

Knot Tying Techniques

Sudhir Kumar Jain, David L Stoker, Raman Tanwar

"Secure knot tying enhances the safety of surgical procedure many fold"

INTRODUCTION

The craft of knot-tying has evolved alongside human civilization, with early cultures mastering both rope making and knotting nearly simultaneously. Historical records indicate that ancient societies recognized the critical role of secure knots in ensuring the effectiveness of ropes. These knotted ropes have been pivotal throughout history, from constructing homes and bridges to navigating the seas. Beyond their practical applications, knots also carry significant religious and symbolic meanings in various cultures. For instance, in Hindu weddings, the act of tying the couple's garments together symbolizes the lifelong union of their souls.

In modern medicine, knots are indispensable for surgical procedures, particularly in approximating tissues or ligating blood vessels. While over 1,400 knots are cataloged in knotting encyclopedias, only a select few are employed in surgery. The choice of surgical knot depends on factors such as suture material, incision depth, and wound stress. Multifilament sutures, with their higher friction, are easier to tie and more stable, whereas monofilament sutures, due to their lower friction and tendency to revert to their original shape, are more prone to loosening. Surgeons must tie knots with precision and patience to prevent slippage and ensure optimal outcomes.

SAFE PRINCIPLES OF KNOT TYING

- *Firmness:* The knot must be secure to prevent slipping.
- *Size:* Keep the knot as small as possible and trim the ends short.
- *Friction:* Avoid excessive friction between strands, which can weaken the suture.
- *Tension:* Apply tension carefully to avoid excessive strain on the suture.
- *Orientation:* Maintain horizontal tension on the final throw.
- *Suture handling:* Prevent damage to the suture material, such as crushing it with hemostats.
- *Maintaining tension:* Keep tension on the knot after the initial loop to prevent loosening.
- *Bulk versus strength:* Additional ties do not increase the strength of a well-tied knot but may add bulk.

METHODS OF KNOT TYING

- Hand-tied knot
- Instrument-tied knot
- Endoscopic knot tying.

A hand-tied knot can be:

- Granny knot
- Square knot or reef knot
- Surgeon's knot
- Reverse surgeon's knot
- Double-double knot.

A hand-tied knot can be created either by one or both hands.

IMPORTANCE OF KNOT TYING

The knot is the weakest link in a tied surgical suture. The consequences of suboptimal and faulty knot construction may be disastrous. For example, massive hemorrhage may result from a poorly tied knot on a large artery. Knot disruption may also lead to wound dehiscence or an incisional hernia. It is important to understand the mechanical performance of a united and knotted suture, and an important complication in a suture's mechanical performance includes knot breakage and knot slippage.

COMPONENTS OF A KNOTTED SUTURE LOOP

A Tied Suture has Three Components

1. The *loop* created by a knot maintains approximation of the divided wound edge.
2. A *knot* is composed of a number of throws snagged against each other. A throw is a wrapping or weaving of two strands.
3. *Ears* or the *cut ends* act as insurance that the loop will not become untied because of knot slippage.

Each throw within a knot can be either a single or double throw. A *single throw* is formed by wrapping the two strands around each other so that the rotation of the wrap is *360°*. In a *double throw*, the free end of the strand is passed twice instead of once around the other strand. The rotation of this double wrap throw is *720°*.

Square knot: When the right ear and the loop of the two throws exit on the *same side* of the knot or parallel to each other.

Granny knot: When the right ear and loop exit or cross *different sides* of the knot.

Surgeon's knot: It is comprised of an initial double throw followed by a single throw.

Reverse surgeon's knot: It is comprised of an initial double throw followed by a single throw and subsequently a double-wrap throw.

Double-double knot: It consists of two double throws.

One handed square knot technique: It can be tied using either hand.

This type of knot is employed if using a suture with a needle attached to it. After passing the needle through the tissue, the thread is pulled until the end of the suture attached to the needle is long. One handed tying of a knot uses two types of throws, i.e., (1) *index finger* throw and (2) *middle finger* throw. If the short end is away from the operator, then the index finger throw is used. If the short end is toward the operator, the middle finger throw is used. If the short end is toward the right-hand side of operator, then one can use either index finger throw by left hand or middle finger throw by right hand. If the short end is toward the left side of operator, then one can use middle finger by left hand or index finger throw by right.

Crossing of hands at the end of each throw is of paramount importance. It means that if the short end is away from the operator, it should come toward the operator at the end of the throw. Crossing of hands is also known as *"squaring the knot"* and ensures that the knot does not become an *unsafe slip knot.*

Steps

1. Hold the short end of suture between the thumb and ring finger of the left hand with the loop over the extended left index finger which has been kept free. Hold the

long end of the suture in between the right thumb and right index finger. Abduct the left index finger, so that short end of suture forms a loop over it **(Fig. 1)**.

2. Bring the long end of suture held in right hand over loop of short end held in left hand, by moving right hand away from you so that it crosses in front of short end **(Fig. 2)**.
3. Bring the index finger of left hand in front of the short end of suture held between left thumb and ring finger **(Fig. 3)**.
4. Pronate the left hand so that the left index finger brings the thread held between left thumb and ring finger inside the loop.
5. Pull the thread out of loop by grasping it between left index and middle finger and complete the throw by bringing left hand toward you and right hand away from you **(Fig. 4)**.
6. Continue to hold the short end of the suture in left hand between thumb and index finger. Flex and abduct left index finger so that it lies at right angle to remaining left hand fingers **(Fig. 5)**.
7. Bring the thread held in the right hand across the left middle finger toward the operator to cross the left-handed thread **(Fig. 6)**.
8. Use the middle finger of left hand to bring short end under the right-handed strand of suture **(Figs. 7 to 11)**.
9. Grasp the short end between left middle and ring finger and bring short end away from you and tighten the knot.

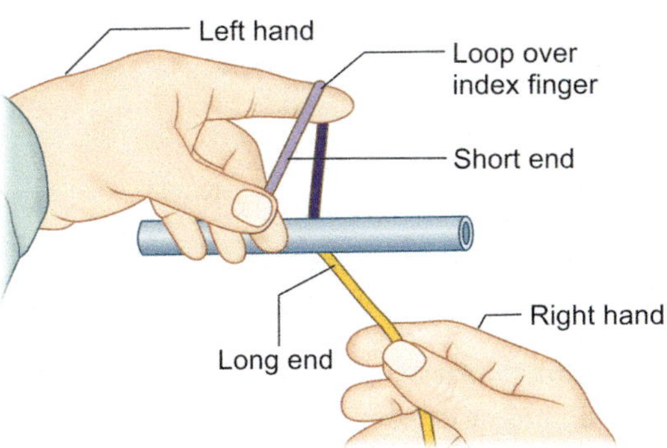

Fig. 1

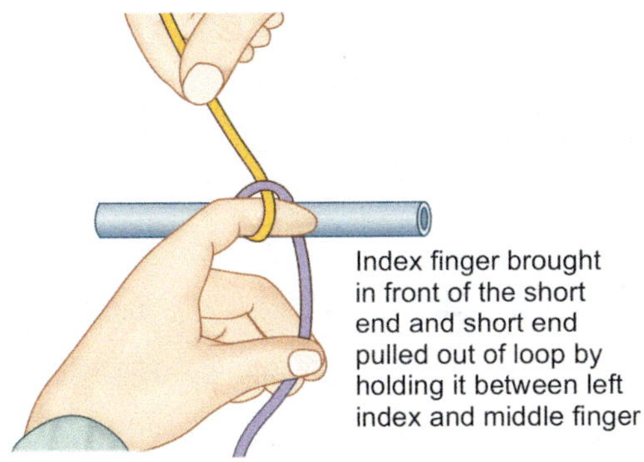

Fig. 3

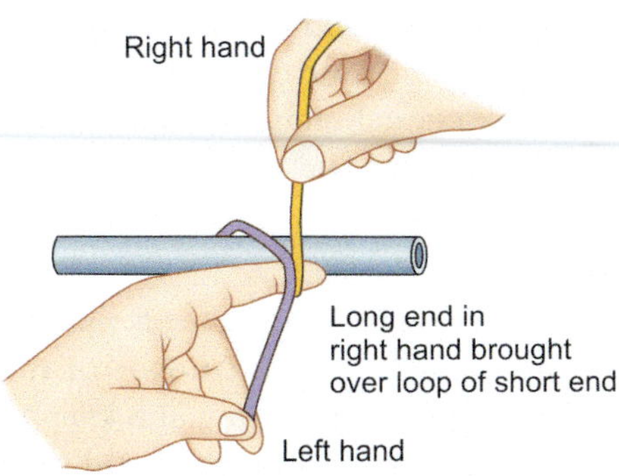

Fig. 2

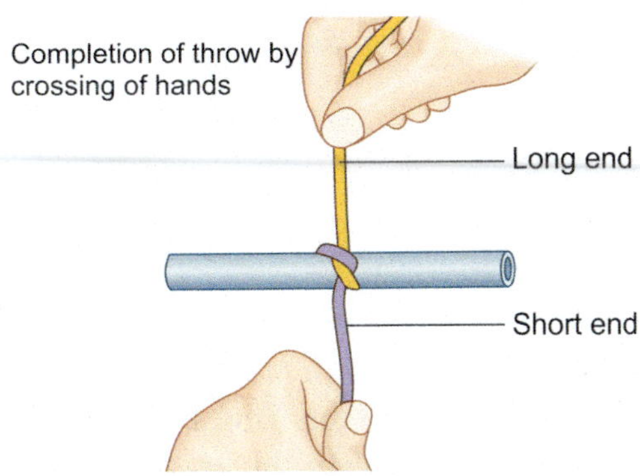

Fig. 4

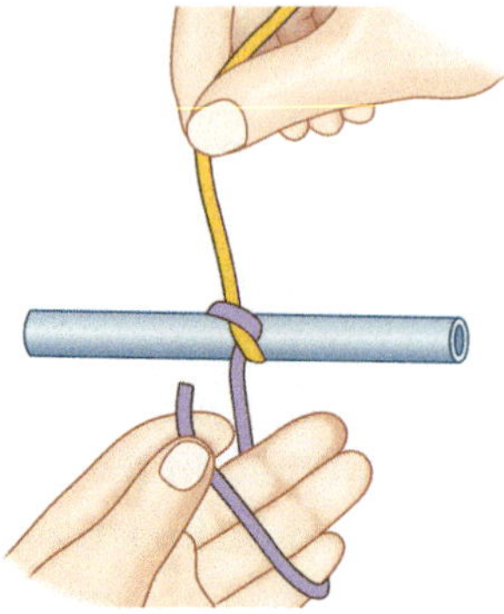

Fig. 5

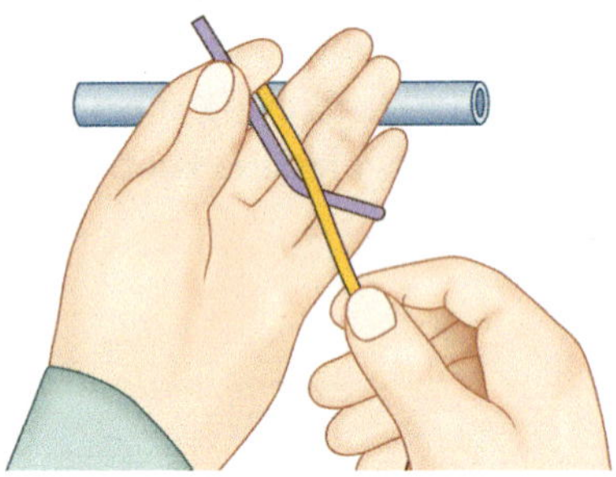

Fig. 6

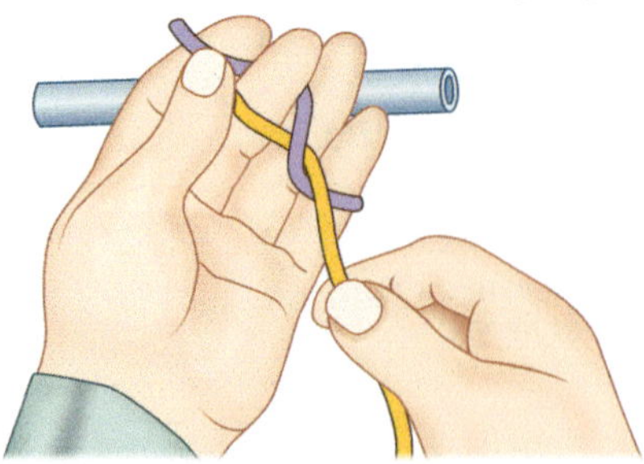

Fig. 7

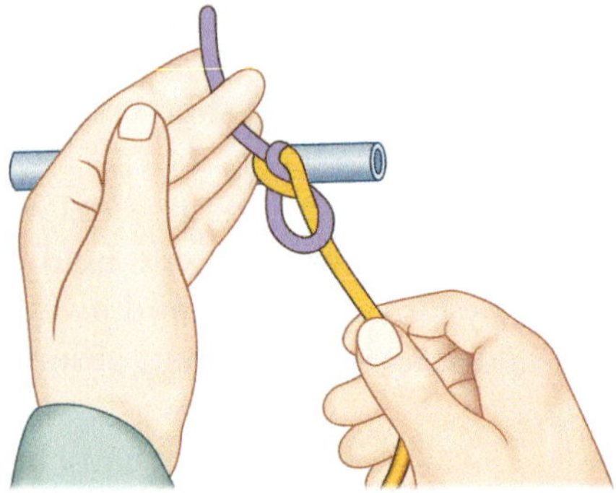

Fig. 8

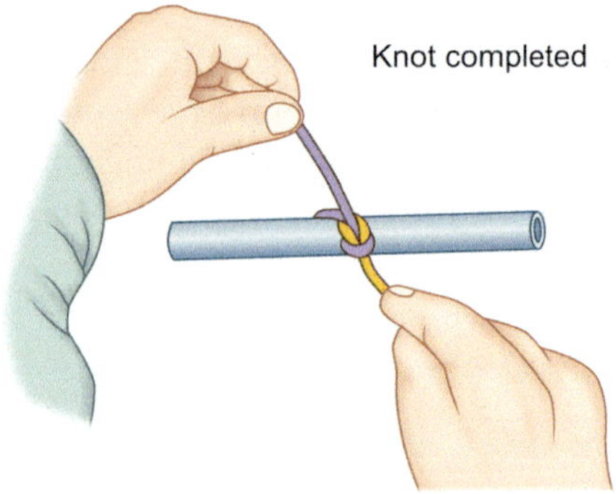

Fig. 9

Figs. 1 to 9: Various steps of single-handed reef knot.

Single-handed Surgeon's Knot

In this knot, there is *double throw* in the *first half knot*. To create this knot the short end is drawn twice through the loop made over index before pulling the short end toward operator. Knot is completed by making a middle finger throw.

Double-handed Reef Knot

A double-handed reef knot is used if there is a free suture without needle attached to it. So instead of the short end and long end, there will be two equal ends. One end away from operator and one end toward the operator.

Steps

1. End away from operator is placed over the extended index finger of the left hand and held in the palm keeping the left thumb free. The other end is held in the right hand **(Fig. 11)**.

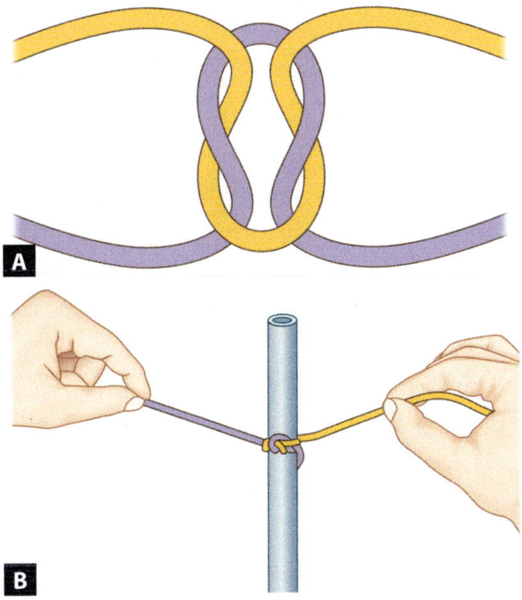

Figs. 10A and B: (A) Cross-section of completed reef knot; (B) Completed reef knot final appearance.

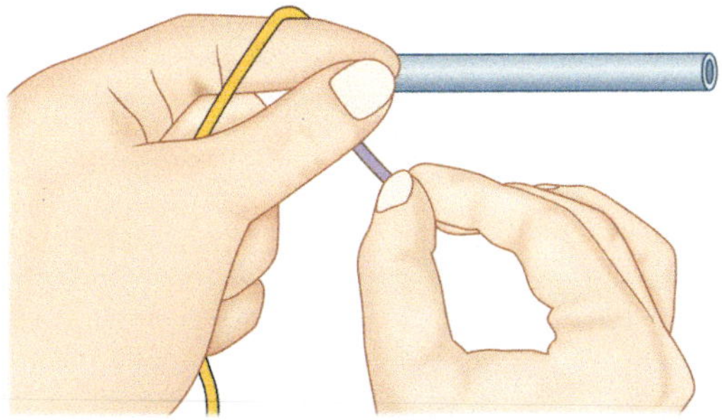

Fig. 12

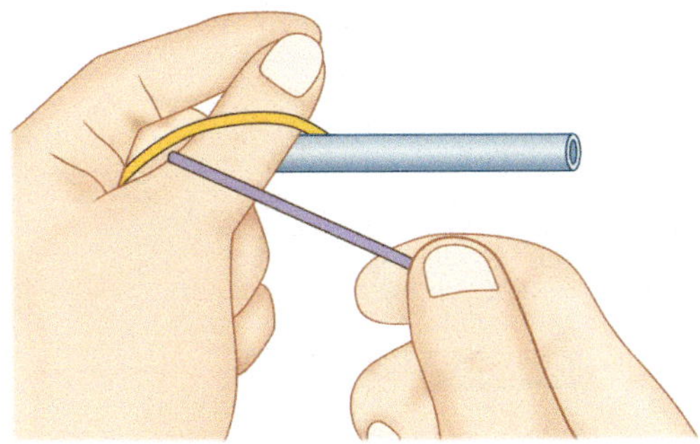

Fig. 13

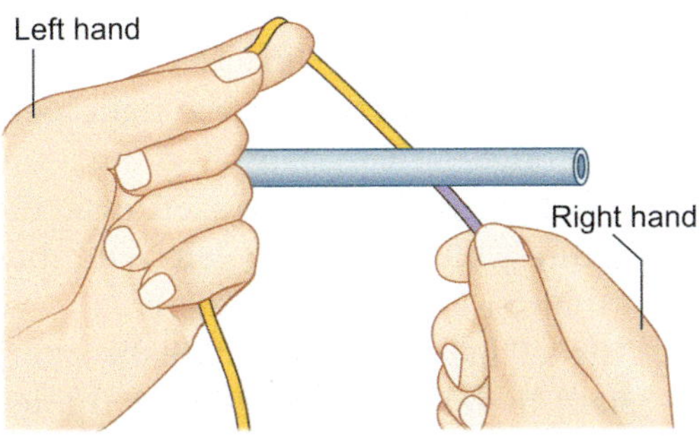

Fig. 11

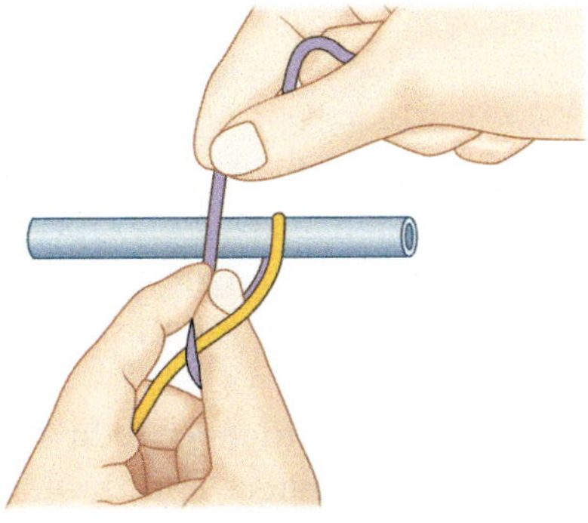

Fig. 14

2. End held in right hand is brought between the left thumb and index finger **(Fig. 12)**.
3. Left hand is turned inward by pronation and thumb is brought under the suture held by the left hand to form the *first loop* **(Fig. 13)**.
4. Suture end held in the right hand is crossed over the loop formed on left thumb and is transferred to be held between thumb and index finger of left hand **(Fig. 14)**.
5. The left hand which is still holding the end between index finger and thumb

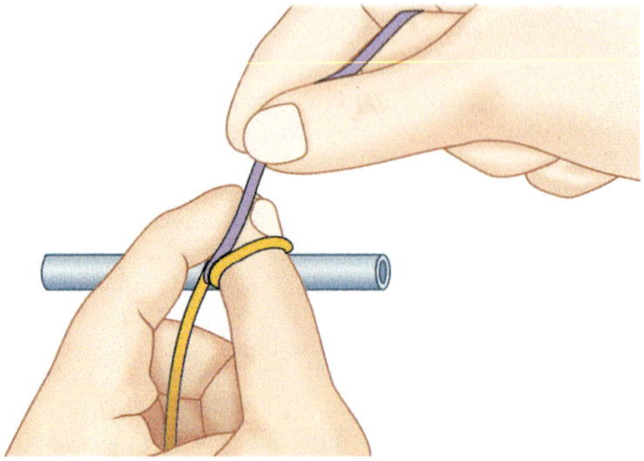

Fig. 15

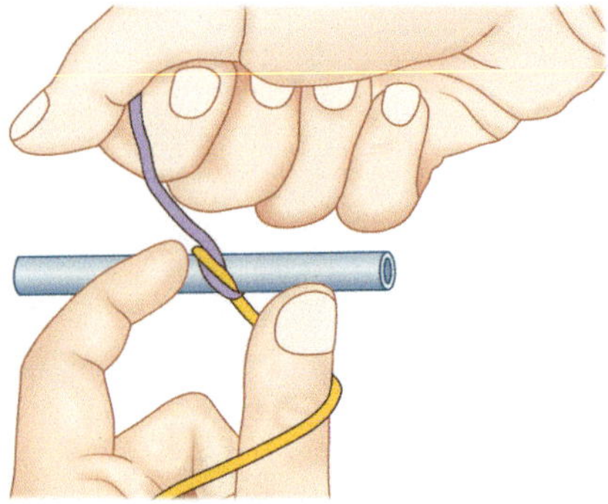

Fig. 17

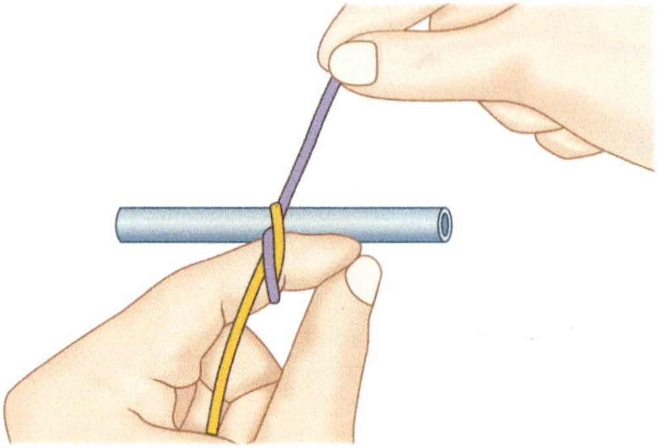

Fig. 16

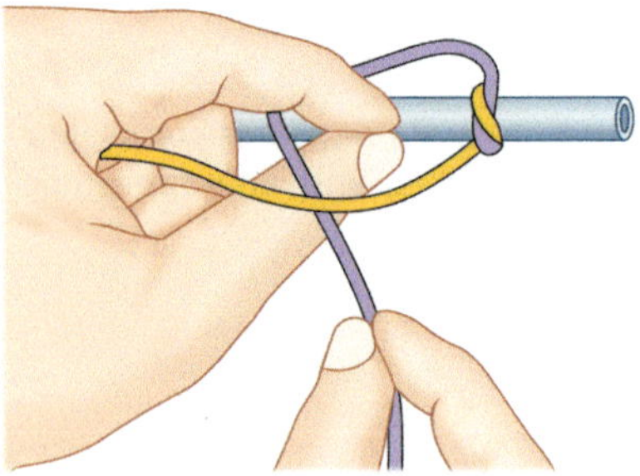

Fig. 18

(which was held by right hand initially) is supinated to bring the end held between the left index finger thumbs through the loop formed over the left index finger **(Fig. 15)**.

6. The end which is held between the left index finger and thumb is brought through the loop formed over the left index finger, released by left hand and then grasped by the right hand.
7. *First half knot* is completed by applying horizontal tension and crossing hands **(Fig. 16)**.
8. The left index finger is freed from the suture held by the same hand. A loop is formed over the left thumb by *supination* of the hand **(Fig. 17)**.
9. The suture end held by the right hand is brought in between left thumb and index finger and is crossed over the suture which is held by left hand thus forming a loop over left thumb.
10. The left hand is supinated till the suture held by left hand slides over the left index finger from left thumb **(Fig. 18)**.
11. The suture end held in the right hand is now held between the left thumb and index fingers **(Fig. 19)**.
12. The left hand is rotated inward by *pronation* thus carrying the end held between the left index finger and thumb through the loop formed by suture end held by remaining fingers of left hand over left thumb **(Fig. 20)**.

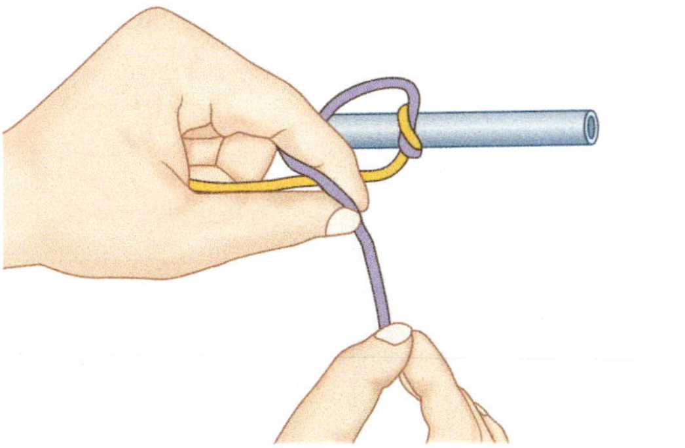

Fig. 19

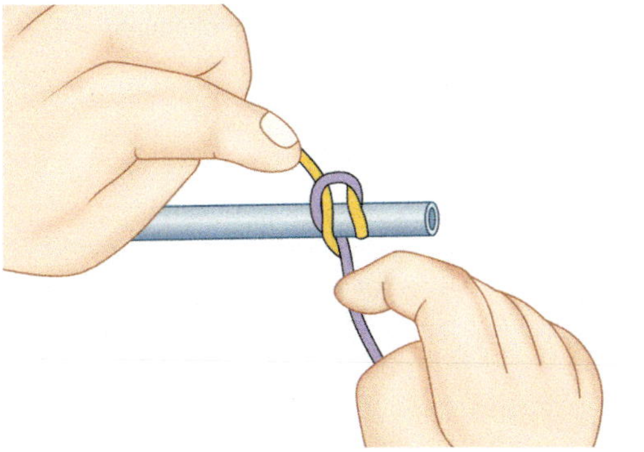

Fig. 21

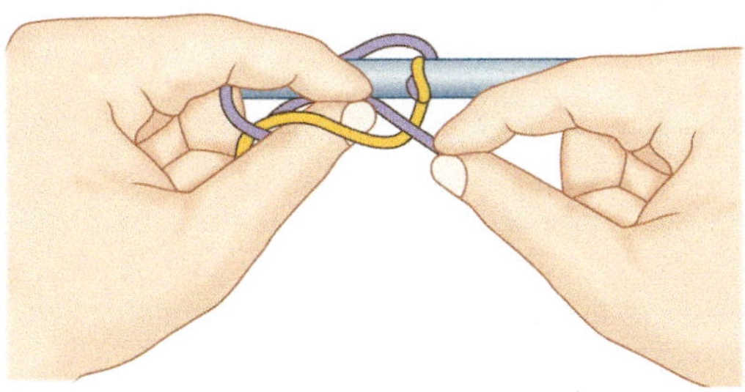

Fig. 20

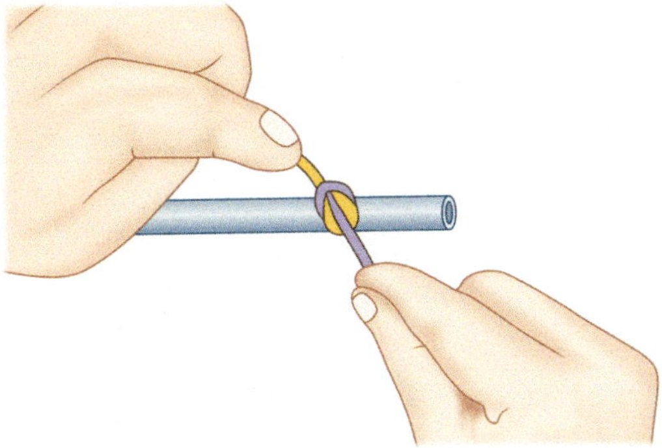

Fig. 22

Figs. 11 to 22: Various steps of two hand tied reef knot.

13. The suture end which was being held by the left index finger and thumb and has been brought through loop is re-grasped between the right thumb and index finger and then released by the left index finger and thumb.
14. *Second half knot* is completed by applying horizontal tension across the two ends **(Figs. 20 to 22)**.
15. Final tension on the final throw should be as horizontal as possible.

Surgeon's Knot by Two Hands (Figs. 23 to 33)

This differs from a two-handed square knot in the first half. The other end held in the right hand is passed through the loop formed over left index finger twice, before pulling the two ends in opposite directions in a horizontal plane.

Instrument tied knot: Instrument tie is useful when one or both ends of the suture material are short.

Steps of instrument tied surgeon's knot:

1. Short end lies freely away from the operator and long end is held between thumb and index finger of the left hand, thus creating an English letter "V" between both ends **(Fig. 34)**.
2. Place the needle holder inside the "V" and make two loops over the needle holder with the long end **(Fig. 35)**.

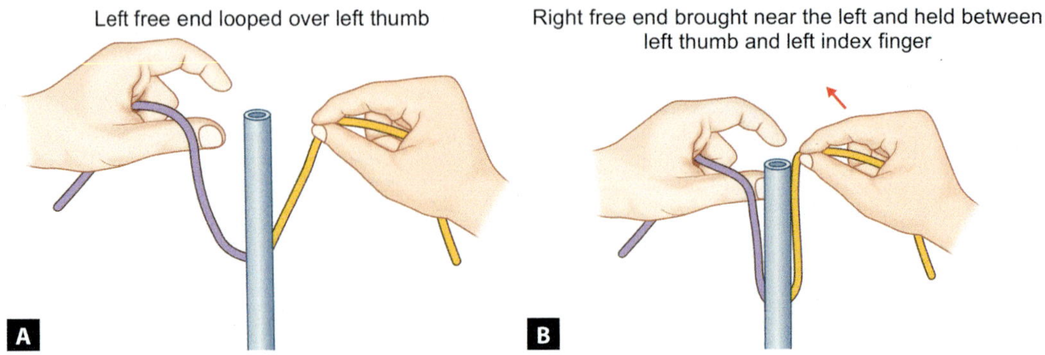

Figs. 23A and B

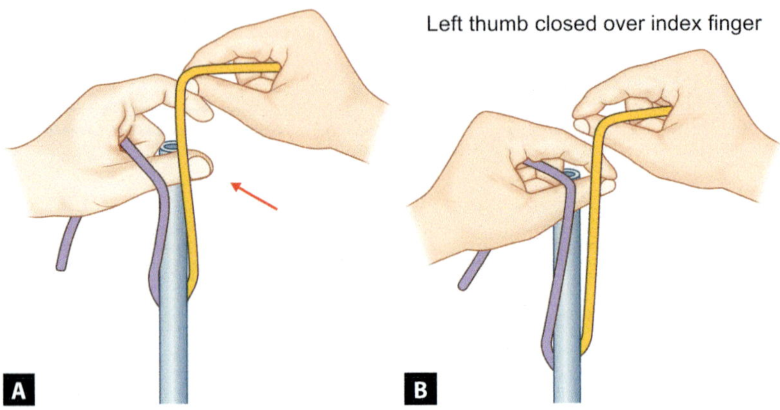

Figs. 24A and B

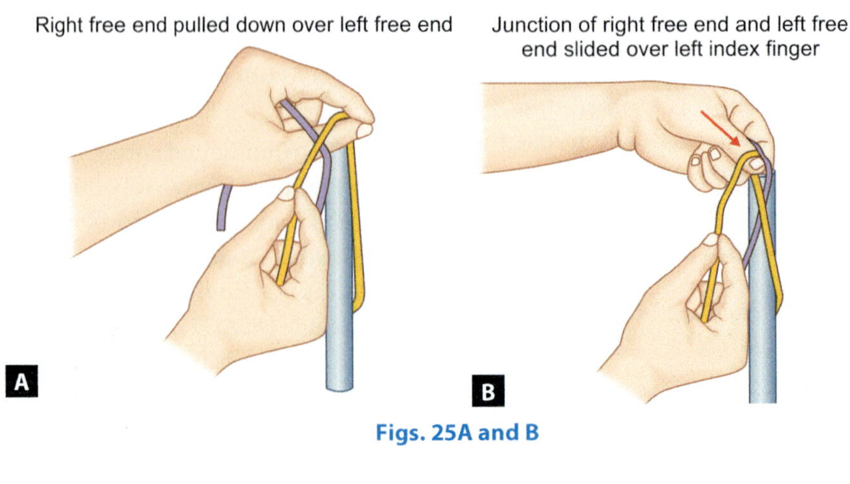

Figs. 25A and B

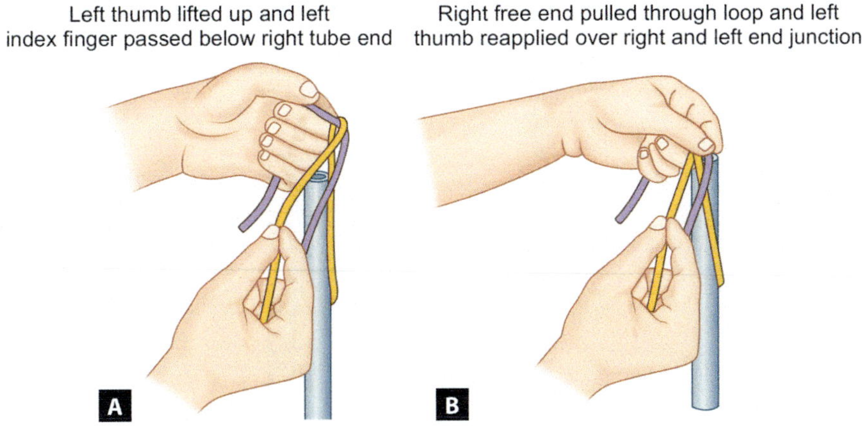

Figs. 26A and B

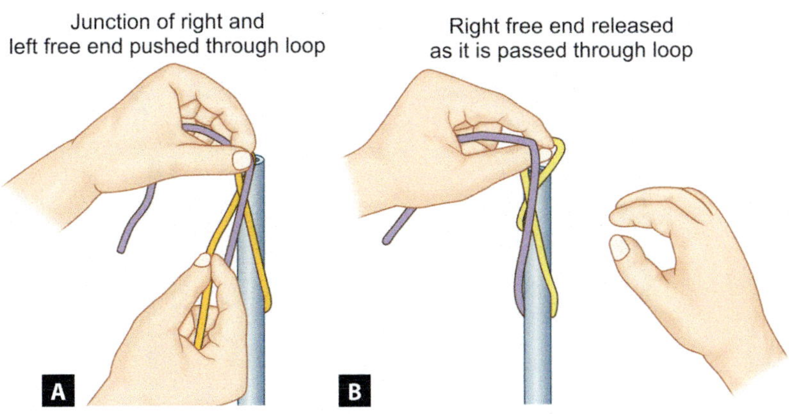

Figs. 27A and B

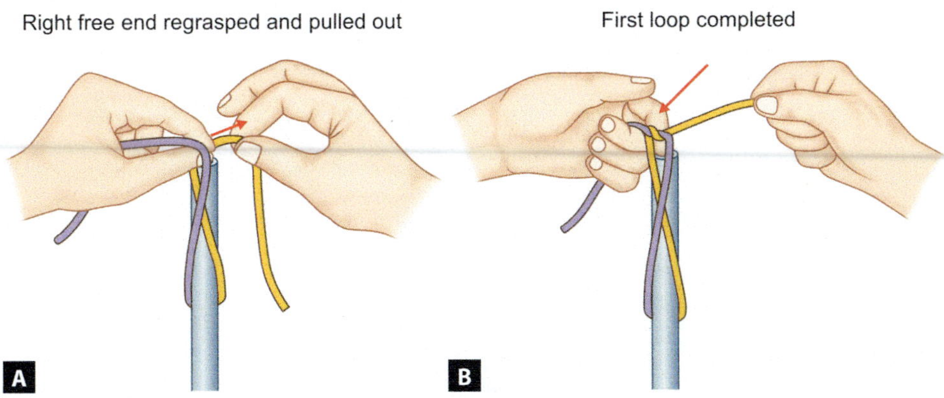

Figs. 28A and B

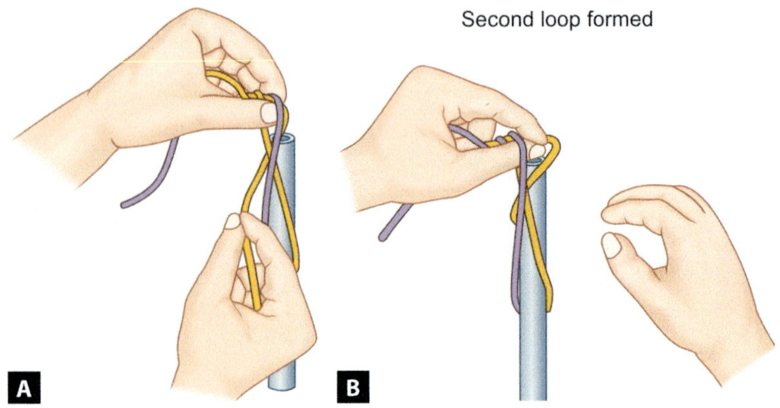

Figs. 29A and B

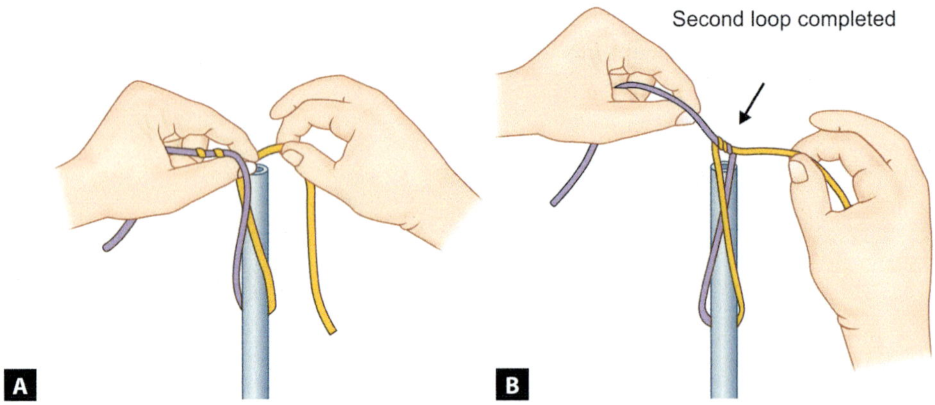

Figs. 30A and B

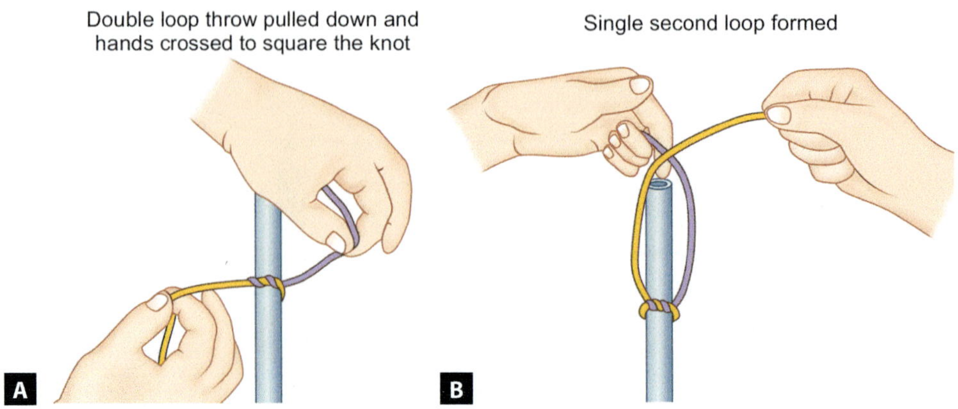

Figs. 31A and B

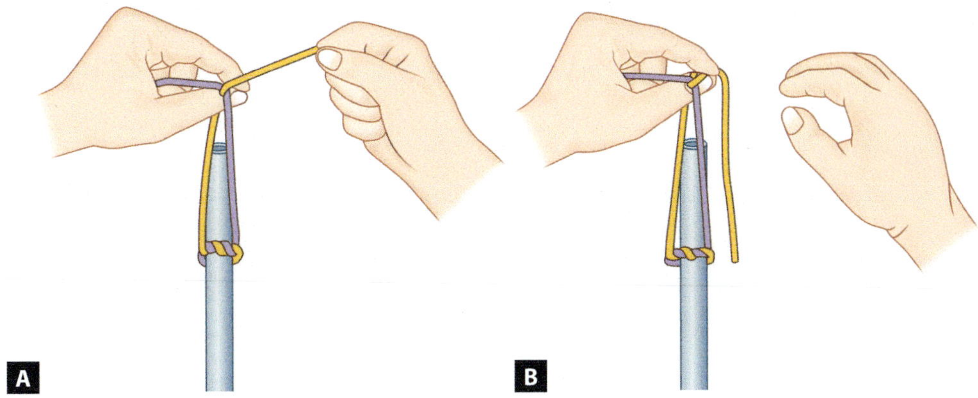

Figs. 32A and B

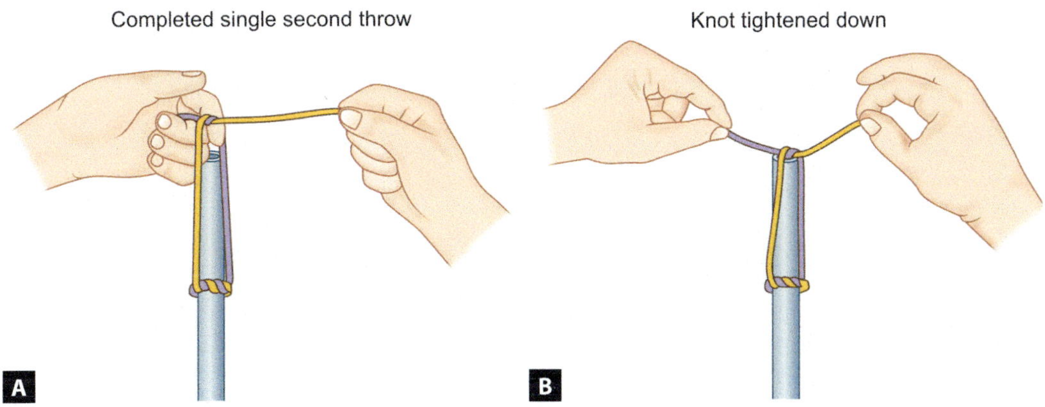

Figs. 33A and B

Figs. 23 to 33: Various steps of two-hand-tied surgeon's knot.

3. The needle holder in the right hand grasps the short end of the thread **(Fig. 36)**.
4. *First half* of the knot is completed by pulling the needle holder toward oneself thus bringing the short end toward the operator **(Fig. 37)**.
5. Long end is again held between left thumb and index finger.
6. The needle holder is held in the right hand and again placed in the "*V*" formed by both ends **(Fig. 38)**.
7. A loop is formed over the needle holder by the long end **(Fig. 39)**.
8. The short end is pulled through the loop away from the operator while pulling the long end in the opposite direction **(Fig. 40)**.
9. The knot is completed by horizontal tension applied by the left hand holding the long end and the right hand holding the short end with the needle holder. Tension should be as horizontal as possible **(Fig. 41)**.

ENDO-KNOTTING

Both intracorporeal and extracorporeal suturing and knot tying techniques are used in laparoscopic surgery.

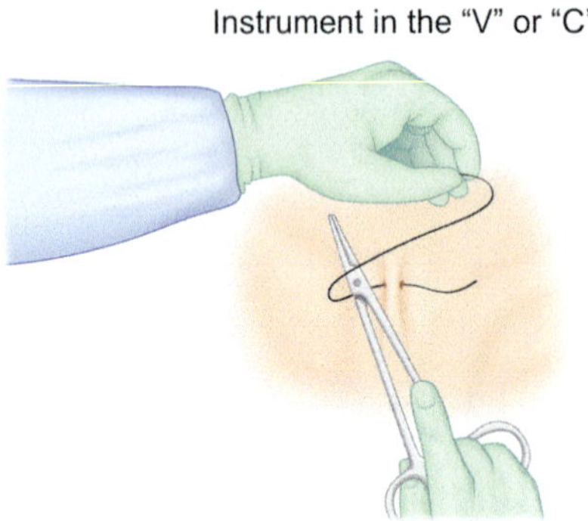

Fig. 34

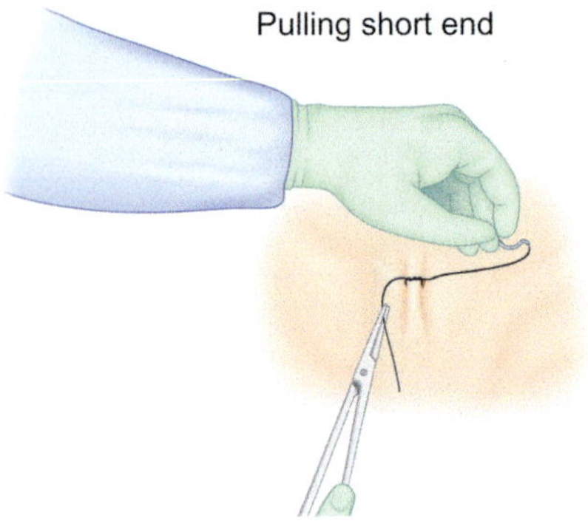

Fig. 37

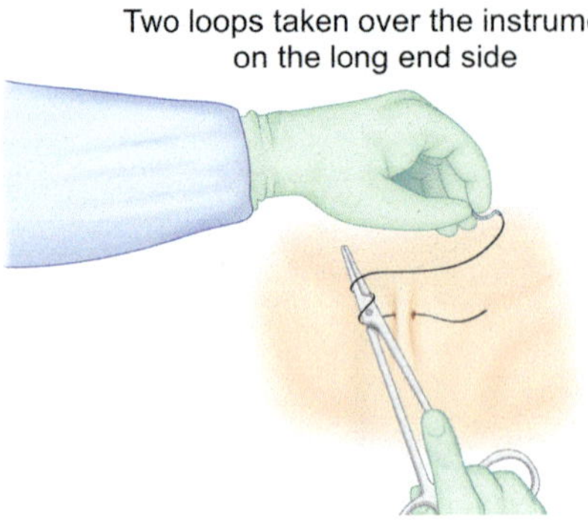

Fig. 35

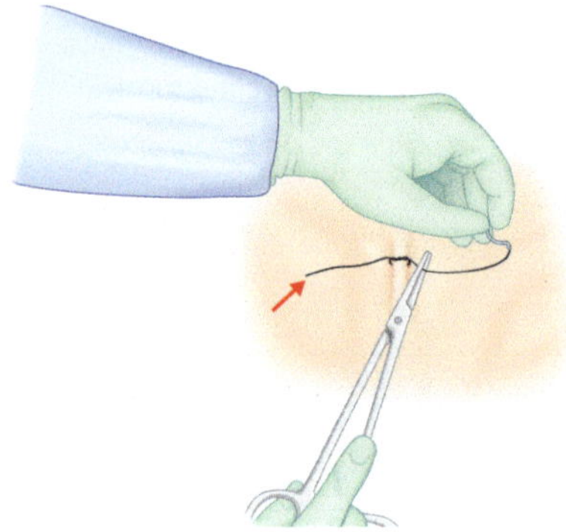

Fig. 38

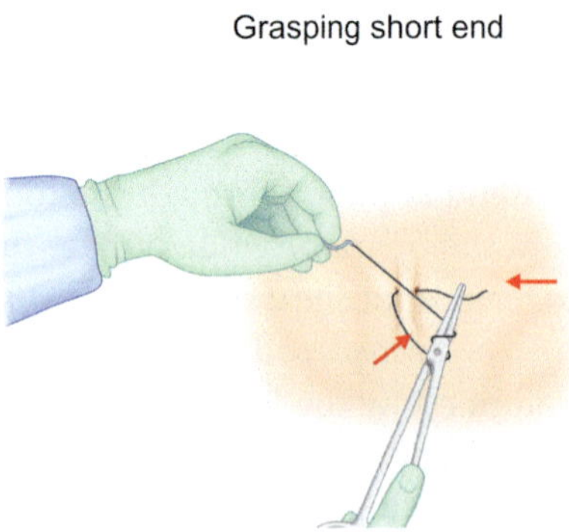

Fig. 36

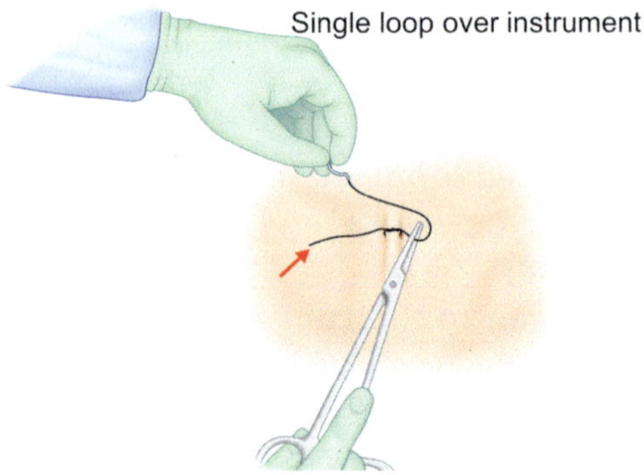

Fig. 39

Extracorporeal Knot Tying

A Roeder's knot is widely used in laparoscopic surgery for extracorporeal tying. Commercially available pretied loops also have a Roeder's knot. *Chromic catgut* or *vicryl* is generally used for making a pretied loop because chromic catgut slips easily. A loop can be made by the surgeon. Self-made loops are cheaper.

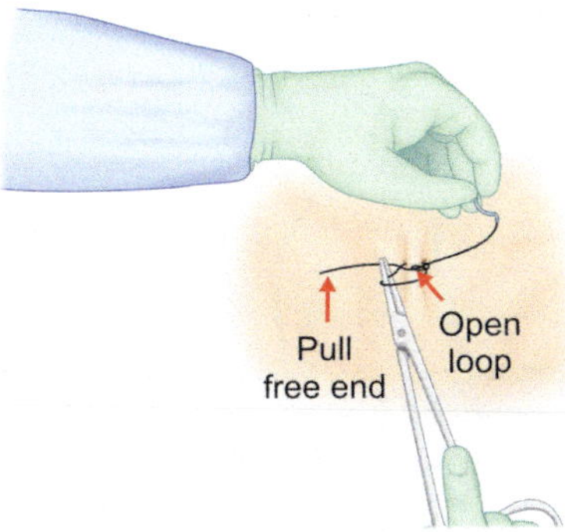

Fig. 40

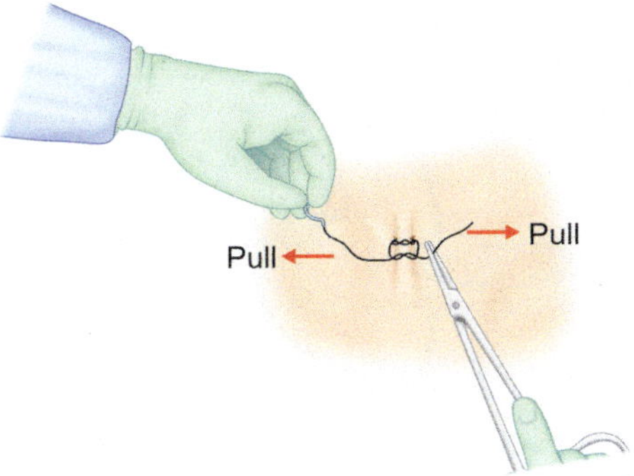

Fig. 41

Figs. 34 to 41: Various steps of instrument tied surgeon's knot.

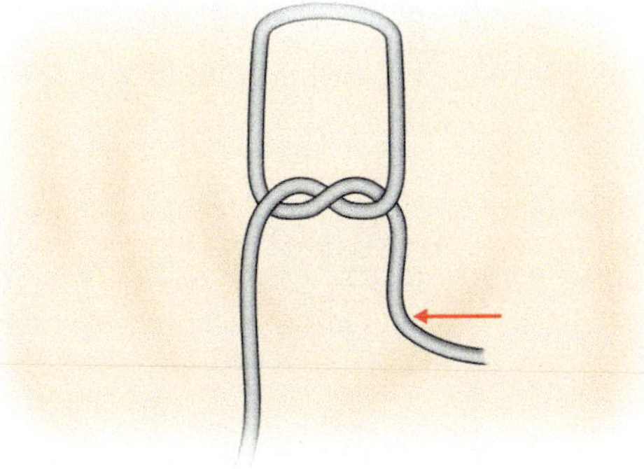

Fig. 42

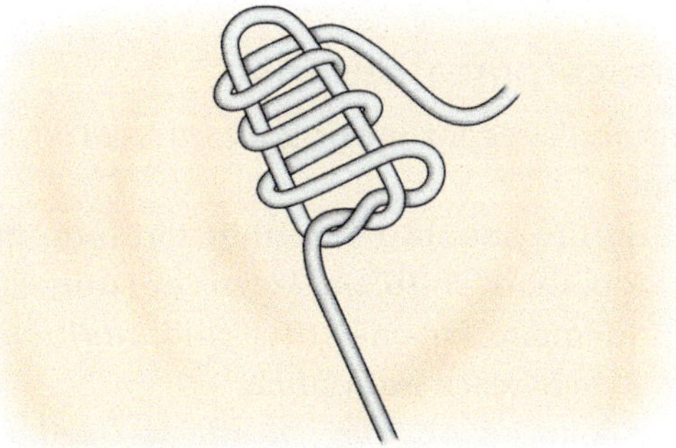

Fig. 43

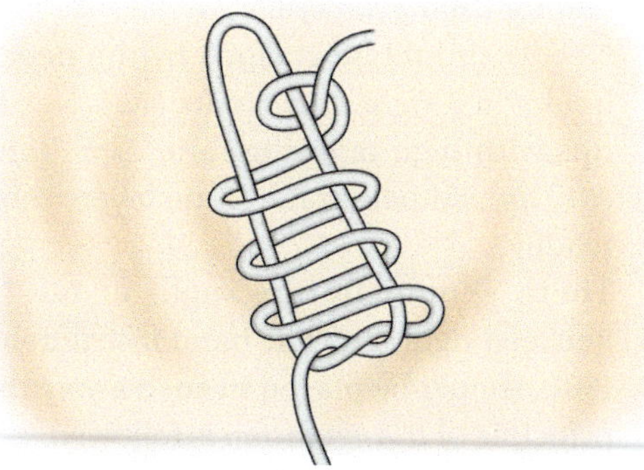

Fig. 44

Steps in Making a Roeder's Knot

1. A loop is formed over the left index finger **(Fig. 42)**.
2. Tail end of the loop is brought out of the loop making a full circle **(Fig. 42)**.
3. Three full circles are thrown on the tail end of the loop **(Fig. 43)**.
4. Tie is closed by encircling both limbs of the loop to complete the final full circle **(Figs. 44 and 45)**.

Indications for Loop Application

- To ligate *pedicles.*
- To ligate of the *base of the appendix.*
- In case of a *wider cystic duct* when appropriate size clip is not applicable.
- To control a *bleeding vessel* which is held by an endograsper.
- To ligate the *hernial sac* in an indirect hernia.

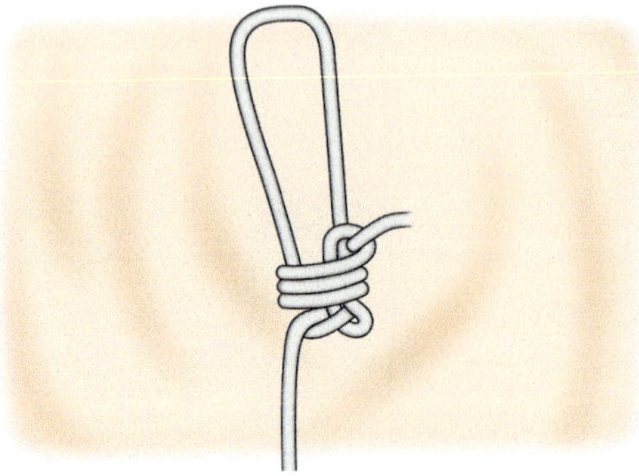

Fig. 45

Figs. 42 to 45: Various steps of tying Roeder's knot.

Intracorporeal Suturing

Prerequisites for making an intracorporeal knot:

- Suture should be neither too long nor too short. *8–10 cm length* of sutures is adequate for one stitch and *additional 3 cm* for each extra stitch.
- A curved or *"ski" needle* is used for endosuturing. Needle is loaded reversely into the reducing sleeve.
- Left hand forceps should be *atraumatic tissue grasping forceps*.
- Needle should be grasped by the needle holder at a *right angle* to its jaws. Needle tips with high tapering ratio or a *"taper cut" tip* will penetrate tissue layers more readily.
- There should be an angle of 60–70° between right- and left-hand instrument.
- Ports should be placed in such a way that principle of *triangulation* is followed.
- *Vicryl* or *PDS* is ideal for endosuturing.

TECHNIQUE OF SQUARE AND SURGEON'S KNOT

Over Hand Flat Knot

- Create a "C" loop held in the horizontal plane **(Fig. 46A)**.

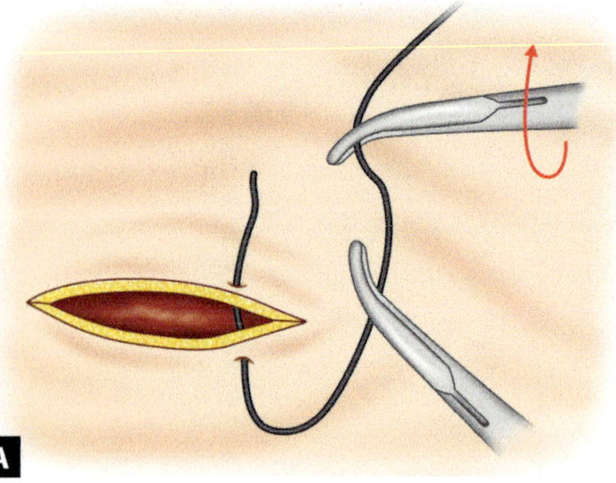

A

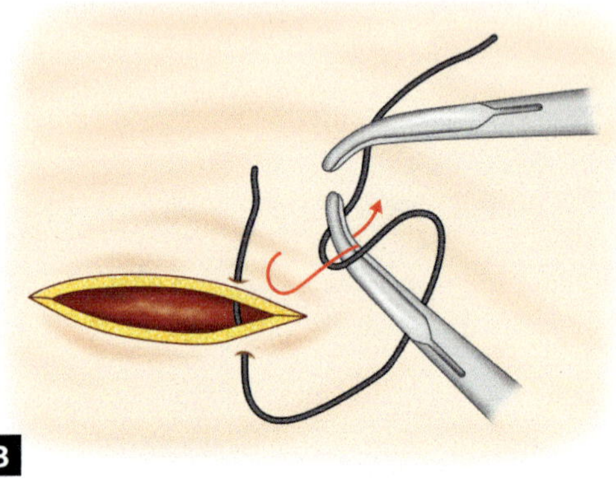

B

Figs. 46A and B

- Thread should lie flat against the tissue.
- Right instrument holds the long tail and left instrument is placed over the loop **(Fig. 46)**.
- The short tail should be long enough to avoid accidentally pulling it out but not so long that its end is hidden.
- Use a large loop to allow sufficient room for movement of both instruments.
- Use the right instrument to wrap the long tail around the stationary tip of the left instrument **(Fig. 46B)**.
- Both instruments move toward the short tail.
- Left instrument is used to grasp the tip of the short tail end and pulled out of the wrap to the right completing the *first flat knot* **(Figs. 47 and 48)**.

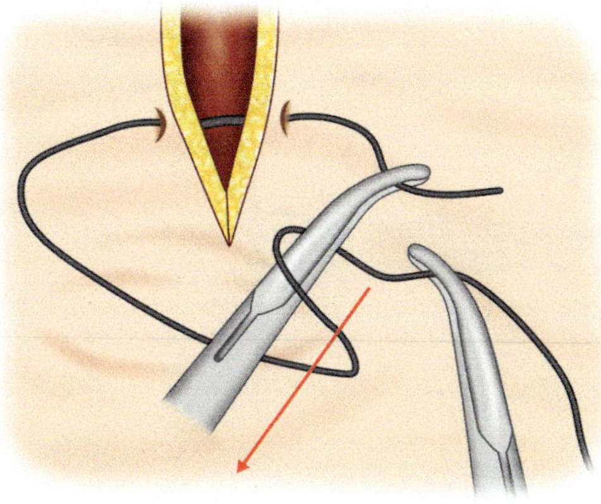

Fig. 47

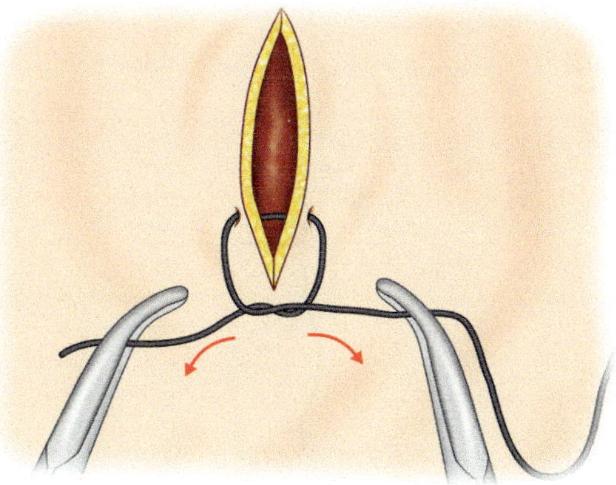

Fig. 48

- Pull the short tail through the loop and adjust it so that there is an equal length left. Pull the two instruments in opposite directions.
- Left instrument then drops the short tail and right instrument keeps its grasp on the long tail **(Fig. 49)**.

Second Opposing Flat Knot

- Right instrument is brought to the left side of the field and rotated clockwise 180°.
- Right instrument transfers the long tail to the left instrument thus creating a reverse "C" loop.

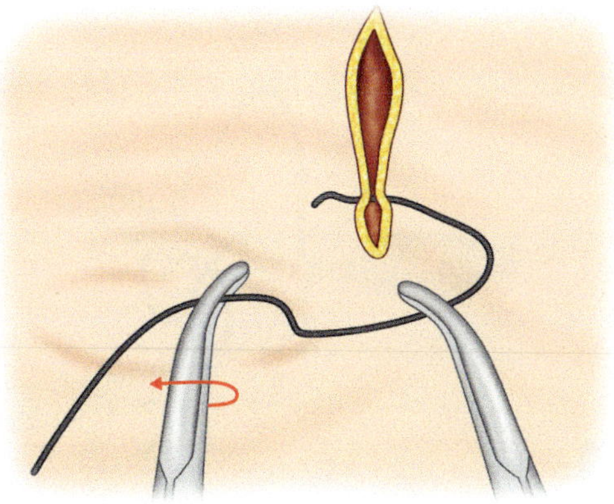

Fig. 49

- Right instrument is placed over the reversed "C" loop and the left instrument wraps the thread around right instrument **(Fig. 50A)**.
- Tips of both instruments are moved together in unison toward the short tail which is grasped with the right instrument.
- Pull the short tail through the loop and then both tails in opposite directions parallel to the stitch with equal tension to configure the knot **(Fig. 50B)**.

Slip Knot Conversion for the Square Knot (Szabo Technique)

This is essential to tighten the first half knot to provide adequate grip **(Figs. 51 to 53)**.

- Both instruments grasp the loop on same side, one below the knot and one above the knot **(Fig. 51A)**.
- Both instruments pull in opposite directions until a snapping or popping sensation can be felt. Conversion is easier in monofilament suture **(Fig. 51B)**.
- Pushing the slip knot. The right instrument maintains its grasp on the tail and pulls it tightly. Left instrument pushes the knot closer to the tissue by sliding on this tail **(Fig. 52)**.

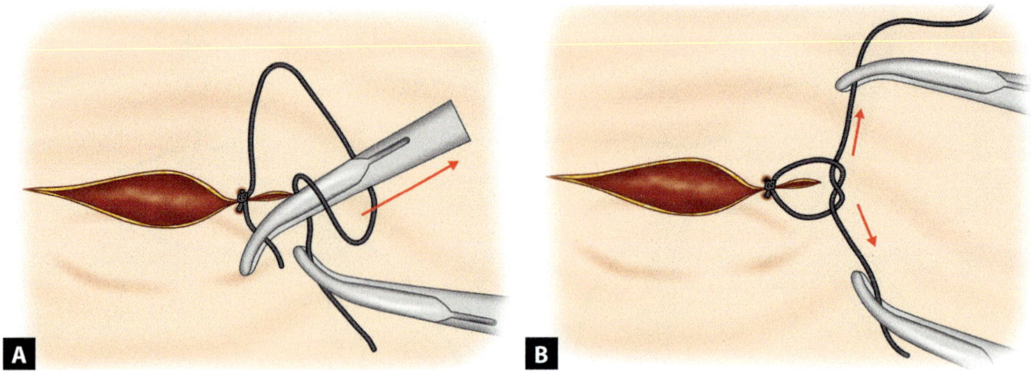

Figs. 50A and B

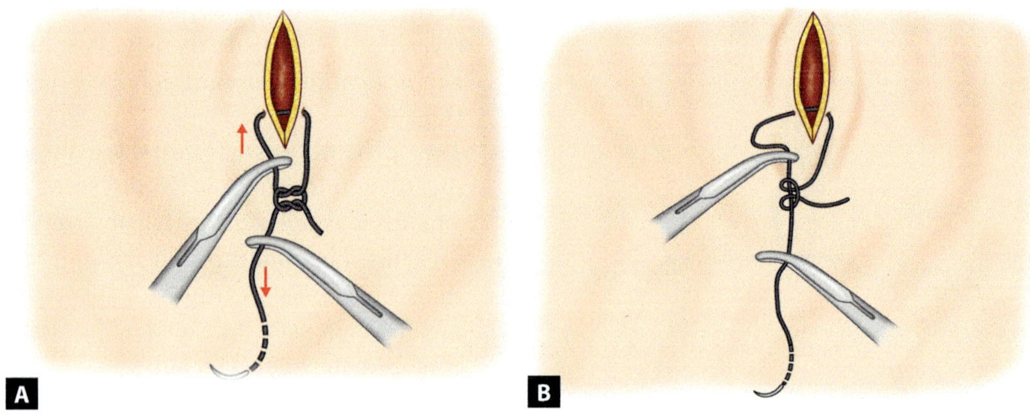

Figs. 51A and B

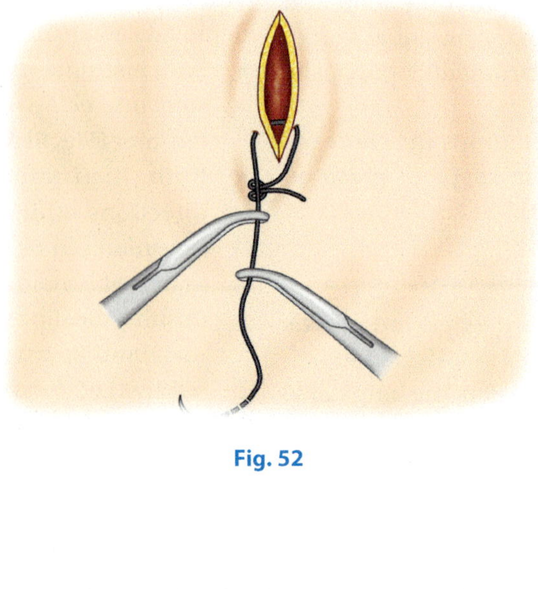

Fig. 52

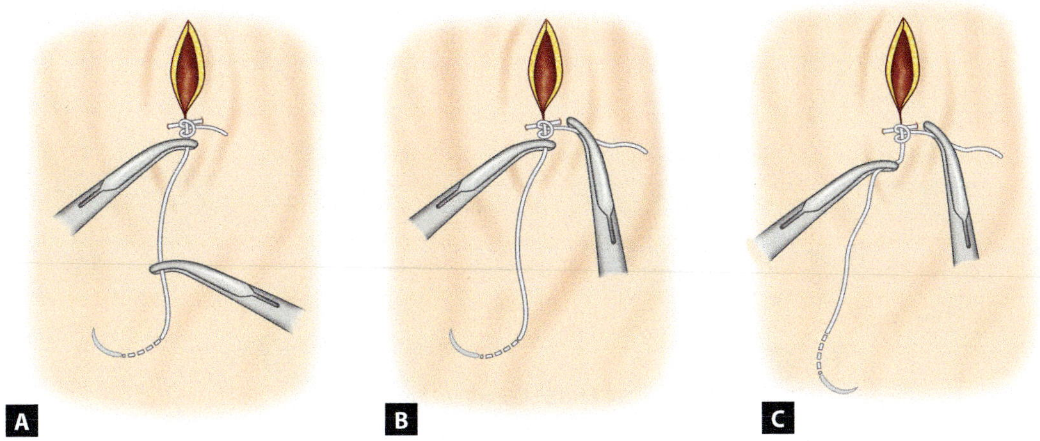

Figs. 53A to C

Figs. 46 to 53: Various steps of intracorporeal knotting.

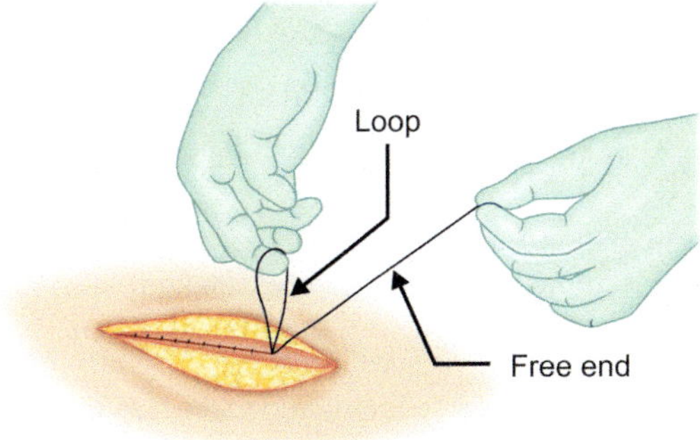

Fig. 54

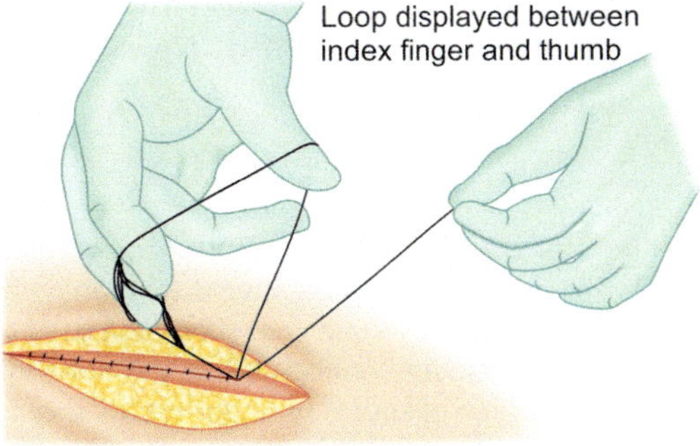

Fig. 55

- Clinch down the slip knot till tissue edges have been approximated **(Fig. 53A)**.
- Reconvert slip knot to square knot by pulling ends in opposite directions **(Figs. 53B and C)**.

ABERDEEN KNOT (FIGS. 54 TO 58)

This knot is applied at the end of a continuous suture, when left with a loop and a free end **(Fig. 54)**. To tie this knot, loop is displayed

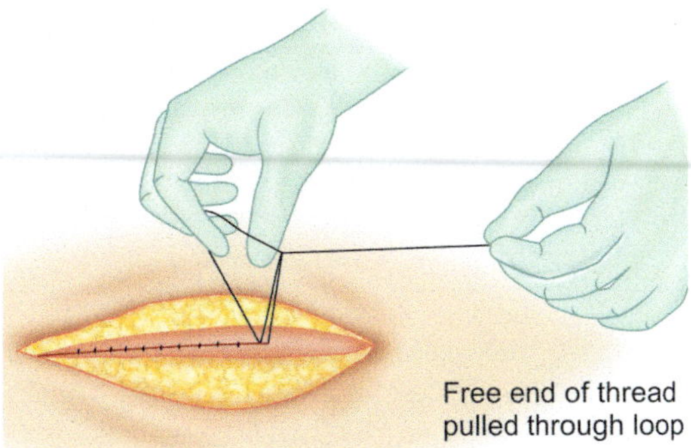

Fig. 56

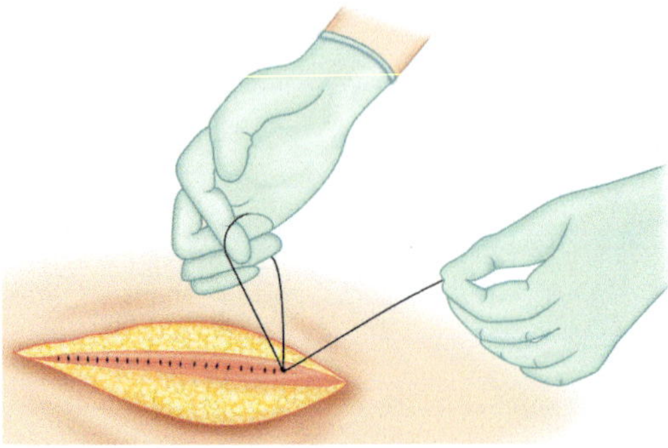

Fig. 57

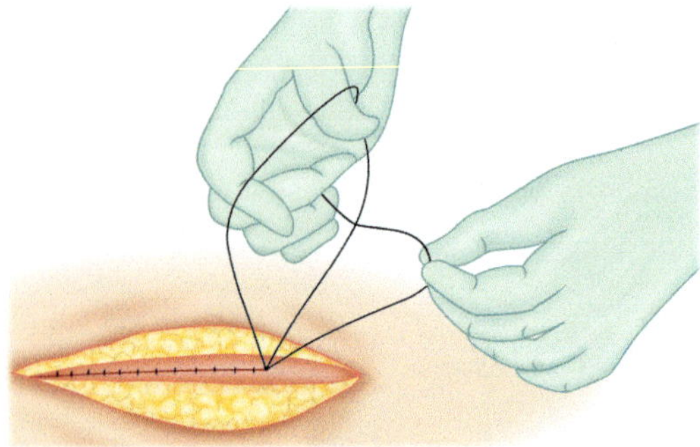

Fig. 58

Figs. 54 to 58: Aberdeen knot.

between the index finger and thumb of left hand and free end is grasped between the index finger and thumb of the left hand through the loop and by pulling it through and releasing the right-hand thread, old loop is eliminated **(Fig. 55)**. New loop is formed again between left index finger and thumb and right-hand thread is pulled again **(Figs. 56 to 58)**. Whole process is repeated 6–7 times using "see-saw" movement. Finally, the free end is passed through the loop and tightened down.

KEY POINTS

- Knots are used for approximation of tissues and ligation of blood vessels.
- Multifilament sutures are easier to tie than monofilament suture and give a more secure knot.
- Surgeon's knot or square knot should be used as far as possible.
- Granny knot should not be used as it is not a safe knot.
- Whatever type of knot is used, the hands should cross after one throw to lock it and make it safe.

CHAPTER 8

Wound Closure Techniques

MD Raihan, Sudhir Kumar Jain, David L Stoker

"Proper wound closure techniques attain optimum functional and cosmetic outcome"

INTRODUCTION

The majority of lacerations can be repaired by primary wound closure.

Primary wound closure has the following advantages:

- Brings wound edges together neatly and evenly.
- Achieves hemostasis.
- Preserves function of the tissue.
- Prevents infection.
- Restores cosmetic appearance.
- Promotes rapid healing by primary intention.
- Decreases patient's discomfort and morbidity.

TIME OF WOUND CLOSURE

There is a direct relationship between the time of wound closure and the risk of infection.

Wounds of the face and scalp can be closed by primary closure up to 72 hours after injury without increasing the risk of infection, due to the high vascular supply in this region. In other areas, there is no significant time-related difference in infection rates for wounds closed within 18 hours.

INCREASED RISK OF INFECTION

There is a high incidence of wound infection after laceration repair in the following situations:

- Diabetes mellitus
- Obesity
- Malnourishment
- Immunosuppression, e.g., human immunodeficiency virus (HIV) infection
- Patient on steroids, chemotherapeutic agents, or immunosuppressive therapy
- Crush injuries leading to devitalized tissue
- Contaminated wounds.

WOUND CLOSURE TECHNIQUES

There are five main options for wound closure available **(Table 1)**.

SUTURING OF LACERATIONS

Suturing of lacerations is generally performed under local anesthesia except in the following situations which may require general anesthesia:

- Large lacerations where the requirement of local anesthesia will exceed the toxic dose.
- Severe contamination requiring extensive cleaning or removal of foreign body or extensive tissue debridement.
- Open fractures, tendon, nerve, or major blood vessel injury.
- Complex structures requiring meticulous repair, e.g., eyelid.

TABLE 1: Five options for wound closure.

Option	*Description*
1. Primary closure by sutures	The most common method used for wound closure. It involves stitching the wound edges together to promote healing
2. Secondary closure or delayed primary closure	Used for wounds that are grossly contaminated, infected, or have been attended to late. The wound is initially left open, cleaned, and then closed once infection is controlled
3. Tissue adhesives (e.g., cyanoacrylate glue)	Adhesive glues applied to the wound edge to bond them together. Useful for smaller wounds and provides a quick closure
4. Staples	Skin staples are used in larger wounds. They are faster to apply than sutures and provide good cosmetic results, though they are more expensive
5. Surgical tapes or steristrips	Adhesive strips that hold the wound edges together. Often used minor wounds or as an adjunct to other closure methods

Equipment Required for Wound Suturing

- Universal precaution kit.
- Suturing tray containing needle holder, toothed forceps, and suture scissors.
- 1 or 2% lignocaine with or without adrenaline for local anesthesia.
- 10-cc syringe and 21–25-gauge needles for infiltrating anesthesia.
- Appropriate sutures.
- Wound preparation and cleaning materials, e.g., povidone-iodine solution, gauze pieces, and normal saline.
- Tetanus immunization serum.

Steps of Laceration Suturing

1. Wound assessment
2. Wound preparation
3. Wound closure
4. Tetanus prophylaxis.

Wound Assessment

- Establish approximate time of injury as after 4 hours, the wound should be scrubbed to remove the protein coagulum.
- Determine exact mechanism of injury which can point toward an underlying fracture, retained foreign body, tendon or nerve injury or wound contamination.
- Ask about tetanus immunization status.
- Test for distal sensory and motor function to rule out nerve and tendon injury.
- Consider imaging studies if there is a radio-opaque retained foreign body such as glass.
- Wound should be accurately described in the patient's record as it may have medico-legal consequences or insurance implications.

Wound Preparation

Hair removal may be required for more precise wound closure. However, shaving might introduce infection. Clipping the hair may be a better approach than shaving. Eyebrows are usually not trimmed or shaved because the hair may regrow in abnormal patterns, and they are a useful guide to correct alignment of a forehead wound.

- Wound cleaning is done either by direct scrubbing or irrigation of the tissue. Vigorous scrubbing may lead to tissue damage which may increase the risk of infection.
- Wound irrigation is another method of wound preparation. It can be achieved either by continuous or pulsatile irrigation. Continuous high pressure

syringe irrigation significantly reduces the bacterial count, and is particularly useful in dense contaminated tissue with limited vascularity such as a lower extremity wound. Irrigation pressures between 5 and 8 psi are appropriate and can be readily obtained with a 30–60 mL syringe and a 19-gauge needle. High pressure irrigation is contraindicated in a well-vascularized location with delicate soft tissues such as eyelid, because it can lead to tissue damage in these areas with an increase in infection rate. A variety of solutions, e.g., detergents, hydrogen peroxide, and concentrated betadine have been used to irrigate wounds, but these are no longer recommended because of their damaging effects on tissues. Normal saline is the solution of choice because it does not damage tissue and is widely available and inexpensive. 100 cc of saline is used for each of wound. If using plain lignocaine for local anesthesia it may be buffered by adding 1 mL of sodium bicarbonate to 9 mL of lignocaine to reduce the pain of injection. Inject slowly, and subdermally, beginning inside the cut margin of the wound. Avoid piercing the intact skin. The maximum safe dose of lignocaine is 3 mg/kg. It can be increased to up to 7 mg/kg when lignocaine is used along with adrenaline.

WOUND SUTURING

Face

Use 4-0 or 5-0 monofilament suture on a cutting needle. Both absorbable and nonabsorbable suture can be used on the face. The type of stitch used is either simple interrupted or subcuticular. Layered closure may be needed if the wound is deep, with a 3-0 or 4-0 polyglactin suture to approximate the muscle. Sutures are removed in 5 days.

Scalp

2-0 or 3-0 nonabsorbable monofilament suture on a cutting needle is used for suturing. Sutures are removed in 10 days.

Lip

4-0 or 5-0 synthetic absorbable suture on a tapercut needle is used for the deeper layers. 3-0 synthetic monofilament on cutting needle is used for the skin. Simple interrupted sutures are applied for deeper layers and for the skin.

Oral Cavity

4-0 absorbable gut or synthetic absorbable suture on tapercut needle is used for suturing employing a mattress technique.

TYPES OF SUTURES

Simple Interrupted Suture

This is the most common suture employed for closure of lacerations. A fine smooth nonabsorbable suture, e.g., nylon or polypropylene is used for this purpose because it causes much less tissue reaction than silk. Cutting needles are used for applying this suture. The needle should pass at a right angle to the incision line and should pass through the whole thickness of the wound **(Fig. 1)**. If the depth of the incised wound is "X", then needle should pass at a distance of one "X" from the cut margin of wound and come out at a distance of "X" from the other margin of the wound, so that the distance between entry and exit point of suture in the skin is "2X" **(Fig. 2)**. This rule does not apply to wounds >1 cm deep, where layered closure is required.

Sutures should be tied with a tension just enough to approximate the edges without causing tissue constriction. If sutures are tied too tightly, they will cause ischemia, delayed

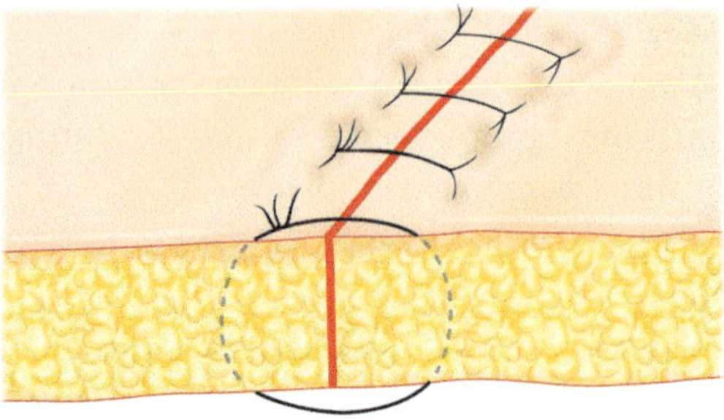

Fig. 1: Suture should be placed at right angle to the wound edge and should traverse whole thickness of the wound.

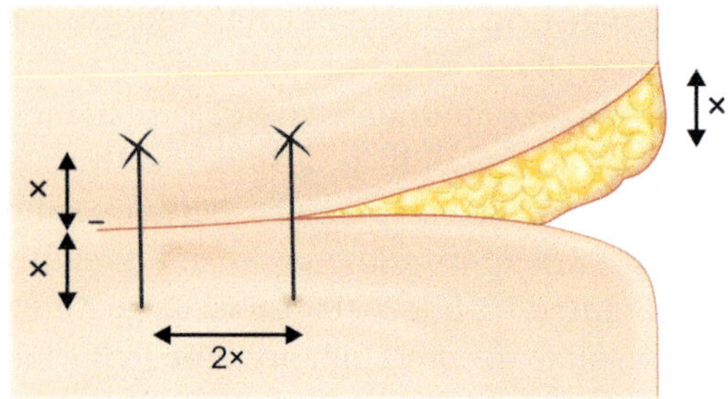

Fig. 2: Bite should be at a distance of "X" from the wound margin and come out at a distance of "X" from the opposite wound margin. "X" is the thickness of the wound. Distance between two sutures should be "2X".

healing, and increased scarring. Knots should be placed laterally and away from the wound. The next stitch should be placed at a distance of "2X" from the previous stitch **(Fig. 2)**. When cutting sutures, the length of left out tails from knot should be just <1 cm. If the tails are too long, they will entangle with the next stitch, and if tails are left too short, there is a danger of knot slippage and difficulty in suture removal later on. Sutures are generally removed around the 7th day except in the face where they are removed on 5th day. Below the knee and on the back, sutures are left for 10–14 days to prevent wound dehiscence.

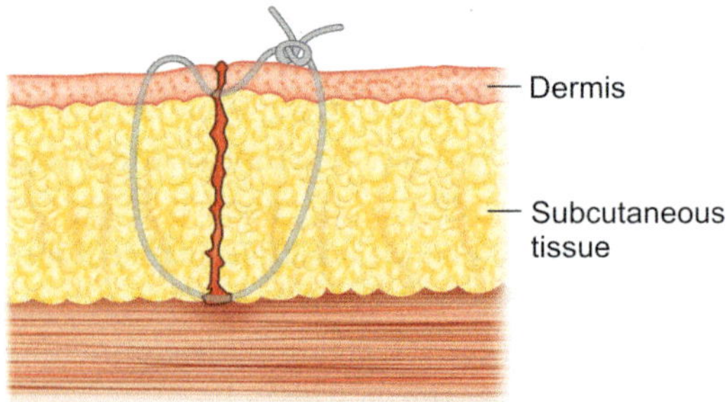

Fig. 3: Method of taking vertical mattress suture.

Vertical Mattress Suture (Fig. 3)

This suture is commonly used for closing surgical wounds. It is useful if there is excess skin or loose subcutaneous fat. There are two entry and two exit points. All points lie in the same line. Firstly, the needle enters the skin at a right angle at a distance from the wound margin of "X" (depth of wound) or about 1 cm if a wound is deep and a layered closure has been performed. It traverses the whole thickness of the wound, and the needle comes out from the other side of the wound at a distance of "X" or 1 cm. Secondly, the direction of needle is reversed. The needle is placed close to the margin of the wound, traversing epidermis only in such a manner that all four points lie in the same line, and the skin edges are everted. The knot is tied to one side. Skin edges may get inverted **(Fig. 4)** as everted by this suture **(Fig. 5)**.

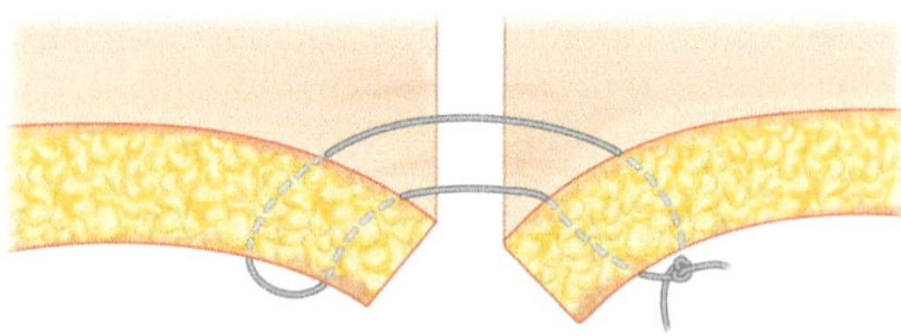

Fig. 4: Inversion of skin edges by vertical mattress suture.

Horizontal Mattress Suture (Figs. 6 and 7)

This is another eversion suture, and may be used where the skin is thick, e.g., on the sole of the foot. There are again two entry and

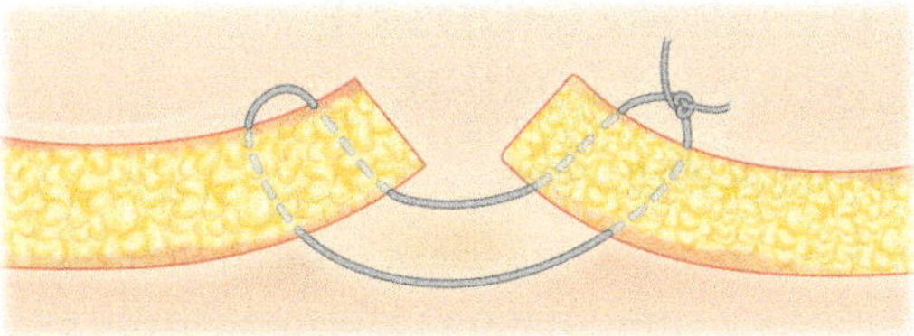

Fig. 5: Eversion of skin margin by vertical mattress suture.

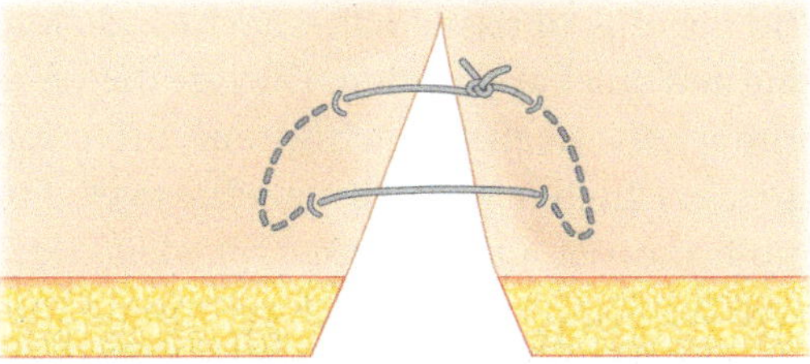

Fig. 6: Horizontal mattress suture.

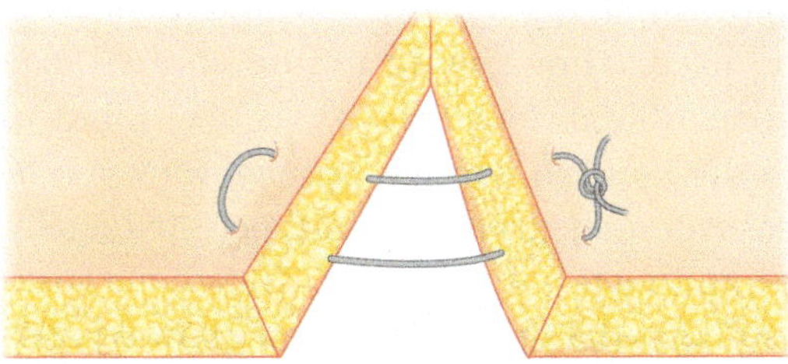

Fig. 7: Eversion of skin margin by horizontal mattress suture.

two exit points. Firstly, the needle is placed 4–8 mm from the wound edge. It then passes through to the opposite wound edge, where it exits the skin at about the same distance on the other side of the wound edge. The needle is reversed in the needle holder, and inserted into the same skin edge 4–8 mm further down the wound, and passed from this side back to the other side of the wound. The needle exits the skin about 4–8 mm down the original wound edge from the initial insertion site. This suture is shown in **Figures 6 and 7**. The main problem with this suture is that skin which is caught between each horizontal bite may lose its circulation when the knot is tied. These areas of ischemia may extend

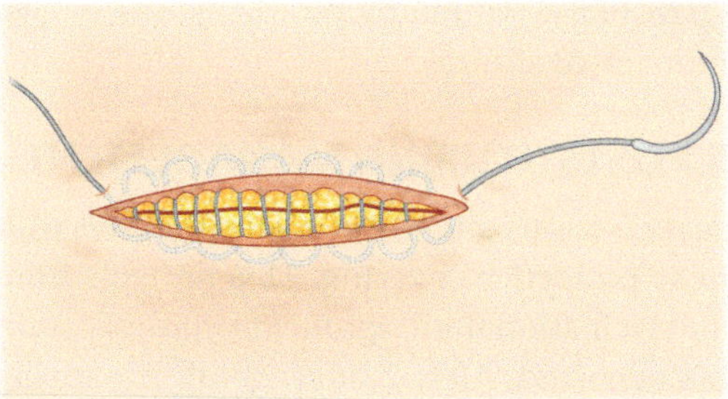

Fig. 8: Subcuticular suture.

up to 50% of the entire skin margin as further sutures are placed. Partial necrosis of the skin margin is therefore quite common.

Subcuticular Suture (Fig. 8)

This suture gives a very fine and neat scar because approximation of skin margins should be perfect. Either absorbable or nonabsorbable suture can be used for this technique. For absorbable sutures, the ends are secured by means of a buried knot. For nonabsorbable sutures, the ends are secured by means of beads or a knot outside. Small bites are taken of the dermis on alternate sides of the wound and these are then pulled together. A continuous subcuticular suture to approximate the dermal layer of the skin is a fast and cosmetically satisfactory method of skin closure. Its main advantage is that additional scarring from sutures is avoided. Its drawback is that it gives no support to the underlying tissue. Surgical gut should not be used for this suture as it produces an intense tissue reaction. If other synthetic absorbable sutures are used, knots should be placed deep and well away from the wound edge. A nonabsorbable nylon or prolene is ideal. Long wounds should have intermittent bridges or external loops of suture to facilitate suture removal. This suture should not be used where there is increased potential for wound infection, as it is not possible to open a part of the wound by removing one or two interrupted sutures.

POSTSUTURING MANAGEMENT

Cover wounds after suturing for 1–2 days with loose protective covering. This protects from contamination until significant epithelization has occurred. After 2 days, gentle cleansing of sutured wound is acceptable. Topical application of antibiotic ointment or petroleum jelly may allow increased rate of epithelization. Prophylactic antibiotics are not indicated after a simple laceration repair but should be given in cases of contamination (including animal or human bites), crush wounds, and in diabetic patients. Antibiotics are also indicated in oral lacerations, open fractures, and where joints and tendons are exposed.

SUTURE REMOVAL

Sutures should be cut as close as possible to the point where it emerges from the skin on the side of incision opposite the knot **(Fig. 9A)**. This enables the surgeon to draw the minimal length of the exposed and possibly contaminated suture material through the skin and tissues. While pulling, suture traction should be toward the incision line, and not away from it **(Fig. 9B)**. If the suture is pulled away from the suture line, a partially healed wound might open up.

OTHER METHODS OF WOUND CLOSURE

Tissue Adhesives

These adhesives consist of a liquid monomer made by a combination of formaldehyde and cyanoacrylate. This reacts with hydroxyl ions found in water and blood, thereby causing a reaction which bonds the edges of the skin. The benefits of tissue adhesive include less pain and quick application. They are therefore potentially useful in children. Infection rates are higher with tissue adhesives. For application of a tissue adhesive, skin edges should be approximated closely and a thin layer of adhesive evenly applied. If there is a significant tension during manual approximation, a tissue adhesive should not be used. They should not be applied over areas of high tension such as over joints or in the hand. If wrongly applied they can be easily removed with acetone, petroleum jelly, or antibacterial ointment. They have some antibacterial property against gram-positive bacteria.

Staples

The benefit of skin staples includes fast application, lower rate of foreign body reaction and decreased infection rate. Staples are particularly useful for wound closure in the scalp, extremities, and trunk wounds.

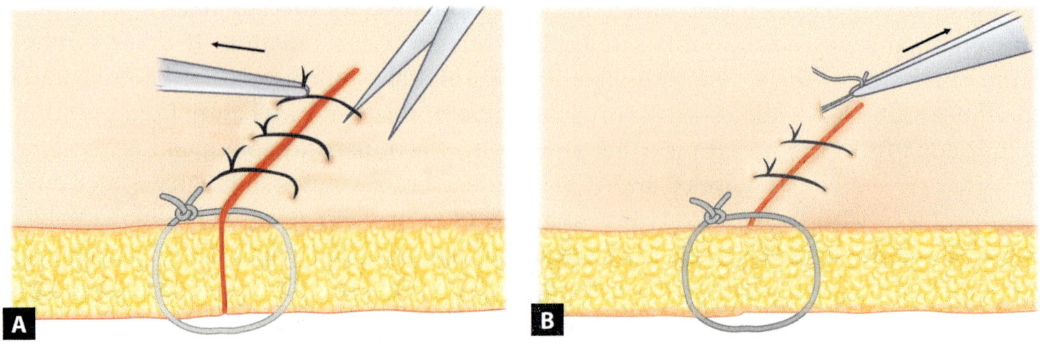

Figs. 9A and B: Proper method of suture removal.

They are also commonly used on long surgical incisions. Their use saves time.

Surgical or Adhesive Tapes (Steristrips)

These cause little skin reactivity, and are useful for very small wounds, and in children. If additional adhesive solution is required, "Opsite" spray is ideal, as tincture of benzoic acid may lead to a local skin reaction or even wound infection. Tapes are not ideal for primary closure of wounds, but can be placed after suture removal and may decrease skin tension. They usually fall away in 7-10 days.

KEY POINTS

- The majority of wounds should be closed primarily to for optimum cosmetic results and for preservation of function.
- Wounds should be closed within 18 hours to avoid wound infection except for wounds of face and scalp where a delay of up to 72 hours is acceptable.
- Wound preparation by hair removal and irrigation by normal saline with irrigation pressure of 5–8 psi is mandatory before wound closure.
- Povidone-iodine and hydrogen peroxide should be avoided for wound irrigation as they have a damaging effect on tissue.
- As far as possible simple interrupted suture should be applied.
- A vertical mattress should be used if there is excess of skin or loose subcutaneous fat.
- A horizontal mattress may be useful for either eversion or inversion of a wound edge but there is a higher incidence of ischemia and necrosis of the skin.
- A subcuticular suture gives a very fine and neat scar, but has the disadvantage of not providing any support to the deep tissues.

CHAPTER 9

Surgery of Common Skin Lesions under Local Anesthesia

MD Raihan, Sudhir Kumar Jain, Raman Tanwar

"A common surgical procedure can lead to significant morbidity if not performed properly"

INTRODUCTION

The indications for removal of skin lesions are as follows:

- Suspicion of malignancy
- Cosmetic reasons
- If the lesion is hampering, the function of a joint or causing compression of a neurovascular structure
- To avoid complications such as infection, bleeding, pain, or irritation.

If a particular lesion is being removed for cosmetic reasons, all efforts should be made to give a neat scar, which is less conspicuous than the original contour of the lesion. Other options for treatment include lasers, cryosurgery, electrocautery excision, curettage, or local applications of skin ointments should be discussed with the patient before offering excision. An accurate clinical diagnosis and dermatology input may be required in these cases. Lasers are particularly useful in arteriovenous malformations and the skin lesions of neurofibromatosis, i.e., Café-au-Lait spots.

Anesthesia

The majority of skin lesions can be removed under local anesthesia. This can be in the form of local infiltration or as a nerve block, e.g., digital, brachial, intercostal, or femoral nerve block or a field block **(Figs. 1 to 3)**. The following agents are commonly used for local anesthesia:

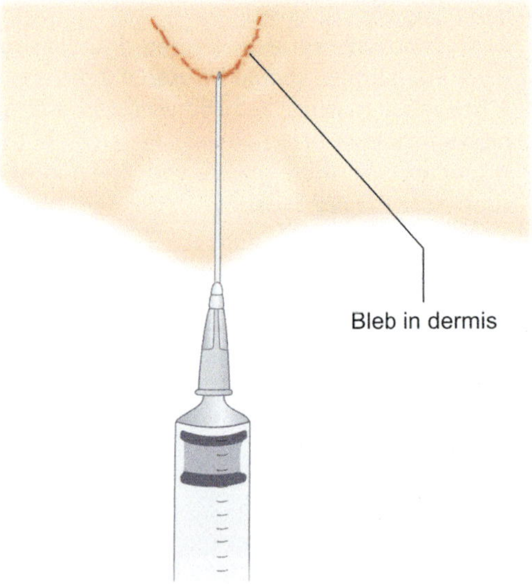

Fig. 1: A bleb should be raised in the dermis by a 24 number needle before starting infiltration of local anesthesia.

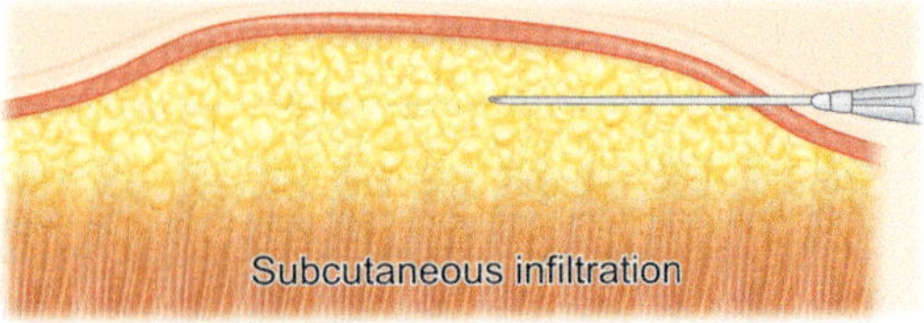

Fig. 2: Method of infiltration of local anesthesia in subcutaneous plane.

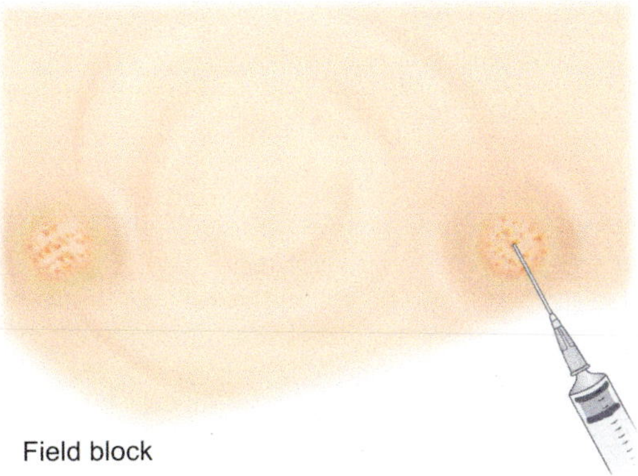

Fig. 3: Field block method of local anesthesia.

Lignocaine 0.5% prepared, or prepared from 1 or 2% commercially available solutions by dilution with normal saline. Maximum dose is 3 mg/kg of body weight without adrenaline and 7 mg/kg body weight with adrenaline. Lignocaine 1 or 2% with 1:200,000 adrenaline gives a longer period of anesthesia because anesthetic washout from the tissues is delayed due to arteriolar constriction. A delay in absorption permits use of lower doses of the anesthetic. Local vasoconstriction also reduces the capillary oozing in operative field. An adrenaline containing solution should not be used in the vicinity of end arteries because vasoconstriction can endanger blood supply particularly in the fingers, toes, ear lobule, tip of the nose, and the penis.

Bupivacaine 0.5% or 0.25% solution is available with or without adrenaline. It is a longer acting agent, but slower in onset of action. Its effect can last up to 6–8 hours, giving a significantly better postoperative pain relief. Injection of local anesthetic agent into skin can be more painful than the surgery itself. 50:50 mixtures of lignocaine and bupivacaine may be used for both quick initial effects, and long-acting pain relief.

Ways to minimize pain during injection of local anesthetic include:

- Explanation of the procedure to the patient with reassurance to allay anxiety is very important.
- Topical application of local anesthetic cream (a combination of lignocaine and prilocaine) avoids pain during infiltration of tissues.
- Prewarming the solution along with the addition of bicarbonate (0.5 mL in 9.5 mL of lignocaine) makes it less acidic.
- Slow injection into subcutaneous tissue first.
- Initial epidermal infiltration by raising a wheal with a fine (26G) needle, prior to using a large (19G) needle for main infiltration decreases discomfort to a great extent.

Field Block (Fig. 3)

In this method, the local anesthetic agent is injected into the tissues at some distance from the actual site of operation, so that a zone of anesthesia is created surrounding the operation area. The skin can be anesthetized first in the area of the block using a small fine needle. The block itself may require a long needle. Injection is made into the subcutaneous plane, and before infiltrating the deeper planes, the syringe should be aspirated to make sure that the needle has not entered a blood vessel. During injection the needle is gradually withdrawn. The advantage of a field block is that the lesion is not obscured by local swelling.

Nerve Block

Local anesthetic agent can be injected around the nerve to anesthetize the area which it serves. Digital nerve block is commonly employed for surgery on fingers or toes. Plain lignocaine is injected at the base of the digit on both sides to block the dorsal and palmar digital nerves. Injection is made in the web space on both sides of the finger. The needle is pushed vertically down until it touches bone, then it is slightly withdrawn, and local anesthetic is injected after confirmation by aspiration that the needle is not in a vessel. 0.5–1 mL of 0.5% lignocaine is often sufficient on each side.

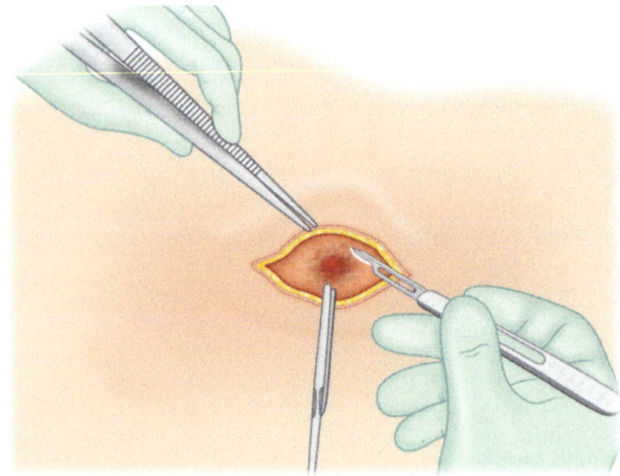

Fig. 4: Raising flaps for excision of sebaceous cyst.

COMMON SKIN PROCEDURES

Excision of Sebaceous Cyst

Excision of sebaceous cyst is advised due to its tendency to grow and become infected. The cyst should be excised completely in order to avoid recurrence. If the cyst is small and the overlying skin is healthy, a linear incision is employed. If the cyst is markedly protuberant or if the skin is thin and unhealthy or if there is an overlying punctum, an elliptical incision is used. The punctum should be in the center of the ellipse which should be equal in length to the diameter of cyst. If the skin overlying the cyst is stretched, the width of the ellipse can be wider to avoid excess skin folds and dog ears when closing the wound. After the skin ellipse is incised, a plane is developed between the cyst wall and the surrounding skin by sharp or blunt dissection, preferable without opening the cyst **(Fig. 4)**. After dissection all around, the cyst is easily shelled out. An alternative method is avulsion of the cyst. This is particularly suited for removal of cysts on the scalp. A comparatively small incision is required and cutaneous scarring is less. A skin flap is raised on only one side. The cyst is then deliberately opened and contents squeezed out. A pair of nontoothed dissecting forceps with one blade outside the cyst and one blade inside, cyst wall is grasped at its deepest part **(Fig. 5)** and by traction on the forceps; the entire cyst wall can be avulsed easily. The cyst wall is held at the deepest portion because the deepest part is tougher than the superficial portion and will not tear easily. The wound is sutured and a pressure dressing is applied to prevent hematoma formation in the cavity.

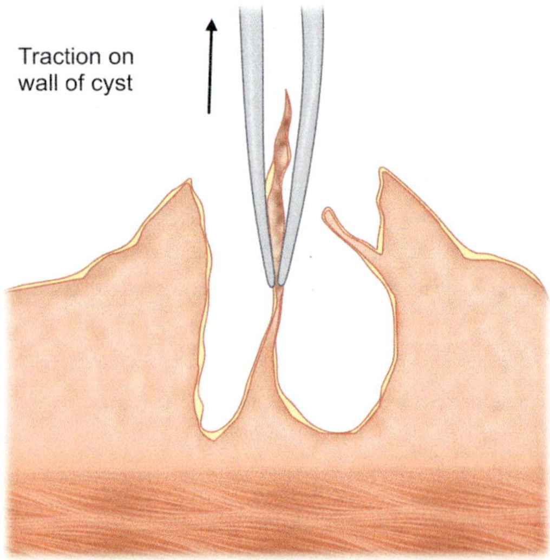

Fig. 5: Avulsion method of removal of sebaceous cyst.

If the sebaceous cyst is infected, removal is deferred until the inflammation subsides. If there is abscess formation, it should be incised and pus drained. Curettage of the abscess cavity or swabbing with pure carbolic acid may prevent the cyst from reforming. Infected sebaceous cysts should not be excised as wound complication rates are high and the resulting scars are unsatisfactory. They often do not recur after incision because infection frequently destroys the lining of the cyst.

LIPOMA EXCISION

Lipomas are slowly growing benign connective tissue tumors derived from adult type fat cells. They can occur anywhere in the body and are therefore known as universal tumors. However, they seldom occur in eyelids, pinna, or penis. They should be excised, if they are rapidly enlarging, painful, unsightly, or if there is a concern about malignant change, or there are associated secondary changes, e.g., myxomatous degeneration, traumatic fat necrosis (suggested by lipoma hardening after trauma) or calcification. Malignant change is suggested by rapid growth over 6–8 weeks, firmness, or early fixity to surrounding tissue. Retroperitoneal lipoma, large lipoma in the thigh or lipomas of shoulder region are more likely to undergo malignant change. They may rarely hamper movement.

For a subcutaneous lipoma excision, a skin incision is deepened through the overlying fat until the capsule of the lipoma is reached. It can be differentiated from the surrounding fat by larger fat globules, color, and a fine capsule. The lesion can often be enucleated after incision of its fine capsule, but larger lesions may need sharp dissection. If a lipoma is adherent to the underlying muscle, it should not be removed under local anesthetic as there may be deep extensions between muscle bellies, with involvement of neurovascular bundles. If a deeper lesion is suspected or if the lesion is >5 cm in diameter, a CT or MRI scan is indicated for accurate anatomical delineation.

BASAL CELL CARCINOMA (RODENT ULCER)

Basal cell carcinoma should be excised with 2 mm of normal tissue all around on all aspects including the deepest plane. Completeness of excision should be verified by histopathology.

Complete excision is associated with a recurrence rate of <2%. Moh has described a technique for recurrent lesions to ensure complete tumor excision. This technique essentially comprises excision in layers with horizontal frozen section control. Radiotherapy is an alternative to surgical excision in difficult situations such as penetrating lesion of eyes, nose, or mouth which would otherwise require major reconstruction after complete excision.

SQUAMOUS CELL CARCINOMA

These should be completely excised with 1 cm of macroscopically normal skin. Skin flaps should be extensively raised so that a still larger area of deep fascia can be excised. This tumor is sensitive to radiotherapy which may be used as an alternative or as an adjunct to surgery.

MALIGNANT MELANOMA

If a malignant melanoma is suspected, the initial surgery should be carried out to excise the lesion with margins reflecting the tumor depth. For a tumor excised with <1 mm depth, a wide excision of 1 cm margin around the tumor is sufficient. If the tumor is between 1 and 2 mm in depth, a 1–2 cm wide margin is adequate. For tumors >2 mm in depth, a 2-cm clearance is recommended. The excision should be carried down to but not through the deep fascia. All patients with tumor depth of >1 cm should be offered sentinel node biopsy at the same time as the wide excision. If the sentinel node is positive, then the patient will need to have complete nodal clearance.

KEY POINTS

- Common indications for removal of skin lesion are cosmetic, concern about malignancy, bothersome symptoms, or limitation in the movement or function of a joint.
- Majority of skin lesions can be removed under local anesthesia.
- Sebaceous cyst should be removed, if there is tendency to grow or if it becomes infected.
- Sebaceous cyst should be removed completely to avoid recurrence.
- Basal cell carcinoma is excised with 2 mm of normal tissue all around.
- Squamous cell carcinoma is excised with 1 cm of normal skin.

CHAPTER 10

Sutures in Surgery

Sudhir Kumar Jain, David L Stoker

"Proper selection of suture is of paramount importance in final outcome of surgery"

DEFINITION

The word "suture" describes any material which is used to ligate blood vessels, tubular structures and ducts or to approximate tissues and close wounds. The suture should be able to hold tissues together until healing is complete. The United States Food and Drug Administration (US-FDA) classify sutures under the Safe Medical Device Act (SDMA).

HISTORICAL ASPECTS

The use of sutures dates back at least 4000 years to the era of the great Indian surgeon Sushruta, the father of ancient Indian surgery. In 2000 BC, Egyptians and Syrians used sutures for various purposes. Archeological records from ancient Egypt showed that Egyptians used linen and animal sinew to close wounds. Linen is the earliest suture which has been described. All sorts of materials ranging from horse's hair, animal tendons, wire, silk, cotton, and linen have been used as suture materials. The use of stainless steel as suture came into vogue after World War II. Some of these are still used today. In the modern era, technical advances have brought us to the stage where specific sutures are available for a particular use. The suture industry currently accounts for >$1.3 billion annually. US Pharmacopoeia (USP), European Pharmacopoeia (EP), and British Pharmacopoeia (BP) are the official bodies which set standards and guidelines for suture manufacture.

IDEAL SUTURE

To date no available suture material meets all requirements but an ideal suture should have the following properties:

- The suture should be able to hold tissues together until healing is complete. The US-FDA classifies sutures under the SDMA.
- It should be devoid of any allergic, carcinogenic, capillary, or electrostatic action.
- It should be easy to sterilize.
- It should not produce any magnetic field around it, as happens with steel wire.
- It should be easy to handle.
- It should cause minimal tissue reaction.
- It should not promote growth of bacteria around it, in other words it should be resistant to infection.
- It should have favorable tensile strength and hold the tissue securely throughout the phase of wound healing.
- It should absorb with minimal tissue reaction after having served its purpose.

- It should hold tissue securely when knotted without cutting or fraying the tissue.
- It should have a consistent diameter.

CLASSIFICATION OF SUTURE MATERIAL (BOX 1)

Suture Size

Suture size denotes the diameter of the suture material. Suture size is generally denoted by 0s. As the number of "0s" in the suture size increases, the diameter of the suture strand decreases. Suture size is directly proportional to the tensile strength of the suture. The smaller the size of the suture, the less is the tensile strength it has. The accepted practice is to use the smallest diameter suture which will hold the tissue securely. The use of small diameter minimizes trauma as the suture passes through tissue and also has advantage that minimum foreign material is left in tissue.

BOX 1: Classification of sutures.

- *Absorbable*
  - *Natural:*
    - Surgical gut (plain or chromic)
    - Collagen (plain or chromic)
  - *Synthetic:*
    - Poliglecaprone 25
    - Polydioxanone
    - Polyglycolic acid
    - Polyglactin 910
    - Polycaprolactone
    - Polysorb
  - Maxon
  - V-Loc™
  - Caprosyn
- *Nonabsorbable*
  - *Natural:*
    - Surgical silk
    - Surgical linen
    - Cotton
    - Surgical steel
  - *Synthetic:*
    - Polyamide
    - Polypropylene
    - Polyester
    - Nylon
    - Polybutester suture
    - Coated polybutester
    - Surgipro II™

Knot Tensile Strength

This is measured by the force, in pounds, which the suture can withstand before breaking when knotted. Tensile strength of the tissue is measured by its ability to withstand stress. Tensile strength of the suture should never exceed the tensile strength of the tissue. The accepted rule is that suture should be as strong as the tissue in which suture is being applied.

Sutures can be classified in many ways:

- Monofilament versus multifilament
- Absorbable versus nonabsorbable
- Natural versus synthetic.

Plasticity and Elasticity of Suture

Plasticity can be defined as the ability of the suture to retain its new shape and length after stretching, thus allowing a suture to accommodate wound edema, and hence decreasing the risk of strangulated tissue and crosshatch marks. However, once swelling subsides, the suture may not continue to adequately approximate the wound edges as it retains its original shape. Elasticity means ability of a suture to resume its original form and length after stretching. After the swelling of a wound recedes, the suture returns to its original length and keeps the wound well approximated. Most sutures are elastic; few are plastic. An ideal suture should have more elasticity than plasticity.

Capillarity of Suture

Capillarity is the process by which fluid and bacteria are absorbed into the intersections of multifilament fibers. Capillary suture materials should not be used in contaminated or infected sites. Coating reduces capillarity of some sutures.

Tissue Reaction

Tissue reaction depends upon the mode of absorption of suture. Natural sutures which are absorbed by proteolysis induce intense inflammatory response. Synthetic materials which are absorbed by hydrolysis cause minimal tissue reaction. Braided sutures which have a high degree of capillary action absorb and retain both fluid and bacteria. These sutures are associated with greater tissue reaction and may promote infection if bacterial contamination occurs during or shortly after surgery.

Monofilament versus Multifilament

Monofilament sutures comprising a single strand of material, encounter less resistance when passing through tissue, and provide poor habitat for harboring organisms. This property makes them suitable for use in vascular surgery. They are easy-to-tie, but are delicate and can break easily. They are also more amenable to crushing or crimping leading to a weak point in suture and breakage. Multifilament sutures consist of multiple filaments and strands, twisted, and braided together leading to greater tensile strength. They are more pliable and flexible. They are usually coated for smooth passage through tissue. They have considerably better knot holding security. They are well suited for intestinal anastomosis. The longitudinal orientation of the individual filaments within the thread results in relatively high capillarity, but the capillarity of braided threads is less than that of twisted threads.

They have a rough surface that impairs passage through tissue.

Pseudomonofilament

The pseudomonofilament comprises core of several twisted materials coated with a layer of the same material as the core. It has low tissue drag, good knotting ability and fair flexibility. It has drawbacks such as low knot security similar to monofilament sutures.

Absorbable versus Nonabsorbable Sutures

Sutures which undergo rapid degradation in tissue, losing their >50% tensile strength within 60 days are known as absorbable sutures. Those which maintain more than half of their tensile strength for >60 days are known as nonabsorbable sutures. Silk loses 50% of its tensile strength in 1 year and has no strength after 2 years. Nylon loses 25% of its original strength after 2 years. Cotton retains 30–40% of its original strength after 2 years.

ABSORBABLE SUTURES

These are either derived from collagen or synthetic polymers.

Catgut Sutures

These are either derived from the submucosa of sheep intestine or from the serosa of beef intestine. Collagenous tissue obtained from gut is treated with an aldehyde solution for crosslinking, which gives the suture more strength and makes it resistant to enzymatic degradation. Sutures obtained in this way are known as plain gut. If plain gut is additionally treated by chromium trioxide, it is known as chromic gut. Chromic gut has more cross linkage and is more resistant to absorption. Reabsorption of gut is by enzymatic degradation, mainly by the lysosomal enzyme acid phosphatase initially, followed by leucine aminopeptidase. Collagenase also plays a significant role in degradation. Plain gut is rapidly absorbed and maintains its tensile strength for 7–10 days and is completely absorbed in 70 days. Tensile strength of chromic gut is maintained for 14–20 days. The drawback of a gut suture is that it may break during knot tying and may vary in its retention of tensile strength. There is also a growing concern regarding transfer of prion disease.

Collagen Sutures

These are derived from homogenized tendo-Achilles of beef cattle and are 100% pure collagen. They are available in plain and chromic form. They are stiffer than surgical gut. Therefore, handling becomes difficult in a large-size suture. Finer size sutures are used in eye surgery.

Fascia Lata

This is obtained from the thigh muscles of beef cattle. Earlier it was used for hernia repair. It is still occasionally used for surgical correction of drooping upper eyelid and for facial palsy.

Kangaroo Tendon

This is obtained from tail tendons of small Kangaroos and varies in length from 10 to 18 inches.

Synthetic Polymer Sutures

Synthetic polymer sutures available are:

- Polyglycolic acid suture (Homomer)
- Copolymers of glycolide and lactide (Polyglactin)
- Poliglecaprone 25 (Monocryl)
- Polydioxanone prepared from polyester.

Polyglycolic Acid Suture (Dexon™ and Dexon 1™)

This is a homomer of polyglycolic acid. It has high tensile strength with retention of 60% strength at day 7 and 35% strength at day 60. This suture is completely hydrolyzed by 90–120 days. This is a multifilament suture with good handling quality and knot security. It has a high coefficient of friction, which gives rise to drag during passage through tissue. This suture has high-tissue reactivity and may potentiate infection. To minimize tissue drag, a coated form of polyglycolic acid is available. Coating is in the form of a copolymer of glycolide and epsilon caprolactone (Dexon 1™).

Polyglactin (Vicryl™)

This is a copolymer of glycolic acid and lactic acid. Polyglactin 910 consists of glycolide and lactide in the ratio of 9:1. For every nine parts of glycolic acid there is one part of lactic acid. The lactide element is more hydrophobic than glycolic acid, and thus slows down the absorption of water by suture material, and hence the breakdown of linkage of copolymer chain is slowed down. Vicryl comes with a coating of 50% polyglactin and 50% calcium stearate. This polyglactin coating consists of 35% glycolide and 65% lactide and is known as polyglactin 370. Calcium stearate is an absorbable organic lubricant. Coating of polyglactin 370 and calcium stearate over polyglactin 910 reduces the surface friction of the suture thus avoiding tissue drag and premature locking. There is minimal absorption until 40 days. After 40 days, there is a rapid absorption and the suture completely disappears between 56 and 70 days. If coated polyglactin 910 is exposed to γ irradiation, it results in a low molecular weight suture in comparison to coated polyglactin and is available as Vicryl rapide. Vicryl rapide has 30% less tensile strength than coated Vicryl. Coated Vicryl retains 80% of postimplantation tensile strength at 14 days, and 30% of tensile strength at 21 days. Vicryl rapide loses all its tensile strength between 10 and 12 days and is totally absorbed within 42 days.

For Secure Knotting of Vicryl

There should be a double throw in the first-half knot, followed by additional two throws (total of four throws). Ends should be cut long. Coated Vicryl sutures are suitable for use anywhere except in the neural or cardiovascular tissue. Coated Vicryl rapide suture is well suited for skin closure, episiotomy closure, and closure of lacerations under plaster casts. Coated Vicryl plus is an antibacterial suture that is covered with a layer of the antibacterial agent Triclosan. The antibacterial agent coating offers protection against bacterial colonization of the suture.

Polydioxanone Suture (PDS and PDS II™)

This monofilament synthetic suture comprises polyester poly (p-dioxanone). It has superior pliability for easy handling and knotting. It is a soft suture and provides support to tissue for 6 weeks. It is almost inert in tissue and elicits almost no tissue reaction. It is absorbed through hydrolysis which is predictable. It retains 70% of tensile strength at 2 weeks, and 50% tensile strength at 4 weeks and 25% at 6 weeks. Absorption is minimal until about the 90th day and is essentially complete within 6 months. It has more flexibility than polyglycolic acid or polyglactin suture. It is basically suitable for procedures which require initial tissue strength. It is used in many types of tissue approximation including pediatric cardiovascular, orthopedic, gynecological, eye surgery, plastic, and gastrointestinal (GI) surgery. Its effectiveness and safety in microsurgery, neural tissue, and adult cardiovascular tissue have not been established. It is available both in undyed (clear) and dyed violet form. The dyed violet form enhances visibility.

Poliglecaprone 25 (Monocryl™)

This is a monofilament suture, which has superior pliability for easy handling and tying. It is a copolymer of glycolide and epsilon-caprolactone. It is composed of 75% glycolide and 25% caprolactone and is available in undyed and dyed violet form. This is the most pliable synthetic absorbable suture. It has a smooth surface which passes through tissue with ease. It is virtually inert, and has good tensile strength. It retains 50–60% of its strength at day 7 and approximately 20–30% at 14 days. All its tensile strength is lost in 21 days. It is absorbed by the mechanism of hydrolysis in 90–120 days. It is used in places where high initial tensile strength for 2 weeks is mandatory, e.g., subcuticular closure, soft-tissue approximation, and ligatures. It is not used in neural, cardiovascular, eye, and microsurgical operations.

Polysorb™

It is a braided absorbable suture produced from Lactomer copolymer. Lactomer copolymer consists of glycolide and lactide in a ratio of 9:1. Glycolide provides initial high tensile strength in tissue but undergoes hydrolysis rapidly. Lactide has a slower and controlled rate of hydrolysis and gives prolonged tensile strength in tissue. Knot construction is easy with polysorb because the knot breaking strength of polysorb is significantly greater than polyglactin 910. The surface of a polysorb suture is coated with mixture of caprolactone/glycolide polymer to reduce the coefficient of friction.

Barbed Suture (Fig. 1)

A *barbed suture* is a type of knotless suture that has barbs on its surface. During suturing of tissue these barbs penetrate inside and lock them into place, eliminating the need

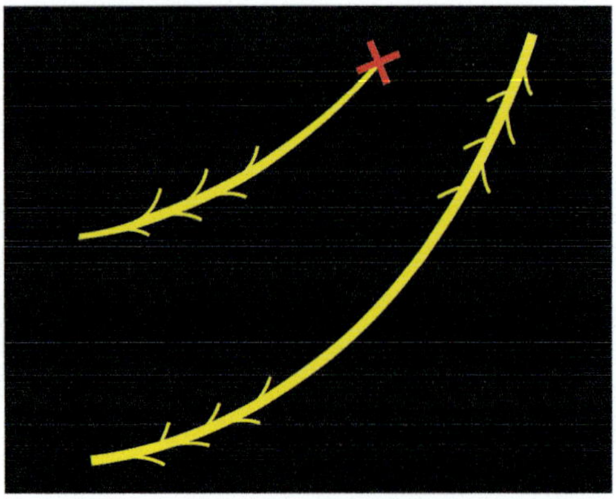

Fig. 1: Barbed suture.

for knots to tie the suture. The various barbed sutures available on the market are Quill, V-Loc, and STRATAFIX™ spiral (Ethicon Endo-Surgery). They are self-anchoring and do not need knotting for wound closure. These sutures consist of axially barbed segments of size 0 polydioxanone. At the midpoint of each side of an axially barbed fiber, there is change in direction. Their use as a wound closure device eliminates the need to tie knots, allowing one to close incisions up to 50% faster without compromising strength and security. These sutures have the potential to reduce knot-related complications. The devices use a unidirectional barbed thread which fixates itself in the tissue, with a loop at the start of the thread which anchors it securely at the edge of the wound. Standard suturing techniques can be used, but without the need to tie knots to fixate the suture. The V-Loc™ device provides evenly-spaced barbs throughout the strand, providing secure closure of the incision by distributing tension across the wound.

Caprosyn

It is rapidly absorbing monofilament absorbable suture prepared from polyglactone 621 synthetic polyester. It is made up of glycolide, caprolactone, trimethylene carbonate and lactide. It retains 50–60% knot strength at 5 days after surgery and minimum of 20–30% at the 10th postoperative day. There is total loss of tensile strength by 21 days. It has superior handling qualities in comparison to chromic catgut. It is much easier to reposition knotted Caprosyn.

NONABSORBABLE SUTURES

Nonabsorbable sutures are classified into three classes:

- *Class I:* Silk or synthetic fibers of monofilament (twisted or braided)
- *Class II:* Cotton or linen fibers
- *Class III:* Metal wire of monofilament or multifilament construction.

Classes I and III are more commonly used in comparison to class II which are prone to contamination and infection.

Silk

Silk sutures are nonabsorbable, sterile, and nonmutagenic, consisting of natural proteinaceous silk fibers called fibroin. This protein is derived from the domestic silkworm *Bombyx mori*. Silk fibers are treated to remove the naturally occurring sericin gum.

Silk sutures are braided around a core and coated with wax to reduce capillary action. They are colored black with logwood extract. Silk, being a foreign protein, causes more tissue reaction than synthetic nonabsorbable sutures. Silk induces a polymorphonuclear type of cellular reaction. Although classified as nonabsorbable, it behaves as a very slowly absorbing suture. It loses most of its tensile strength in about 1 year and usually cannot be detected in tissues after 2 years. Encapsulation of the silk with a fibrous capsule occurs in 14–21 days. Handling properties are good, and it knots easily and securely. Surgical silk loses tensile strength when exposed to moisture and should be used dry.

Linen

This is made from flax and is a cellulose material. It is twisted to form a fiber to make a suture. It can be used for general surgery, gynecology, cardiovascular surgery, gastrointestinal surgery, and plastic surgery. The linen suture is not absorbed and, hence, it does not lose the tensile strength. Its tissue reaction is similar to silk, and handling and knotting properties are very good. It has a unique property that it gains 10% more tensile strength when wet. It is still widely used for tying pedicles and as a ligature. Another variant treated with silicone and polyvinyl solution (Linatrix™) is also available.

Cotton

Cotton was first used as a suture material in 1939 during World War II to replace silk sutures. It is derived from the hairs of the seeds of the cotton plant. It gains tensile strength and knot security when wet. It comprises twisted, long, and staple cotton fibers, and slowly loses tensile strength after implantation, with 50% loss of tensile strength at 6 months, and 70% at 2 years. However, it is not an absorbable suture. It has better knot security than silk. The disadvantages of cotton suture are capillarity, tissue reactivity, inferior handling ability due to electrostatic properties, and ability to potentiate infection. It becomes encapsulated within the body tissue. It is weak in comparison to linen and is rarely used in the present time.

Surgical Steel Suture

It is made up of stainless steel (Iron-Chromium-Nickel-Molybdenum alloy). It is available in monofilament and twisted multifilament form. It has high tensile strength with little loss over passage of time. It holds knots well and does not show any tissue reaction. Surgical steel can be used in sternum closure, abdominal wall closure, and orthopedic surgery. Surgical steel is difficult to handle because of its tendency to get kinked, fragmented, and barbed. It can also pull, cut, or tear tissues.

Nylon

This is composed of a long chain of polyamide polymers. It has a high-tensile strength and low-tissue reactivity. Because of its elasticity it is well suited for abdominal and skin closure. Nylon has a low coefficient of friction and tissue reaction is minimal. It loses 15–20% of tensile strength in 1 year by hydrolysis. It has a memory, and knot security is lower than that of other sutures. It is available as monofilament (Ethilon™) or multifilament strands known as Nurolon™. Monofilament nylon in a wet state is more pliable than dry nylon. Multifilament nylon sutures have more strength and elicit less tissue reaction than silk. Multifilament nylon sutures generally lose 15–20% of their tensile strength per year in tissue by hydroxylation.

Polyester Fiber

This comprises untreated fibers of polyester braided into a multifilament strand. This is also known as terylene or Dacron. It has a very high-tensile strength and relatively low-tissue reactivity. It retains tensile strength for an indefinite period. Dacron in a wet or damp state is more pliable and easier to handle than in dry state. It has become the suture of choice for cardiovascular procedures, blood vessel anastomosis, and for placement of prosthetic material. Polyester sutures have a tendency to cut through tissue and to obviate this tendency, a coating of Teflon or polybutylate is provided over the polyester suture. Polyester coated with polybutylate is known as "Ethibond." The polybutylate coating does not increase the diameter of the suture in contrast to Teflon coating and also does not flake in the tissue.

Polypropylene

This is also known as Prolene. It is monofilament and has extremely high-tensile strength which is retained for an indefinite period. It has very low-tissue reactivity. It can stretch up to 30% before breaking and hence is useful in situations where postoperative swelling is anticipated. Knotting is extremely secure because the suture deforms on knotting and allows the knot to bend down on itself. It has a low coefficient of friction and slides through tissue readily. In comparison to silk it is less thrombogenic. It is very smooth and does not saw through the tissues. As it does not adhere to tissue, it is useful as a "pull out" suture, e.g., subcuticular suture. Polypropylene is recommended for use where minimal suture reaction is desired, such as in contaminated and infected wounds to minimize sinus formation and suture extrusion.

Polybutester

The Polybutester suture (Novafil™) is a copolymer that comprises butylene terephthalate (84%) and polytetramethylene ether glycolterephthalate(16%).Polybutestersuture has unique performance characteristics. This is a monofilament synthetic nonabsorbable suture. This suture yields significantly greater elongation than other sutures even with low forces and has elasticity which is superior to that of other sutures, allowing the suture to return to its original length once the load is removed.

The Polybutester skin suture diminishes the risk of hypertrophic scar formation because of its special properties allowing it to adapt to changing tensions in the wound. The clinical performance of Polybutester suture has been enhanced by coating its surface with a unique absorbable polymer of polytribolate (Vascufil™).

This polymer is composed of three compounds: (1) Glycolide, (2) e-caprolactone, and (3) poloxamer 188. Coating the polybutester suture markedly reduces its drag forces in musculoaponeurotic, colonic, and vascular tissue. Knot security with the Vascufil™ suture is achieved with only one more extra throw than with comparably sized, uncoated Polybutester sutures.

Surgipro II™

Surgipro II™ is basically a polypropylene suture which has been developed with increased resistance to fraying during knot run down especially with smaller diameters. This suture retains its tensile strength for 2 years in tissue and is extremely inert. It has a lower drag coefficient in tissue in comparison to nylon thus making it ideal for continuous suture closure.

Hexafluoropropylene-VDF (PRONOVA™ POLY)

This is nonabsorbable monofilament suture. It is copolymer of vinylidene fluoride and hexafluoropropylene. This suture does not get involved in infections and hence can be used in infected and contaminated wounds as it reduces incidence of sinus formation and suture extrusion. This suture does become adherent to tissues, and so can be used as a pull-out suture.

Recent Advances in Sutures

The following advances have taken place in suture manufacture:

- Sutures modified with antimicrobial.
- Sutures modified with bioactive molecules such as DNA.
- Sutures modified with antibodies.
- Sutures modified with proteins, growth factors and silver.

Antimicrobial Sutures

Antimicrobial sutures prevent adherence of bacteria to sutures and reduce surgical site infection. Triclosan-coated sutures and sutures coated with amphiphilic polymer poly (PAMBAM) or chlorhexidine are available. Triclosan is bacteriostatic but PAMBAM and chlorhexidine bactericidal. Triclosan-coated Polyglactin 910 (Vicryl plus™) and Poliglecaprone 25 (Monocryl plus™) are available. Triclosan has activity against *S. aureus* and *S. epidermidis*. Use of triclosan-coated sutures has been shown to reduce surgical site infection (SSI).

TIPS FOR PRESERVATION OF TENSILE STRENGTH OF SUTURE

Absorbable Sutures

- Protect them from heat and moisture. Store them at room temperature. Avoid storage in hot areas, e.g., near steam pipes, and in sterilizers.
- Do not soak absorbable sutures.
- To restore pliability surgical gut can be dipped in water at room temperature or saline.
- Synthetic absorbable sutures must be kept dry.

Nonabsorbable Sutures

- *Silk:* Store silk in dry environment. Dry strands are stronger than wet strands. Wet silk loses up to 20% of its strength. Avoid kinking, nicking, or instrument damage.
- *Polyester fiber:* It is unaffected by moisture. It can be used either wet or dry. Handle it carefully to avoid abrasions, kinking, and nicking or instrument damage.
- *Nylon:* Straighten kinks or bends by passing strands between gloved fingers a few times. Avoid kinking, nicking, or instrument damage.
- *Polypropylene:* Unaffected by moisture. It can be used wet or dry. Thread should be straightened with a gentle, steady, and even pull.

RECENT ADVANCES IN SUTURES

Recent studies have revealed that sutures coated with growth factors or stem cells can be used as a mode of delivery for these biologically active factors to the desired tissue. The stem-cell-coated sutures increase the number of stem cells at the injured site to enhance tissue regeneration and repair. Pluripotent stem-cell-coated or L-lysine or bone marrow-derived mesenchymal stem-cell-coated braided sutures are being studied for mechanical repair of tendons. A stem-cell-seeded biological suture material has been developed for cardiac surgery. This is a human mesenchymal stem-cell-seeded suture developed by loading quantum dot nanoparticles which can track the seeded cells within the myocardium.

SURGICAL NEEDLES

Composition

Surgical needles are made up of stainless-steel alloy, which is resistant to corrosion and contain a minimum of 12% chromium. When a needle is exposed to oxygen in air it forms a thin protective layer of chromium oxide.

An ideal needle should have following characteristics:

- Made of high-quality stainless steel.
- As thin and slim as possible without compromising strength
- Should have a stable grasp on the needle holder.
- Should cause minimal trauma to tissue.
- Should be able to penetrate tissue with minimal resistance.
- Should resist bending.
- Should be resistant to breaking under a given amount of bending. An ideal needle should bend before breaking if excessive force is applied.

Anatomy of the Needle

Components

Every surgical needle has three basic parts: (1) Swage, (2) Body, and (3) Point.

Swage

The swage is the site of attachment of the suture to the needle. It is usually round in section. Swaged needles produce smaller holes in tissue in comparison to threaded eye needles.

Body

The body of the needle is the portion which is grasped by the needle holder during the surgical procedure. It is often *square* in section. The diameter of the body of the needle should be as close as possible to the diameter of the suture material to minimize bleeding and leakage. This is especially important for cardiovascular, gastrointestinal, and bladder procedures.

Point

The needle point extends from tip of the needle to the level of the maximum cross-section of the body.

Types of Needle Point

Cutting needles have two opposing cutting edges.

Conventional Cutting-edge Needle

This has two opposite cutting edges and a third cutting edge on the inside of the concave curvature of the needle. The inside cutting edge produces linear cuts perpendicular and near to the incision. When the suture exerts a wound closure force, it can cut through this hole. It is primarily used for closure of skin and sternum.

Reverse Cutting-edge Needle

This has a cutting edge on the outer convex curvature of needle. It has more strength than a conventional cutting needle. The danger of tissue cut out is much less because the hole produced by it has a good support of tissue contrary to the linear cut produced by a conventional cutting needle. The wide wall against which the suture is tied prevents suture cut through.

Spatula Needle

This is a side-cutting needle, flat on both bottom and top, with cutting edges on the side. It is primarily used for eye surgery. It can also be used for repairing lacerations of the nail matrix. Side-cutting edges split or separate the tissue without cutting them. These allow maximum ease of penetration and control as they pass between and through tissue layers.

Taper Point Needle

This needle tapers to a sharp tip, with a round body. It spreads the tissue without cutting it, and is used where the surgeon wants to make the smallest hole possible without cutting tissue. It is used in soft tissue, e.g., vessels, abdominal viscera, and fascia which do not resist needle penetration.

Taper Cut Needle

This combines the unique features of taper point and cutting-edge needles. Cutting edges extend only for a short distance from the needle tip and blends into a round taper body. The taper cut needle is used for anastomosis of calcified and fibrotic blood vessels, to graft, and for closure of defects in the oral mucosa. The penetrating point needle is a type of taper cut needle with a diamond-shaped point.

Blunt Point Needle

This has a taper body with a rounded blunt point that will not cut through tissue. It is used for suturing the liver and kidney, and also to prevent needle stick injury in patients with human immunodeficiency virus (HIV), or hepatitis B/C infection.

TYPES OF NEEDLES ACCORDING TO SHAPE (TABLE 1)

- *Straight needle:* This can be used for suturing easily accessible tissue, where direct manipulation can easily be performed by the fingers (*see* **Fig. 1**).
- *The Keith needle:* It is a straight-cutting needle for skin closure of abdominal wounds and for arthroscopic suturing of the meniscus in the knee.
- *Bunnell needle (BN):* It is used for tendon repair.
- The *half-curved needle or "Ski" needle* is used for laparoscopic anastomosis.
- *Curved needle:* These needles have predictable needles that turn out from tissue. They require less space for maneuvering than a straight needle but require a needle holder for manipulation. The curvature of the needle may be 1/4, 3/8, 1/2, or 5/8 of a full circle. 3/8 circle is used for large superficial wounds. The curve of the needle can be manipulated with slight pronation but then has a larger arc of manipulation, so it is not suitable in a deep body cavity or restricted area. 1/2 circle needle is used in a confined space. 5/8 circle needle is used for hemorrhoidectomy, in the nasal cavity, oral cavity, and pelvis **(Fig. 2)**.

TABLE 1: Types of needles and their uses.

Needle type	***Description***	***Common uses***
Straight	Can be used for suturing easily accessible tissue; direct manipulation is performed by fingers	Accessible tissues; straightforward suturing
Keith needle	A straight-cutting needle	Skin closure of abdominal wounds; arthroscopic suturing of the meniscus in the knee
Bunnell needle (BN)	Used for tendon repair	Tendon repairs
Half-curved needle/ "Ski" needle	Used for laparoscopic anastomosis	Laparoscopic anastomosis
Curved needle	Requires less space for maneuvering compared to a straight needle; needs a needle holder. The curvature may be 1/4, 3/8, 1/2, or 5/8 of a full circle	• *1/4 circle:* Large superficial wounds • *3/8 circle:* Superficial wounds • *1/2 circle:* Confined spaces • *5/8 circle:* Hemorrhoidectomy, nasal cavity, oral cavity, and pelvis

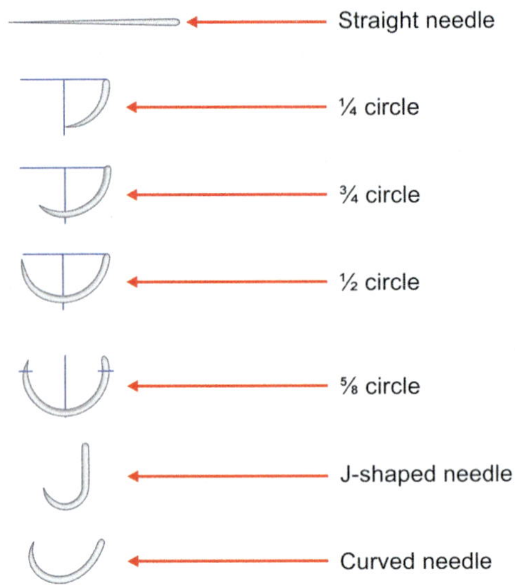

Fig. 2: Different shapes of surgical needles.

KEY POINTS

- Ideal sutures having all the desirable properties do not exist.
- One should choose a suture carefully, keeping in mind the type of operation being performed.
- Tensile strength of suture and ease of knotting is an important aspect to be considered while selecting suture material.
- If selecting a nonabsorbable suture, one should choose a suture which maintains its tensile strength for 90–120 days, i.e., the time required for healing.
- Surgical silk loses tensile strength when exposed to moisture.
- Monofilament sutures are preferred for vascular surgery because of minimal tissue drag and resistance against harboring organisms.
- Multifilament sutures have more tensile strength, pliability, flexibility, and are well suited for intestinal anastomosis.

CHAPTER 11

Patient Positioning During Surgery

Sudhir Kumar Jain, David L Stoker

"Faulty positioning in operating room can result in significant injuries and litigations"

INTRODUCTION

Proper positioning of the patient during surgery is very important for the proper exposure of the operative field. The poor positioning leads to following:

- Poor access
- The increased risk of complications in both the operative and postoperative period such as pressure area damage and nerve injuries.

In this chapter, positioning of patients during common surgical procedures will be described. The surgical team is responsible for proper patient's position on the table. No part of the patient's body should be in contact with a metal surface if electrocautery is to be used, to avoid leaking of current from the point of contact. Excessive abduction of the upper limbs or pressure over bony prominences should be avoided to prevent neuropraxia or skin damage.

GOALS OF PROPER POSITIONING

- The patient's airway should be maintained.
- The surgeon should avoid constriction or pressure on the chest cavity.
- The circulation should be maintained, e.g., like in lateral position, there can be pressure on inferior vena cava (IVC) or aorta.
- The nerve injuries should be avoided due to pressure.
- It should provide adequate exposure of the operative site.
- To provide comfort, safety, and dignity to the patient
- To promote access for the administration of intravenous fluids and anesthetic agents.

The following criteria should be met to prevent injury from pressure, obstruction, or stretching during positioning:

- No interference with respiration
- No interference with circulation
- No pressure on peripheral nerves
- Minimal skin pressure
- Accessibility to operative site
- Accessibility for anesthetic administration
- No undue musculoskeletal discomfort
- Maintenance of individual requirements.

Effects of positioning in obese patients are as follows:

- *In supine position:*
    - Normal blood flow may be impeded due to compression of vena cava and aorta by heavy abdominal contents.
    - There is impairment of diaphragmatic movement as the domes of the diaphragm ascend up in supine position, leading to reduction in lung capacity.

- *Trendelenburg position:*
    - It is tolerated less well than supine position.
    - Shifting of abdominal contents leading additional weight on the diaphragm may lead to atelectasis and hypoxemia to reduce movement of diaphragm.
- *Prone position:*
    - It is problematic as the patient has to be shifted from supine to prone after induction of anesthesia.
    - It requires additional support and monitoring of the patient and pressure on the abdomen.
    - Ventilation may be markedly more difficult.
- *Lateral position:*
    - It is well tolerated.
    - In this position, correct sizing and placement of axillary roll are important.
- One should ensure that pendulous abdomen does not hang over side of operation table.
- *Head-up position*: (Reverse Trendelenburg/semirecumbent)
    - It is the safest position.
    - Weight of abdominal contents is unloaded and taken away from the diaphragm.
    - Well-padded footboard is used to prevent sliding.

Desired features of operating table to have proper positioning are as follows:

- It should have stable base.
- It should have easy to maneuver mechanisms for different positions and lock into place.
- It should have easy adjustments for arm boards, stirrups, kidney rests, move head section to foot of OR table.
- It should be radiolucent to allow taking X-rays or using fluoroscope.
- One should purchase heavyduty operating tables, which can support up to 1,000 pounds.
- Mattress should have following characteristics:
    - It should be easy to clean.
    - It should have gel mattress or foam covered with nylon or vinyl.
    - It should be made of resilient, long-lasting material, including no breakdown when cleaned with disinfectant agents.
    - Radiolucent (if surgery department performs procedures that require intraoperative imaging studies)
    - Moisture resistant
    - Fire retardant
    - Nonallergenic, in particular, no presence of latex in material.

Even if the surgery department does not perform bariatric surgical procedures, it is still required that the department be prepared for performing other types of surgical procedures on obese patients.

SUPINE POSITION FOR LAPAROTOMY (FIG. 1)

It is the most commonly used position during abdominal surgery. In this position, the head is padded and stabilized with various positioning aids, e.g., closed head ring or gel head cushion or double wedge cushion with padding under the shoulders. Purpose of this head stabilization is to keep the cervical spine in the neutral position (awake) so that any pressure on the back of the head is avoided.

In abdominal surgery, both arms are abducted to the side either in pronation or supination. In prone position, the arms should be abducted to approximately 60°, flexed at the elbows, and fixed with the arm positioning device. Support with a short armrest should always be provided for the

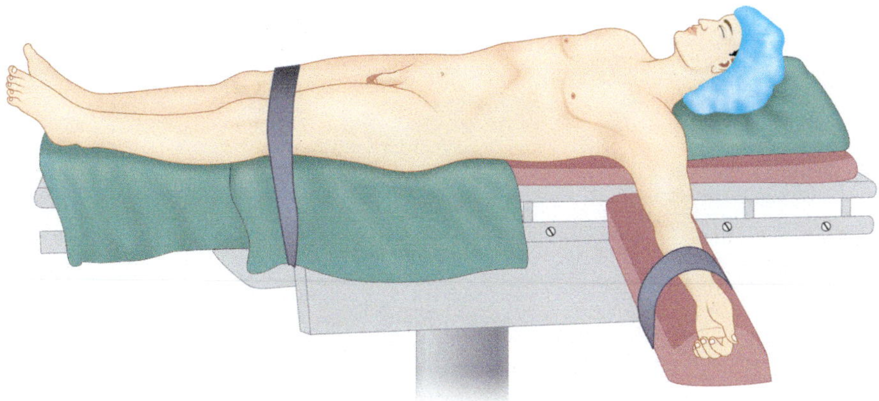

Fig. 1: Supine position.

lower arm and hand. This positioning of the arm prevents wrist drop. In case abduction of the arm is required between 60° and 90°, the patient arm should be adjusted to supine position (Texas position). A pad is placed under the wrist in this position to keep nerves in the elbow free of pressure. The shoulder elevation from the level of the table enlarges the gap between clavicle and the first rib and reduces the risk of compressing the nerves. The arm must be elevated over the level of the shoulder.

The rule of thumb for positioning the arm in supine position is to elevate the shoulder from the level of the table and keep the distal joint higher than the proximal joint resulting in the elbow is higher than the shoulder and the wrist higher than the elbow.

Hips and knees should be preferably mildly flexed with pads placed under the lumbar spine. Hips are parallel to the spine.

The pads can be in the form of a small rolled/folded towel. If necessary, a half-rolled towel is placed under the knees at the distal thigh. Pressure on the heels should be reduced to a minimum. One of the methods for this can be the use of small gel mats placed under the lower leg. Spinal column should be in alignment with legs parallel to the operation table. Safety belt is placed 2″ above the knees while not impeding circulation.

PRONE POSITION (FIG. 2)

- The patient is anesthetized supine, usually on the stretcher, prior to turning. A minimum of four persons should assist in transferring the patient from the supine to the prone position to provide full support to the patient and avoid injuries to care givers and patient. The anesthesiologist is responsible for supporting the head and neck of the patient, and ensuring the endotracheal tube is not dislodged. Two persons should position themselves alongside the operation table and the other two persons should take a position opposite on the far side of the operation table.
- The tuning of patient is synchronized and supported.
- The patient lies with face down, resting on the abdomen and chest.
- The two chest rolls are placed lengthwise under the axilla and along the sides of the chest from the clavicle to iliac crests (to relieve the weight of the body off of the abdomen and thorax).

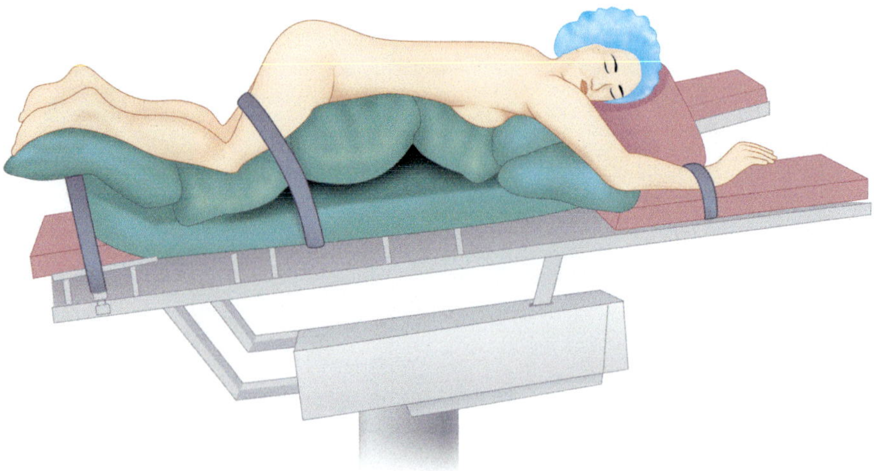

Fig. 2: Prone position.

- One roll is placed at the iliac or pelvic level.
- The cervical spine should be in alignment with the rest of the spine, with no torsion or twisting, and the legs parallel to each other.
- The breasts of females should be positioned laterally to avoid compression or torsion injury.
- The male genitalia should be confirmed to be in a downward natural position to avoid compression or torsion injury.
- Arms lie at the sides or over head on arm boards (must lower arms slowly to the ground then bring them up in an arc to place on arm boards).
- Head is face down and turned to one side with accessible airway.
- Forehead, eyes, and chin are protected. The eyes are at particular risk for compression injuries. Direct pressure on the eyes should be avoided by not using a horseshoe-shaped headrest. The eyes should not be padded but gently taped shut.
- Padding is used to bilateral arms and under knees. A pillow should be placed under the ankle joints to elevate the foot to relieve tension on the sciatic nerve and prevent the toes from resting on the OR table mattress.
- Pillow is placed under bilateral feet (for maintenance of foot extension)
- Safety strap placed 2″ above knees.

Prone Concerns

- Greatest concerns are to the respiratory and circulatory systems and pressure points.
- *Most common nerve damage:* Brachial, radial, median, and ulnar
- *Vulnerable bony prominences:* Temporal, acromion, clavicle, and iliac
- *Vulnerable vessels:* Carotid, aorta, vena cava, and saphenous
- Susceptible to hyperextension of the joints.

NECK SURGERY

Thyroid Surgery

Patient is placed supine with the table tilted up at an angle of 15° at the head end to reduce venous engorgement. A ring is placed underneath the occipital region to stabilize the head. The neck is extended by placing a sand bag transversely across the shoulders. Neck extension makes thyroid gland, skin, platysma, and strap muscles more prominent and facilitates dissection. Precautions should be taken in elderly patients and in patients with pathology of the cervical spine, and hyperextension of neck should be avoided in these cases during positioning.

Parotid Surgery

Position of the patient is supine with head resting on a ring and turned away from the side of the pathology.

POSTEROLATERAL THORACOTOMY (FIG. 3)

Patient is turned on the unaffected side in the lateral decubitus position with the hips secured to table by means of wide adhesive tapes. The lower leg is flexed at the knee with a pillow between the upper and lower legs. The upper leg is extended. The shoulder and upper thorax are supported by a rolled sheet or blanket placed under the axilla. Table supports are used to maintain the position, and additional strapping is used at the hip for stability. The upper arm is supported by a bracket in a position of 90° flexion. The lower arm is flexed and positioned underneath the head.

LUMBAR APPROACH FOR KIDNEY (FIGS. 4 AND 5)

Patient is turned on the unaffected side in the lateral position toward the edge of the operating table. Hip and knee next to the table are fully flexed with a pillow between the two legs. Patient is maintained in this position with a back support or by strapping. To increase the space for access, the trunk should be flexed on the lower side by breaking the table, or by the use of an inflatable cushion under the loin. A support for the arm

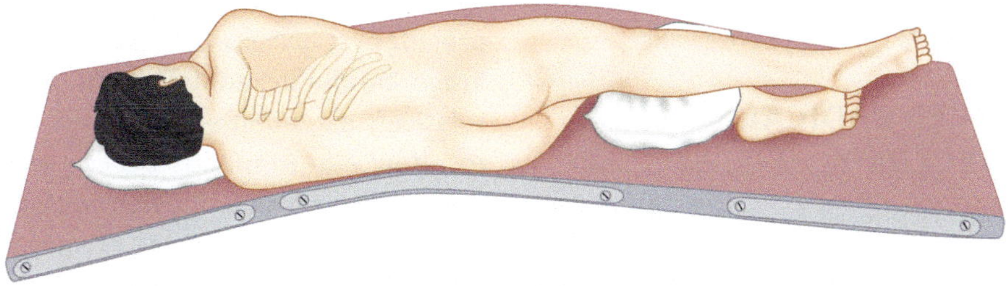

Fig. 3: Patient position for posterolateral thoracotomy.

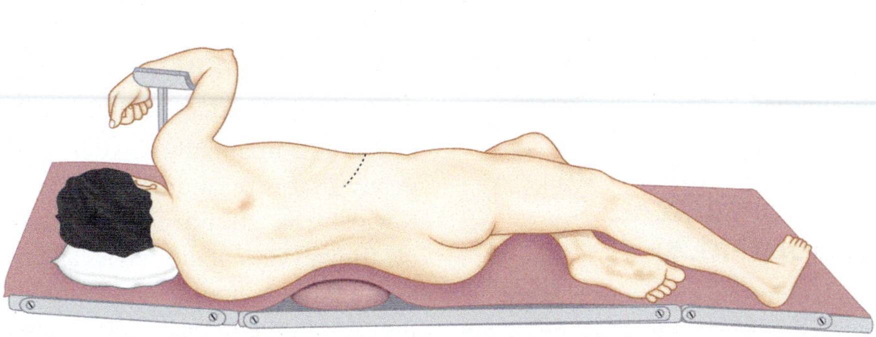

Fig. 4: Patient position for kidney exposure.

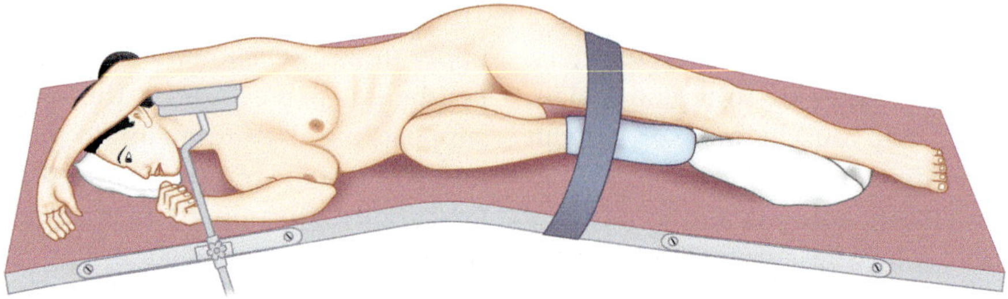

Fig. 5: Position of patient for kidney operation through flank approach.

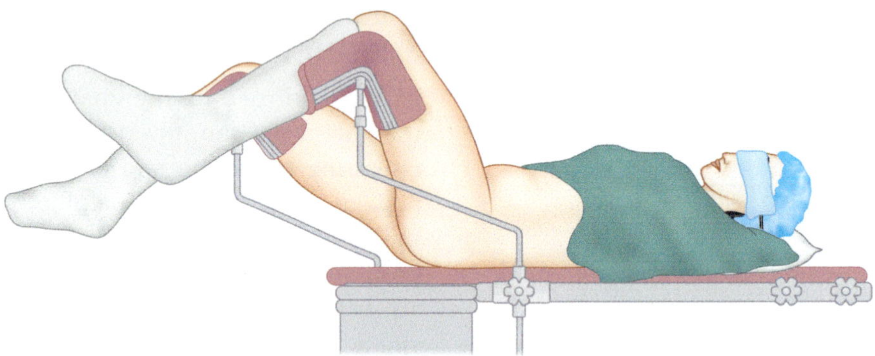

Fig. 6: Lloyd–Davis position for abdominoperineal resection.

prevents the shoulder from sagging forward with consequent rotation at the waist.

MODIFIED RADICAL MASTECTOMY

The patient is placed near the edge of the operating table on the side of the surgeon. The patient lies supine with the arm and forearm on the side of the surgery outstretched on an arm board to which the wrist is secured by a bandage. The forearm is supinated so that the palm faces upward.

ANTERIOR RESECTION OR ABDOMINOPERINEAL RESECTION (FIG. 6)

The patient is placed in the perineal lithotomy position with the legs in stirrups. The patient should be brought down to the edge of the table with a sand bag under the buttocks to provide proper exposure of the anal canal. The knees can be flexed, but the hips should be relatively extended and the thighs abducted to allow simultaneous access to both the abdomen and the perineum. A moderate degree of head down tilt (Trendelenburg) aids in dissection.

TRENDELENBURG POSITION (FIG. 7)

In this position, the head is tilted downward by 30°. It is frequently used in surgery of the pelvis. In this position, mobile gut gravitates toward the diaphragm, so that a less obstructed view of the pelvis can be obtained. Well-padded shoulder rests are attached to the table in such a manner that the pressure is exerted over the region of acromioclavicular

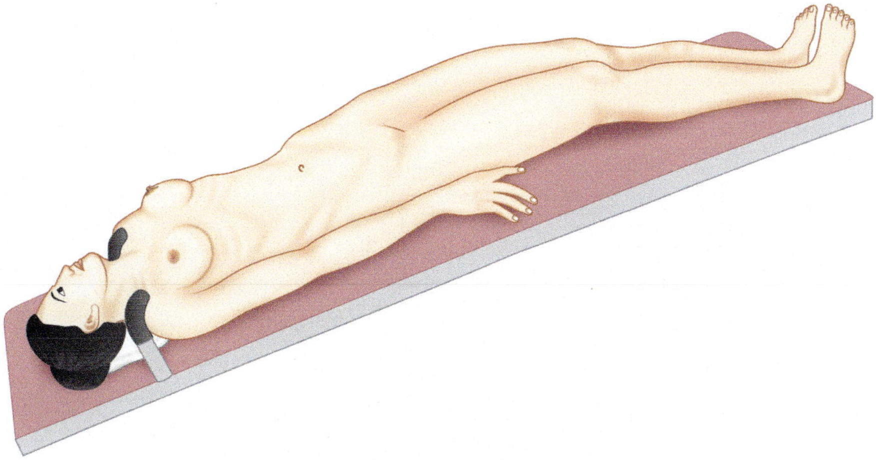

Fig. 7: Trendelenburg position.

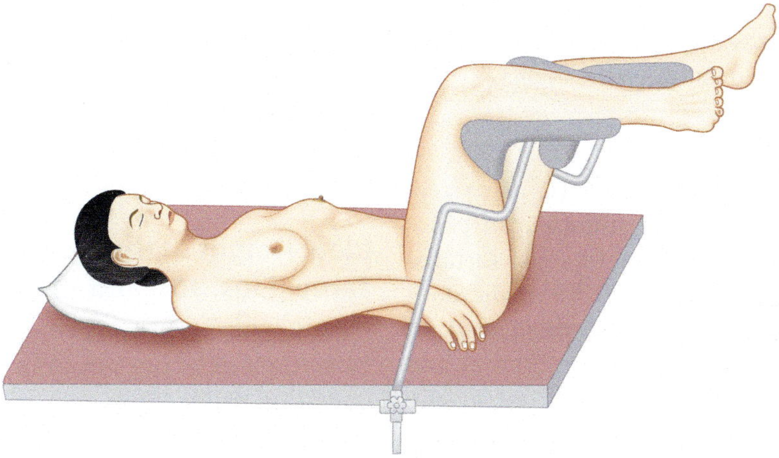

Fig. 8: Patient position for cystoscopy.

region to prevent the patient sliding headward. If the pressure of shoulder head is applied on the root of the neck, brachial plexus injury may occur.

Position for Cystoscopy (Fig. 8)

Patient is placed with his buttocks near the end of the table with legs abducted. The thighs should be maintained at angle of 45° with the trunk. In this position, the axis of the telescope is approximately horizontal when the bladder base is being examined.

VAGINAL OPERATIONS (FIG. 9)

Lithotomy position is used for transvaginal procedures. In this position, the patient's buttocks are on the edge of the table and rising upward with a sandbag placed across the sacrum. The knee and hip joints are flexed at an angle of 90° with legs supported on leg

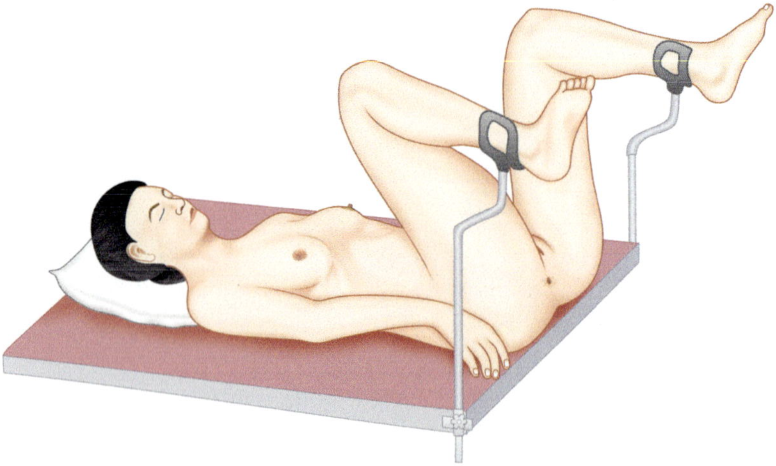

Fig. 9: Lithotomy position for vaginal operations.

rests. The thighs may be slightly abducted to generate space in between the thighs.

Surgeon's Position

The operating table should be at correct height according to the operating surgeon. The surgeon should work in a comfortable and relaxed posture so that he or she does not sustain back or neck muscle strain after long hours of operating. Elbows and shoulders should be kept relaxed by the proper adjustment of height of the operating table as explained later. The surgeon should stand on the side which permits the operating hand and arm to reach the area of pathology most easily. The surgeon should stand in a position with his left foot forward and right foot backward. In this position, the surgeon's shoulder, arm, and wrist are free of strain. In this position, the needle is directed toward the left foot, and the surgeon is able to perceive proprioceptive sensation as the needle passes through the tissue. He is able to feel the depth of tissue bites. Suturing in this position is known as forehand suturing and needs a strong biceps muscle for pronation and supination. Back hand motion is when an instrument is directed toward the right foot and is required when cutting by scalpel or by electrocautery or during insertion of Lembert sutures.

Ideal Height of the Operation Table (Figs. 10A and B)

Ideal height of the operating table should be at the level of the surgeon's elbow, while operating on the abdomen or chest. If the operating table is at the level of the surgeon's elbow, the wrist is in slight dorsiflexion, which is a position of ideal function. If the height of the operating table is higher than the level of the surgeon's elbow, there will be flexion of both elbow's and wrist. In the position of wrist flexion, long extensors of the forearm and hands will be in contraction and long flexors of the forearm and hands will be in a relaxed position, but no longer in tonic balance. This imbalance increases small muscle fatigue of the hands and reduces performance of small muscles of the hand. Eye stereopsis is more appropriate if the operating field is at a distance of 18″ from the eyes. If the operating

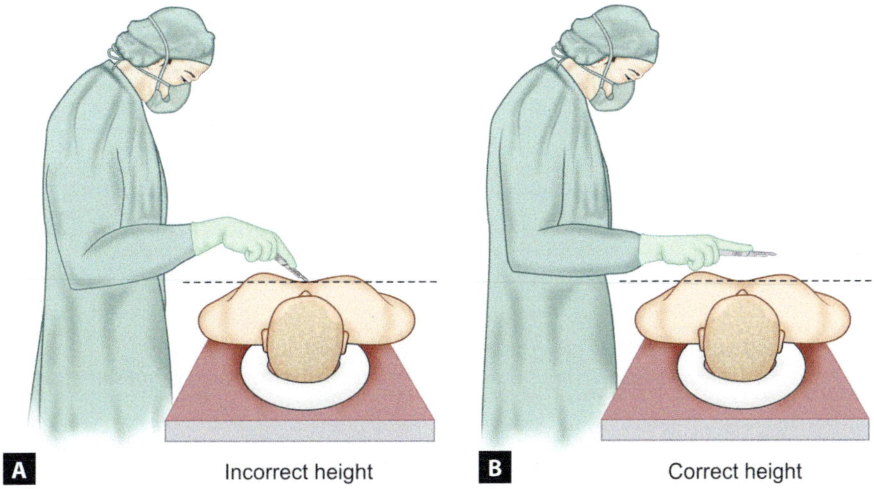

Figs. 10A and B: Ideal height of the operation table.

field is a depressed body surface, within oral cavity or within pelvis, the operating table should be below surgeon's elbow, so that the wrist is in a position of mild ulnar deviation and relatively straight. This is the functional position of the wrist, which greatly improves dexterity and strength in the fingers.

POINTS TO REMEMBER FOR PROPER POSITIONING

- Good positioning starts with an assessment of patient.
- The surgical team members should abstain from leaning against patients.
- The surgical arm board pads should be in level with table pads.
- Cushioning of all pressure points should be performed as the correct use of padding can protect the patient.
- Procedures longer than 2½ to 3 hours significantly increase the risk of pressure ulcer formation.
- During a longer procedure, one should assist with shifting the patient, adjusting the table, or adding/removing a positioning device.
- The nurse must assess extremities at regular intervals for signs of circulatory compromise.
- Documentation of the positioning process should be performed accurately and completely.

KEY POINTS

- Proper positioning of patient during surgery helps in the proper exposure of the operative field and facilitates the completion of a procedure with minimal stress and fatigue.
- Improper position can complicate the surgery.
- Avoid pressure on bony prominences.
- Avoid excessive abduction of the upper limbs.

CHAPTER 12

Anastomosis in Surgery

Raman Tanwar, Sudhir Kumar Jain, David L Stoker

"The enemy of good is better: The first layer is the best—why spoil it?"
"Staplers are not a substitute for sound surgical technique in carrying out gut anastomosis"

INTRODUCTION

The term "anastomosis" is derived from a Greek word meaning "without a mouth". Galen (AD 131–201) was one of the earliest surgeons who used this term.

In modern day surgical practice, the term anastomosis can be defined as a joining of two hollow viscera or tubular structures with an intention to restore continuity.

The need for anastomosis arises if a portion of hollow viscus has been surgically removed or destroyed by trauma, or there is a distal obstruction.

In general surgery, an anastomosis may involve:

- Gut—intestinal anastomosis
- Vessel—vascular anastomosis
- Urinary tract
- Biliary tract or pancreatic duct.

HISTORICAL ASPECTS

In 1826, Antoine Lembert, a French surgeon, described the seromuscular suturing technique which proved to be the mainstay of gastrointestinal surgery. Nicholas Sen from USA in 1893 described a two-layered technique of intestinal anastomosis, using silk with ordinary sewing needles. The celebrated 19th century American surgeon Halsted described a single-layer closure without incorporating the mucosa. Connell from Chicago in 1963 described an interrupted single-layer technique of gut anastomosis with knots lying intraluminal and bites going through all the layers. Kocher described a two-layered technique using silk and catgut. The current method of single-layer extramucosal anastomosis was advocated by Matheson of Aberdeen. Alexis Carrel in 1926 described his technique of end-to-end vascular anastomosis which proved to be a revolution in the field of vascular surgery.

IDEAL ANASTOMOSIS

An ideal anastomotic technique should have the following features:

- Zero leak rates
- Should promote early recovery of function
- No vascular compromise at the incised or divided margins of a viscus
- Should not narrow the lumen of a viscus
- Easy to learn, teach, and perform
- Technique should preferably be quick to perform.

Such an ideal technique is still to emerge.

TYPES OF ANASTOMOSIS

- End-to-end anastomosis
- End-to-side anastomosis
- Side-to-side anastomosis.

INTESTINAL ANASTOMOSIS

Intestinal anastomosis may involve:

- Joining two ends of similar type of gut, i.e., jejunojejunal, ileoileal, or colocolic.
- Joining two different types of gut, i.e., esophagus and jejunum, stomach and jejunum, and ileum and colon or rectum.
- Joining of gut with another hollow tubular structure, e.g.,
    - Common hepatic duct and jejunum—hepaticojejunostomy
    - Common bile duct and duodenum—choledochoduodenostomy
    - Common bile duct and jejunum—choledochojejunostomy
    - Gallbladder and jejunum—cholecystojejunostomy
    - Pancreatic duct and jejunum—pancreaticojejunostomy
    - Ureters may be implanted into an ileal conduit or into the sigmoid colon.

Healing of Intestinal Anastomosis

Intestinal healing process can be divided in following phases:

- Acute inflammatory phase (lag phase)
- Proliferative phase
- Remodeling or maturation phase

Intestinal healing is different from healing at other sites because of presence of shear stress resulting from peristalsis and transit of intestinal contents as well as presence of aerobic/anaerobic bacteria.

Degradation of mature collagen starts in first 24 hours and continues for 4 days. This degradation occurs due to activation or upregulation of matrix metalloproteinase (MMP) which is involved in collagen metabolism.

By postoperative day 7, collagen synthesis starts in the gut proximal to the anastomosis and continues for 5–6 weeks. After 6 weeks, there is no significant increase in collagen in the anastomosis, and the tensile strength increases by orientation and the cross-linkage between collagen fibers.

Early anastomotic strength in the first 7–10 days is dependent upon the suture or staple holding capacity of existing collagen. New collagen is synthesized by both fibroblast and smooth muscle cells.

Vascular Anastomosis

Vascular anastomosis may involve the aorta, a peripheral artery or vein, coronary arteries, or cerebral arteries.

Techniques of Anastomosis

Anastomosis can be:

- Hand sewn using sutures
- Stapled
- Sutureless anastomosis using laser (Nd:YAG) or tissue glue, e.g., fibrin glue. These are still experimental. Fibrin glue has been used to reinforce anastomotic suture lines.

Table 1 shows the factors which increase the rate of anastomotic leak.

Emergency surgery, if associated with a hypovolemic condition, as in abdominal trauma with intra-abdominal bleeding. Hypovolemia compromises the splanchnic circulation, which may result in ischemia at the site of an anastomosis.

Peritonitis is a major risk factor. Most patients with peritonitis have septicemia with a systemic inflammatory response syndrome (SIRS). Here, there are high circulating levels of inflammatory mediators, which induce excessive inflammation (more than required for wound healing) at the site of the anastomosis, rendering it friable and prone to leak.

TABLE 1: Factors which increase the rate of anastomotic leak.

Factor	*Description*
Emergency surgery with hypovolemia	Hypovolemia from abdominal trauma or bleeding compromises splanchnic circulation, leading to ischemia at the anastomosis site
Peritonitis	Peritonitis often involves septicemia and SIRS, which cause excessive inflammation at the anastomosis site, making it prone to leaks
Low-hemoglobin concentration	Decreased oxygen-carrying capacity of the blood leads to relative ischemia at the anastomosis site
Malnutrition	Low-serum protein and albumin levels cause tissue edema, increased suture tension, and poor healing
Previous irradiation	Irradiation for malignancy induces fibrosis and reduces blood supply, increasing the risk of anastomotic leak
Immunosuppressive drugs	Steroids and other immunosuppressive drugs impair tissue healing and increase leak risk
Unprepared gut	Performing an anastomosis on an unprepared colon with high fecal bacterial load increases the chance of leak
Malignancy, infection, and inflammation	These conditions impair healing and increase the likelihood of anastomotic leaks
Distal obstruction	Ongoing obstruction increases tissue tension and ischemia, increasing the risk of leak
Ongoing tension	Mechanical twists or a narrow lumen causing insufficient fluid passage can lead to ischemia and anastomotic dehiscence

Low hemoglobin concentration may cause decreased oxygen carrying capacity of the blood, inducing relative ischemia at the site of an anastomosis.

Malnutrition leads to low levels of serum protein and albumin, causing interstitial tissue edema, increased suture tension, and poor healing.

Previous irradiation: Patients who have been irradiated for malignancy have a higher incidence of anastomotic leak because irradiation induces fibrosis and reduces blood supply.

Immunosuppressive drugs including steroids cause poor tissue healing.

Unprepared gut: An anastomosis performed on unprepared colon with a high fecal bacterial load has an increased chance of leak.

Malignancy, infection, and inflammation will all impair healing.

Distal obstruction should be excluded before joining two ends. Ongoing obstruction will lead to increased tissue tension and ischemia.

Ongoing tension on an anastomosis may be seen due to mechanical twists and may also occur secondary to a narrow lumen, not wide enough to allow passage of fluid. This also leads to ischemia and the possibility of anastomotic dehiscence.

The Hand-sewn Anastomosis: Technical Issues (Figs. 1 and 2)

Choice of Suture Material

One should choose a suture material, which induces the least inflammatory reaction. The majority of sutures available today act as a

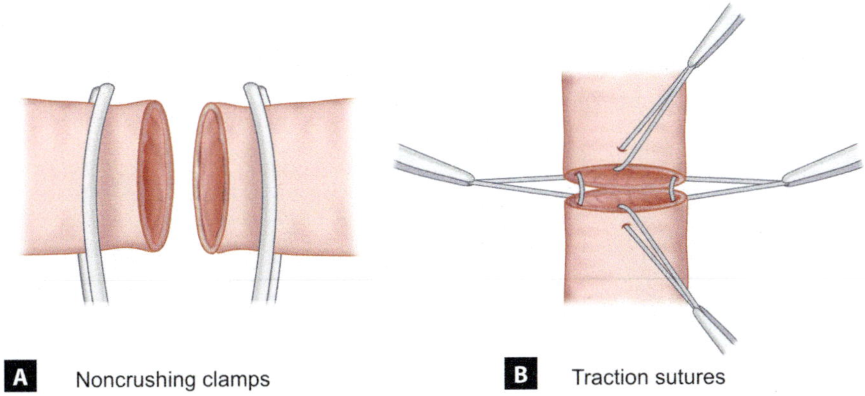

Figs. 1A and B: Preparation of gut to form an anastomosis. Noncrushing clamps are applied to prevent leakage, and ends are held together by traction sutures.

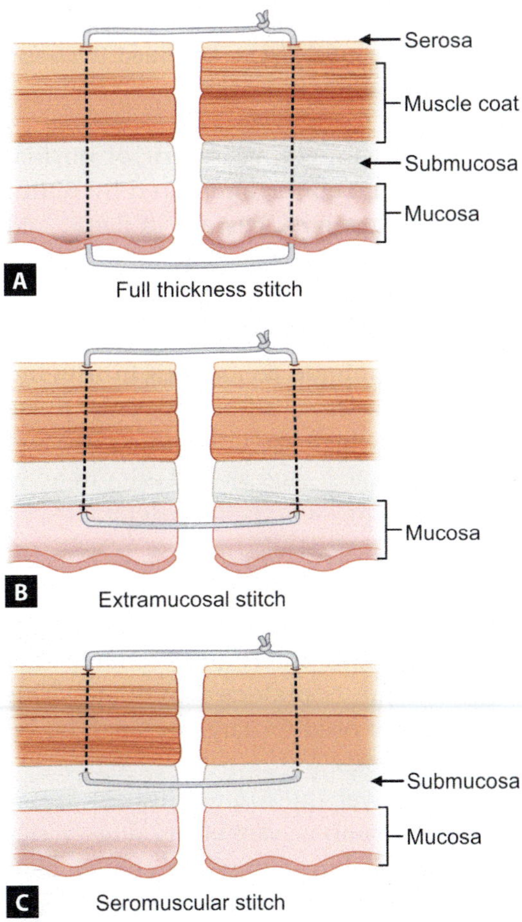

Figs. 2A to C: (A) Full thickness stitch (above); (B) Extramucosal stitch; and (C) Seromuscular stitch.

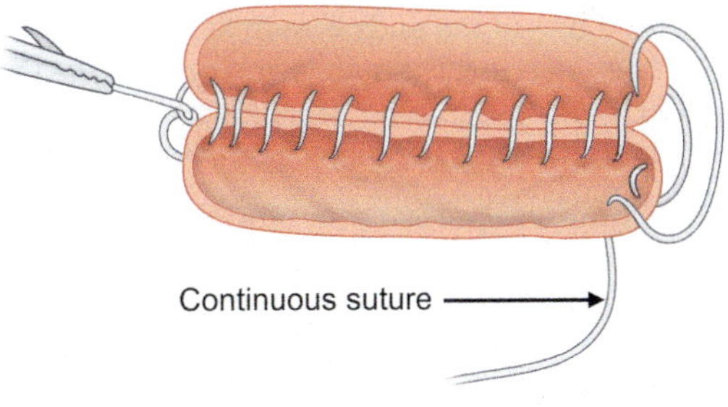

Fig. 3: Anastomosis by continuous suture.

foreign body and induce inflammation. It has been seen that silk induces a significantly greater cellular reaction at the site of anastomosis, which persists up to 6 weeks in comparison to polypropylene, polyglycolic acid, or polyglactin. An ideal suture material for anastomosis should cause minimal inflammation and tissue reaction and should provide maximum strength during the lag phase of wound healing. Monofilament and coated braided sutures are most effective but still not ideal.

Continuous versus Interrupted Sutures (Figs. 3 and 4)

To date, no randomized trial has established the superiority of one technique over the

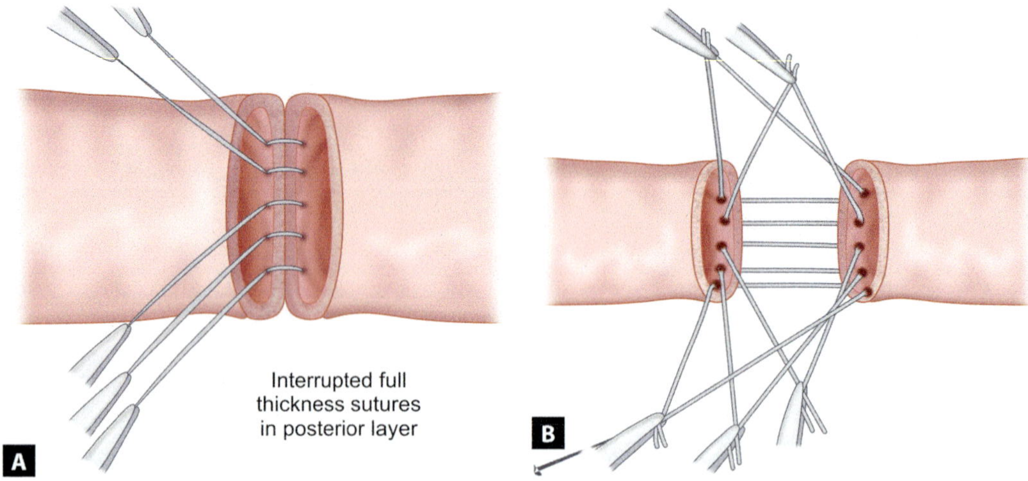

Figs. 4A and B: (A) Method of anastomosis of bowel if the ends are fixed. Posterior layer stitches are applied first; (B) If one of the ends is mobile, stitches are left with ends separated until all posterior wall sutures have been inserted. The mobile end can then be railroaded along the sutures and the knots tied. This is also known as the "telescoping" technique.

other, but in experimental studies using a rat model, perianastomotic oxygen tension was found to be lower with continuous sutures. Narrowing of the lumen may occur with continuous sutures, especially in the early phase when postoperative edema tends to tighten the suture. There may sometimes be a drawstring effect also.

Single-layer versus Double-layer Anastomosis

Double-layer anastomosis which came into vogue before single-layer anastomosis was traditionally thought to be more secure. However, studies have clearly shown the advantages of single-layer anastomosis due to:

- Decreased operative time
- Less narrowing of intestinal lumen
- More rapid vascularization and mucosal healing
- Rapid increase in the strength of the anastomosis in the first few postoperative days
- Early postoperative return of normal bowel function as measured by return of bowel sounds, passage of flatus, and resumption of oral feeding.

Types of Sutured Anastomosis

There are multiple techniques in use, but the authors have described only those techniques which are in common use and widely accepted. One should adopt one of these techniques and try to master it.

Single-layer Anastomosis

There are three types:

1. A single-layer interrupted extramucosal technique is preferred by many. This is mainly used for large or small bowel anastomosis.
2. Single-layer interrupted full thickness. This is mainly used in biliary surgery, e.g., hepaticojejunostomy and choledocho-duodenostomy.
3. Single-layer full thickness continuous technique is commonly employed

for gastrojejunal anastomosis. The continuous suture gives the advantage of hemostasis, as the gastric wall is very vascular. It also reduces intraoperative time.

Two-layer Anastomosis

The two-layered anastomosis consists of an inner layer taking a bite through the full thickness of the viscus. This inner layer can be continuous or interrupted depending upon the portion of the viscus to be anastomosed. For the small bowel, the inner layer can be continuous, but for colon, the inner layer can be interrupted or continuous depending on the surgeon's choice. The outer layer takes a bite through the seromuscular layer only and is usually interrupted in colonic surgery. In the small bowel or stomach, it is usually continuous.

Stapled Anastomosis

Surgical stapling devices were first introduced by Hulti in 1908 but did not gain popularity because the instruments were cumbersome, unreliable, and difficult to use. The past three decades have seen the development of reliable, disposable surgical stapling devices, which produce consistent quality staple lines with rare technical failures. With the help of these stapling devices, anastomoses at difficult sites such as low rectum, or high esophagus, have become safer and more technically feasible. The drawbacks of stapling devices are that they are costly, and the surgeon is as much reliant on technology as on his surgical skills. The main advantage of these devices is that they save time and may have a place where multiple anastomoses have to be created, e.g., in Whipple's procedure, or in radical cystectomy with ileal conduit reconstruction.

Staplers

Three types of staplers are in vogue for creating intestinal anastomosis:

1. *Transverse anastomosis (TA) stapler:* It is the simplest type of stapler. This device places two staggered rows of B-shaped staples across the bowel but does not cut them. The surgeon needs to divide the gut separately.
2. *Gastrointestinal anastomosis (GIA) linear cutter:* This gastrointestinal stapler places two double staggered rows of staples and simultaneously cuts between the double rows.
3. *Circular or end-to-end anastomosis (EEA) stapler:* This places a double row of staples in a circle and then cuts out the tissue within the circle of staples with a built-in cylindrical knife. These staples are used for LAR, for gastroesophageal anastomosis, or for stapled hemorrhoidopexy.

There is also an Endo GIA gun, which is used for laparoscopic surgery. Staples are made up of titanium, which causes little tissue reaction, and is nonmagnetic, thus enabling future magnetic resonance imaging (MRI) scanning.

Staplers can produce:

- Functional end-to-end anastomosis
- Anatomical end-to-end anastomosis
- Side-to-side anastomosis.

Functional Stapled End-to-end Anastomosis

The steps of a functional EEA are:

- Place two cut ends of the bowel side to side, maintaining the orientation of mesentery.
- Insert the two limbs of GIA stapler, one each into the lumen of each bowel end either through an enterotomy or through the open end of the bowel. Engage the

two limbs of the stapler into each other, making sure that the mesentery of the gut does not become caught in the staple line. This can be ensured by putting a finger in between the mesenteries when the stapler is engaged.

- The stapler is then fired to fuse the two bowel walls into a single septum and to create a cut between the two rows of staples.
- Wait for 1 minute before removing the stapler for hemostasis to occur (This is not always necessary but is a useful precaution).
- Inspect the staple line for completeness and hemostasis. Underrun bleeding vessels if necessary.

A noncutting linear stapler (TA) or a suture can be used to close the defect in the gut through which GIA was inserted. Alternatively, the initial enterotomies may be placed in that part of the bowel which is to be resected.

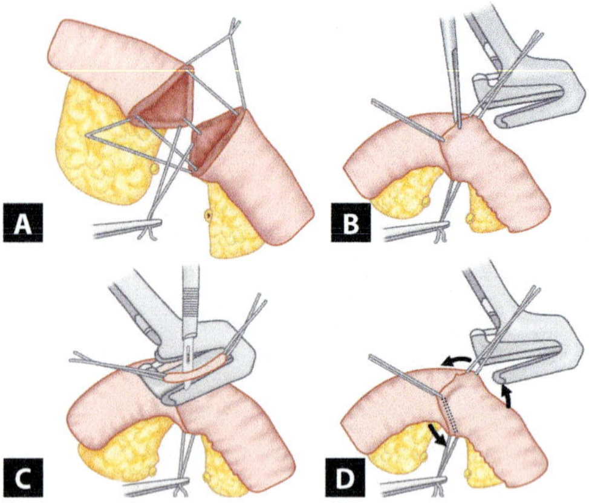

Figs. 5A to D: Triangulation technique of end-to-end anastomosis by stapler: (A) Three stay sutures at three corners of divided ends of gut to triangulate the ends; (B) Linear staplers applied between two stay sutures; (C) Excess tissue above staple line excised; (D) Gut rotated and similar process repeated between remaining stay sutures.

True Anatomical End-to-end Anastomosis by Stapler

- *Triangulation technique:* Cut ends of bowel are triangulated together by taking stay sutures, and three linear staplers are fired in intersecting vectors to achieve a complete closure. Drawback of this technique is that staple lines are everted **(Figs. 5A to D)**.
- Two cut ends of the bowel can be united together by using an EEA stapler, which produces a directly apposed, inverted stapled end-to-end anastomosis. This is not used much now as more often end-to-side technique is used.

Advantages of Stapled Anastomosis over Hand-sewn Anastomosis

- Titanium staples used in anastomosis provoke minimal inflammatory response.
- They provide support to the cut surfaces in lag phase (weakest phase of healing).
- Stapling may shorten operating time, especially in low pelvic anastomosis, or in the thorax, or in high abdomen.
- After resection of tumor, recurrence at the staple line is theoretically much less than at the suture line because suture materials produce a more pronounced cellular proliferation than staples.
- Stapled anastomosis heals by primary intention but sutured anastomosis heals by secondary intention.

Inverted Suture Line versus Everted Suture Line

An inverted suture line is found to be better than an everted suture line in terms of bursting pressure, rate of healing, and degree of inflammation. An inverted suture line has a greater aesthetic appeal although this has little relevance to healing.

Testing the Anastomosis

In certain situations where an anastomosis is performed in a difficult situation, e.g., low anorectal anastomosis, esophagogastric anastomosis or where the anastomosis is complex as in the creation of an ileoanal pouch, testing of anastomosis is important. Anastomosis can be tested by following methods discussed here.

Underwater Test

This test is performed in cases of LAR or in cases of esophagogastric anastomosis. A soft noncrushing clamp is applied on gastric side or on the sigmoid colon just distal to the anastomosis. Pelvic cavity or left subdiaphragmatic space is filled with saline. Air is insufflated from the anal opening in case of LAR or nasogastric tube in case of esophagogastric anastomosis. If there is no bubbling of air into the saline, the anastomosis is airtight and presumed to be safe.

Methylene Blue Test

This test is performed in cases of gastric pouch surgery for obesity. After completion of the anastomosis, methylene blue is injected through a nasogastric tube. There should not be any leak of methylene blue from the gastrojejunostomy.

Protecting an Anastomosis

Nasogastric Decompression

Routine nasogastric decompression is not mandatory after lower intestinal anastomosis unless there is a significant paralytic ileus with abdominal distension, gastric dilatation, or excessive emesis.

In upper gastrointestinal anastomosis, e.g., gastrojejunostomy or gastroduodenal anastomoses, nasogastric suction is essential for 3–5 days to avoid any tension on the suture line caused by retention of gastric secretions. Gastric motility takes around 72 hours to recover and a nasogastric tube may prevent acute gastric dilatation. Stents are left across an anastomosis following hepaticojejunostomy and pancreaticojejunostomy to prevent bile or pancreatic leaks. A nasogastric tube is left after every emergency laparotomy. An unwanted side effect of nasogastric tube placement is discomfort in the pharynx, and difficulty in coughing, along with increased risk of upper airway tract infection.

Abdominal Drains after Intestinal Anastomosis

The ability of abdominal drainage to "protect" an anastomosis has been challenged by Yates. The peritoneal cavity cannot be drained effectively by a single drain due to the rapid development of adhesions and sealing of the drainage tract. Severe inflammatory reactions have been shown to occur around the drains. An intra-abdominal drain after anterior resection or ileo-anal anastomosis is kept in the pelvis because there is higher than usual incidence of fluid collections in the pelvis after these operations.

General Principles of Intestinal Anastomosis

- There should not be any disparity between the two ends of lumen to be joined together. If one end is narrower than other, it can be enlarged by giving a cut along the antimesenteric border sometimes also known as "fish mouthing" of the end.
- To prevent leakage of contents and to steady the two ends, either noncrushing

clamps can be applied across the gut or stay sutures can be taken at the end.

- Three types of sutures can be used for anastomosis of the gut:
  1. All coat stitches in which bites are taken through all layers of the gut. This was advocated by William Halsted (1852–1922) **(Fig. 2A)**.
  2. In extramucosal or serosubmucosal technique, all layers are included except mucosa. Submucosa is the strongest layer, as it contains plenty of collagen tissue **(Fig. 2B)**.
  3. In seromuscular stitch bites are taken through the serosa and part of the muscular layer. This was described by a surgeon from Paris (Antoine Lembert). This stitch is also known as a Lembert stitch. It is generally used as a second layer to strengthen the first layer.

BASIC ARTERIAL SURGICAL TECHNIQUES

Arterial surgery is generally undertaken to:

- Repair arteries after trauma
- Reconstruct arteries which are diseased or blocked.

Arterial surgery like all other anastomoses should be undertaken in optimum conditions with good light, good exposure, and good control of bleeding.

Precautions during Arterial Anastomosis

- Handle arteries gently, and veins with extreme gentleness.
- Vessels should be held by the adventitial tissue whenever possible to avoid trauma to the vessel wall.
- If one needs to handle the arterial wall directly, use the tip of closed dissecting forceps.
- Use a suture which passes easily without causing trauma and which causes least tissue reaction. A monofilament suture such as prolene is an excellent choice.
- Round-bodied needles are used for the majority of vessels, but taper cut needles are better for dense graft material or for heavily diseased arteries.
- The needle should be passed from inside outward—from intima to adventitia. This pins down atherosclerotic plaques to prevent the formation of intimal flaps, which may lead to dissection, embolization, or thrombosis.
- Suture material should not be held with dissecting forceps, needle holders, or forceps, all of which can damage the thread.
- Knots should be hand tied.
- When a needle has to be passed from adventitia to intima (from outside to inside), the intima should be supported against the vessel wall as the needle is inserted.
- The needle should pass at right angles to the arterial wall and should be passed through the wall along the arc of the needle without deploying excessive force, to avoid splitting or tearing the delicate vessel wall.
- The suture line should be smooth and everted. This provides good intimal apposition and prevents platelet aggregation on the suture line.
- When suturing a transverse defect in an artery, start from the outside in on the upstream side and from inside out on the downstream side, in order to avoid dissection of intima from the arterial wall by turbulent blood flow. This technique helps in preventing a dissecting aneurysm, especially in the aorta.

- Vascular sutures may be:
    - *Unlocked continuous:* Continuous unlocked sutures form a spiral around the artery, which tightens with each distending pulsation of the vessel. A tightened spiral reduces the likelihood of leakage. If a continuous suture is locked, the spiral effect will be lost, and the suture will not become tightened with arterial pulsations.
    - *Interrupted sutures:* These are used for small vessels to reduce the risk of stenosis. They are also used in children, to permit the growth of vessel circumference along with the growth of child. A drawback of interrupted sutures is increased risk of bleeding when the sutures separate with distension of vessels.
    - *Mattress sutures:* Mattress sutures are not generally used in vascular surgery because they tend to narrow the lumen. Sometimes a single mattress suture may be used to initiate eversion or in case of diseased arteries when there is danger of simple sutures cutting out.

Arteriotomy (Fig. 6)

An arteriotomy should be longitudinal to permit visualization of the vessel lumen and to permit approaches to branches of the artery. In cases of vessels <4 mm in diameter, where an arteriotomy has been made only for embolectomy, a transverse incision can be made which has the advantage of less narrowing of the lumen.

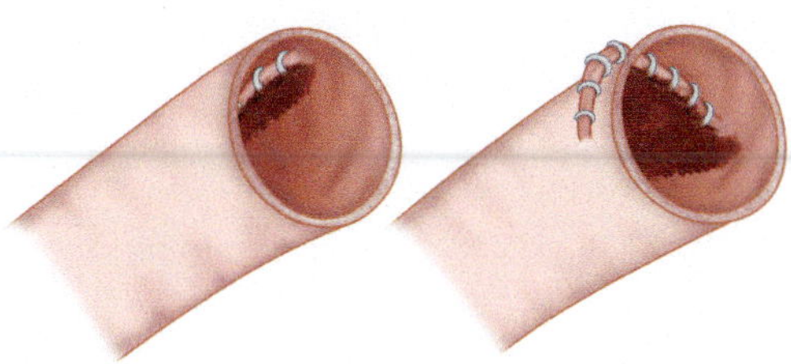

Fig. 6: Arteriotomy in a small size vessel should be longitudinal, because clot if formed on suture line will cause less narrowing of lumen if formed around longitudinal suture line in comparison to a transverse suture line.

Closure of an arteriotomy is performed by a continuous unlocking suture with intimal apposition and eversion of cut edges. The nonintimal layer of the arterial wall should not come in contact with flowing blood unless an endarterectomy has been performed. As it may be difficult to include all layers in the suture at the end of the arteriotomy, two appropriately sized double-ended arterial sutures are used. Closure is started from either end with both needles passing from inside out. Sutures are tied and secured in a pair of rubber shod forceps.

Suturing is continued from both ends using fine, evenly spaced stitches, until one reaches the apex of the vessel. The two sutures from both ends are then tied at the apex.

Vein Patch Graft

Vein patch grafts are used to close an arteriotomy if it is likely that simple closure will result in narrowing of the lumen of the artery. The chances of narrowing after simple closure of an arteriotomy are greater if the artery is smaller than the diameter of the common femoral artery or if the closure of a diseased segment of artery is performed. Vein patches are usually from autologous long saphenous vein taken from the ankle or from one of the groin tributaries. Proximal long saphenous vein should not be sacrificed as it may be utilized for future vascular reconstructive procedures. If suitable vein is not available, then a patch of Dacron or expanded polytetrafluoroethylene (e-PTFE) can be used.

Steps of Arteriotomy Closure Using Vein Patch Graft (Fig. 7)

- A suitable vein patch graft or synthetic graft patch is prepared by trimming one end to form an ellipse that will fit into the end of the incision. Do not cut the other end, because the excess portion can be used to handle the patch without damaging the intima.
- Take a suitable size double needled prolene suture on a round bodied needle. Insert both needles from outside in, at one end of the vein patch. Pass needles from inside to outside through one cut end of the incision in the artery in such a manner that the suture is divided into two halves to cover each side of the incision.
- Continue taking continuous over and over sutures on the back wall and front wall using one needle each.
- Once the halfway point is reached, trim the end of the vein patch to a rounded ellipse to fit in the remaining defect. While trimming the other end of vein patch, make sure that tension on the suture is not loosened.
- After trimming the vein patch, continue suturing on such that suture from one side is carried back around the other end, and two ends of suture are tied at the midpoint of the front side.

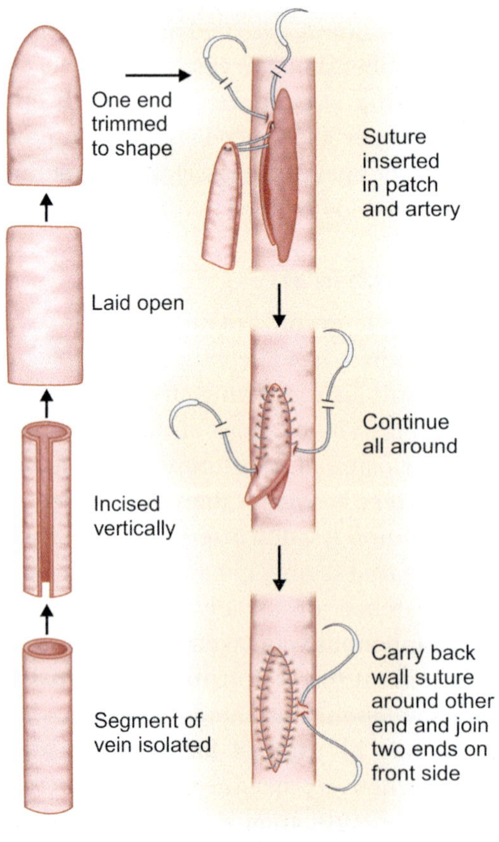

Fig. 7: Steps of vein patch insertion to close an arteriotomy.

End-to-end Anastomosis (Figs. 8 and 9)

General Principles

- Bevel the ends of the arteries to be united to avoid narrowing except in large vessels. Beveling can be done by cutting the ends obliquely.

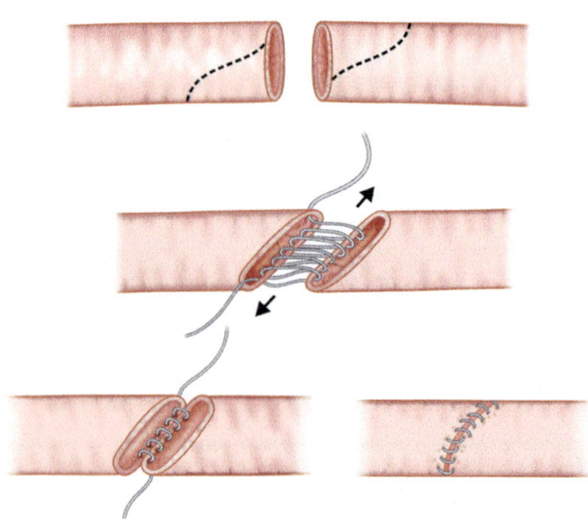

Fig. 8: Method of performing end-to-end arterial anastomosis. Ends are beveled by cutting obliquely before performing anastomosis to prevent narrowing.

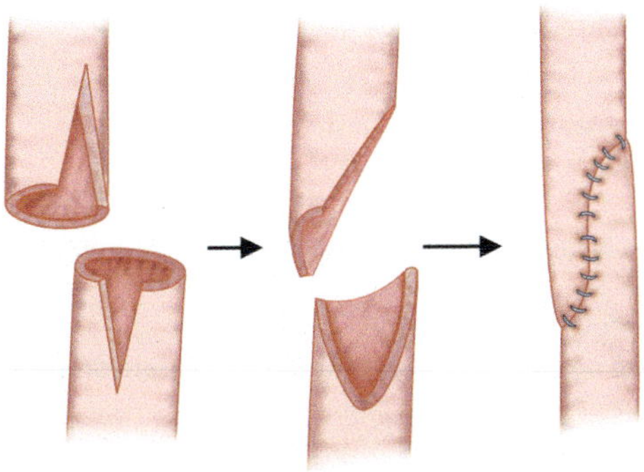

Fig. 9: End-to-end arterial anastomosis. Ends are beveled to avoid narrowing.

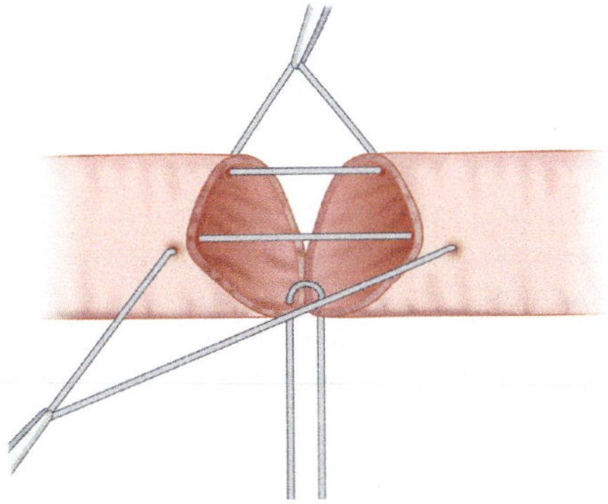

Fig. 10: Anchoring suture technique for vascular anastomosis.

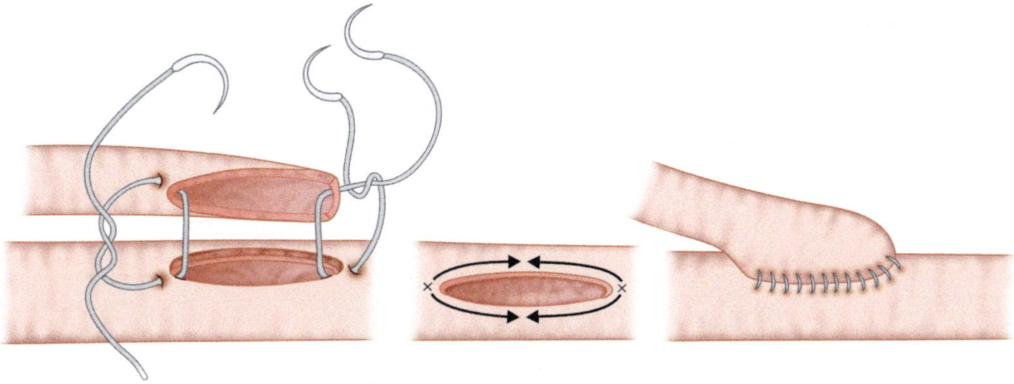

Fig. 11: Parachuting technique.

- Use continuous unlocked sutures except in children to avoid hampering of growth and in very small or delicate vessels.
- Pediatric vessels are more prone to go into spasm, so handle them gently.
- Place sutures from outside to inside on the upstream side and from inside to outside on downstream side. There are two techniques of performing vascular anastomosis:
    1. Anchoring suture technique
    2. Parachuting technique.

Anchoring Suture Technique (Fig. 10)

Three anchoring sutures are placed at equal distance around the whole circumference of the vessels. These sutures are used for rotating the vessel for the purpose of gaining access. This technique is very good where mobility of vessels is not restricted.

Parachuting Technique (Fig. 11)

This is useful if the mobility of vessels is restricted by branches. In this technique, the vessels are kept apart. A posterior row of continuous unlocked sutures is applied first using a double needled suture starting from the posterior midline and working outward alternatively on each side, continuing around up to the front. Ends of the vessels are then gently drawn or parachuted together. Parachuting is only possible if a frictionless polypropylene suture is used.

KEY POINTS

- The ideal anastomotic technique is still to emerge.
- Every surgical trainee must learn and master hand-sewn anastomotic techniques.
- A stapled anastomosis is not superior to a hand-sewn one, but it may save time.
- Staplers add to the cost of surgery.
- There is no difference in leak rate between continuous and interrupted sutures following intestinal anastomosis.
- Vascularity of resected ends of gut should be ensured before joining them.
- Abdominal drainage after intestinal anastomosis should be avoided except in cases of peritonitis or trauma.
- Single-layer anastomosis scores over double-layer technique in terms of time saving, less luminal narrowing, and early return of postoperative bowel function.
- During arterial anastomosis, hold arteries by periarterial or adventitial tissue to avoid trauma to arterial wall.
- Monofilament suture, i.e., prolene with round-bodied needle is the suture of choice for arterial anastomosis.
- For an arterial anastomosis, the needle should pass from inside to outside to prevent formation of intimal flaps and to fix any atherosclerotic plaque.

CHAPTER 13

Art of Instrument Handling

Sudhir Kumar Jain, David L Stoker

"The beauty of an art lies in the proper handling of instrument by the craftsmen"

INTRODUCTION

Every surgeon must know and understand their instruments properly used in day-to-day surgical practice, especially laparoscopic and robotic instruments in order to avoid injury to the surgical team or the patient and to prevent malfunctioning of instruments. In an infamous case, patient died on table while performing robotic coronary artery bypass graft (CABG) as there was malfunctioning of robotic machine, and operating surgeon did not know how to correct the malfunctioning. In this chapter, basic instrument handling techniques have been described.

BROAD CLASSIFICATION OF INSTRUMENTS

Classification of instruments is as follows:

- *Instruments for cutting:*
  - Scissors
  - Scalpel
- *Instruments for grasping:*
  - Thumb forceps (toothed/nontoothed)
  - Artery forceps
  - Babcock forceps
  - Ellis forceps
- *Instrument for suturing:* Needle holders
- *Instruments for retraction:* It includes various types of retractors for superficial and deep retraction as described later in this chapter.

SCALPEL

This is the most basic surgical instrument, comprising of a handle and a blade. Blades are disposable, and the handle is reusable. The handle is commonly known as a BP handle after Bard Parker, the inventor. It comes in two sizes: 3 and 4. The number 3 handle will accommodate a small-sized surgical blade from numbers 10 to 15 **(Figs. 1 and 2)**. The number 4 handle will accommodate larger blades ranging from sizes 18 to 24. Scalpel can be used for making deliberate controlled cut into the tissue, e.g., for opening peritoneum, for making skin incision, for raising skin flaps as in thyroid surgery or mastectomy (although many surgeons use electrocautery for this purpose).

Handling

A surgical knife or scalpel should be transferred from scrub nurse to surgeon and vice versa in a kidney tray, not from hand to

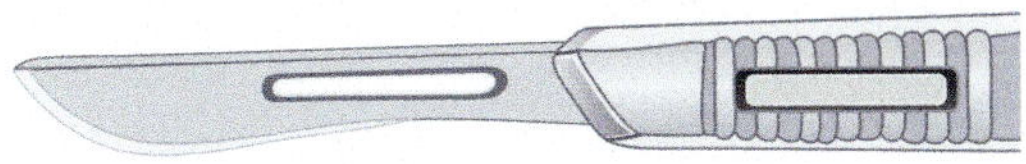

Fig. 1: Number 10 surgical blade.

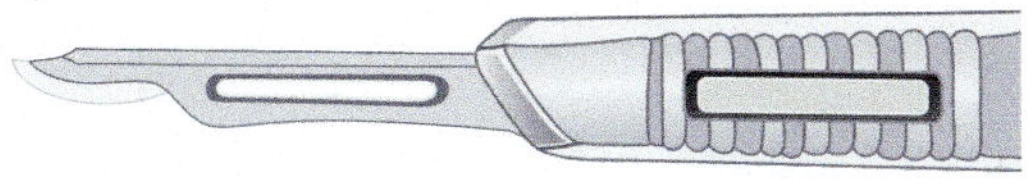

Fig. 2: Number 15 surgical blade.

hand, so as to avoid injuries from the very sharp blade.

Never try to load or unload the blade on to the handle by hand. This should only be attempted with the blade being held in forceps. To load the blade onto a scalpel handle, hold the blade in artery forceps near the base of cutting edge and advance it into the scalpel, until the lower end of the blade fits into a groove on the handle and you hear a click **(Fig. 3)**. To unload the blade, hold the base of the blade and then lift it up and pull it out of the groove, again using a pair of forceps **(Fig. 4)**.

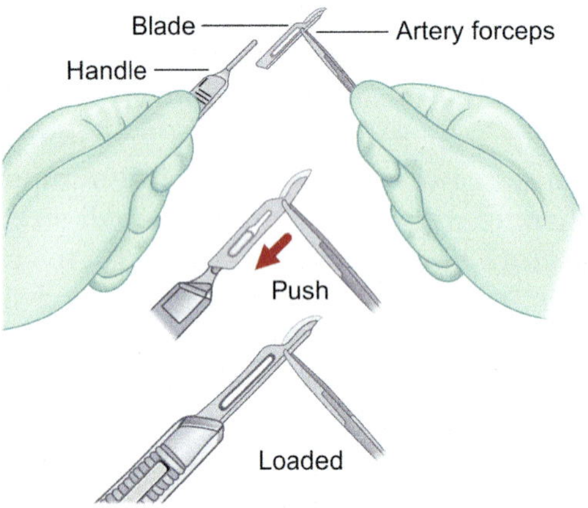

Fig. 3: Steps for loading a blade on scalpel handle.

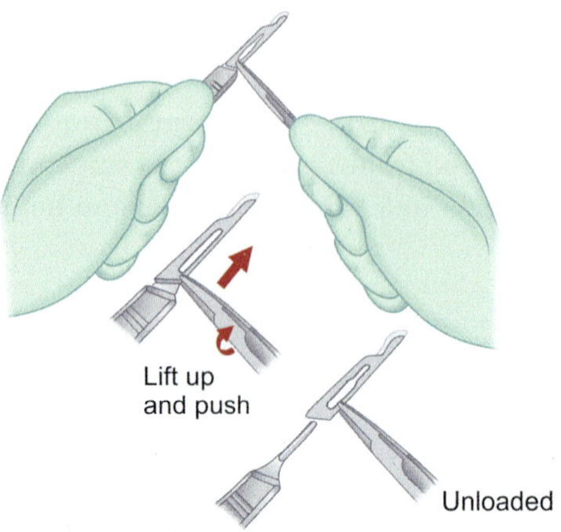

Fig. 4: Steps for unloading a blade from a scalpel handle.

The scalpel can be held as a table knife for a skin incision. The knife is held at 30° or less from the horizontal in a pronated hand, between the thumb and middle finger with the index finger at the base of the blade on the upper surface to apply and control pressure. Grip is strengthened by wrapping the ring and little finger around the handle, which rests on the hypothenar muscles **(Fig. 5)**.

For a small, precise cut, the scalpel is held like a pen **(Fig. 6)**. It is a good surgical practice to mark the incision with a skin marking pencil or with the back of the blade before actually incising it. Blade numbers 20–24 have a wider shaft and are used for larger incisions and dissection. Number 15 blades have a narrower shaft and are used for

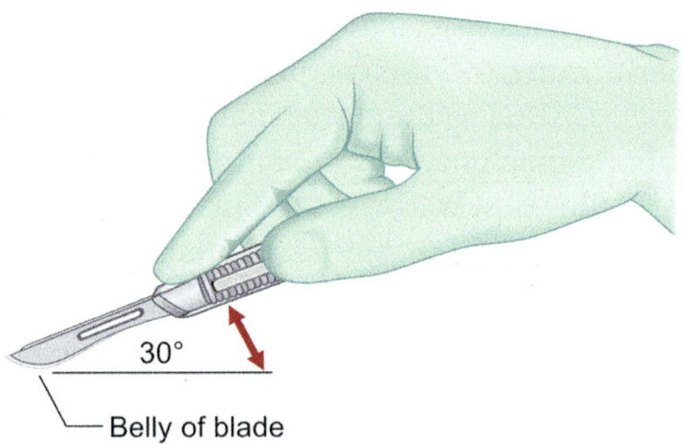

Fig. 5: Method of holding scalpel as a table knife.

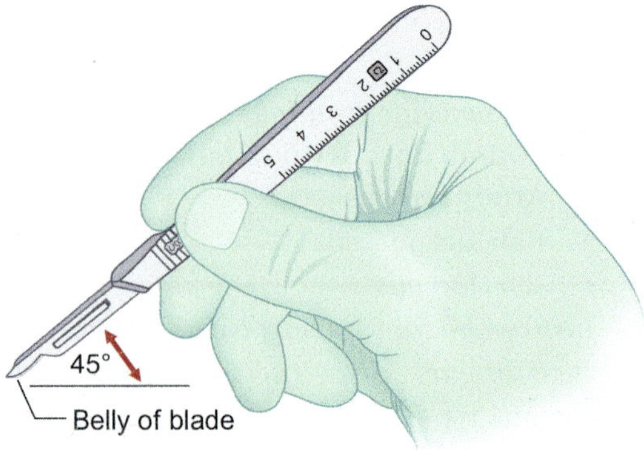

Fig. 6: Method of holding scalpel as a pen.

smaller incisions, for example, when making port sites for laparoscopic surgery, or when removing small skin lesions. The number 11 blade is also known as a stab knife and is used for incision and drainage of abscesses and to incise skin for inserting drains.

SCISSORS

Scissors are essential and versatile instruments. They can be used for:

- Tissue dissection
- Undermining skin or raising skin flaps
- Dividing tissue
- Cutting sutures
- Cutting gauze, meshes, or other surgical materials
- Spreading and opening tissue planes
- Assisting the surgeon in the palpation of tissues
- Probing cavities
- The closed scissors may be swept from side to side and used as a tissue elevator and blunt dissector.

Types of Scissors

- Dissecting scissors with a blunt tip
- Cutting scissors with a sharp tip.

Scissors have two blades—one is a moving and cutting blade, while the other is stationary. Scissors can be straight or curved. Cutting scissors are known as Mayo's scissors and are used for cutting heavy fascia and sutures. Lighter dissecting scissors such as Metzenbaum or McIndoe's scissors are used for dissecting and cutting delicate tissue. They have a longer handle-to-blade ratio. A typical pair of scissors measures 6 inches, which is designed and balanced for a normal size adult hand. Longer-sized scissors are only to be used if one is working inside the depth of body cavity or in large surgical wound which requires extra length of handle to reach the tissue. The tip of scissors can be sharp or blunt. If dissecting in dense scar tissue, sharp pointed pairs of scissors are required, which can penetrate the collagen bundles easily. If the surgeon is dissecting in loose tissue planes without fibrous tissue, blunt-tipped scissors are used which make dissection fast and safe. Scissors with curved blades give flexibility of approach angle and makes it possible to lift and palpate tissue to greater extent in comparison to straight scissors.

Straight blade scissors are ideal for cutting ends of sutures or ligatures. Straight blade scissors allow rapid and accurate positioning of scissor tip before cutting.

Handling (Fig. 7)

Each blade has a ring at the end, also known as a bow. For holding scissors, the hand should be in a mid-pronated position. The distal phalanx of the thumb should go into the ring of the moving blade and the distal phalanx of the ring finger into the other ring. The ring should never go beyond the distal interphalangeal joint. The tip of the index finger should rest over the joint of the blades,

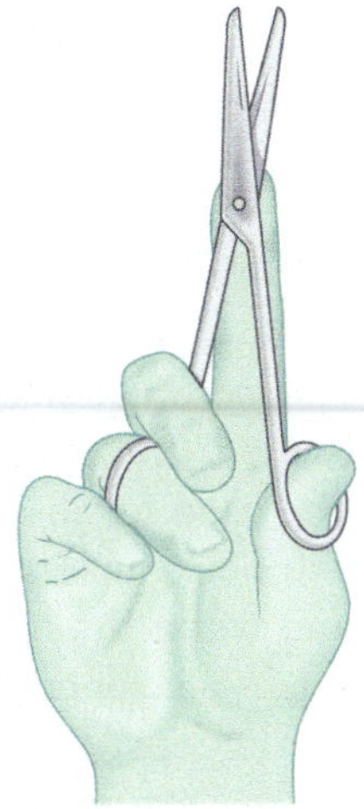

Fig. 7: Method of holding scissors.

and middle finger should wrap around the handle to steady it. While dividing tissues or sutures in a cavity, the scissor blades should rest over the index finger of the nondominant hand to steady them, and to minimize tremors.

In a vertical direction, cut with scissors from near to far and in a transverse direction from dominant to the nondominant side. If you want to cut from nondominant to dominant side or from far to near, it is advisable to use a scalpel unless skilled in using scissors in either hand. Some surgeons point the direction of blades toward the elbow while cutting from left to right with the right hand.

THUMB FORCEPS AND TISSUE HOLDING FORCEPS

These consist of two shafts held together at one end with a spring device that holds the shafts open. The tips of forceps can be smooth, serrated, or have teeth. All these forceps should have very light springs to open their jaws. In case of strong spring, the surgeon is unable to appreciate how firmly he or she is grasping the tissue. For holding skin, tough fascia or tendon, thumb forceps with a toothed tip are used. For holding delicate structures, thumb forceps with smooth tips or serrated tips are used. The main use of forceps is to retract, stabilize, or grasp tissue. Forceps are held like a pen between the thumb and middle finger in the nondominant hand with index finger to stabilize the forceps **(Fig. 8)**. Nontoothed thumb forceps with round tips may be used for dissection. The closed forceps tips are inserted into the desired plane and when the blades spring open, the tissue plane also opens.

Beside thumb forceps, there are other tissue holding forceps, e.g., Babcock forceps, Allis forceps, and Lane's tissue forceps.

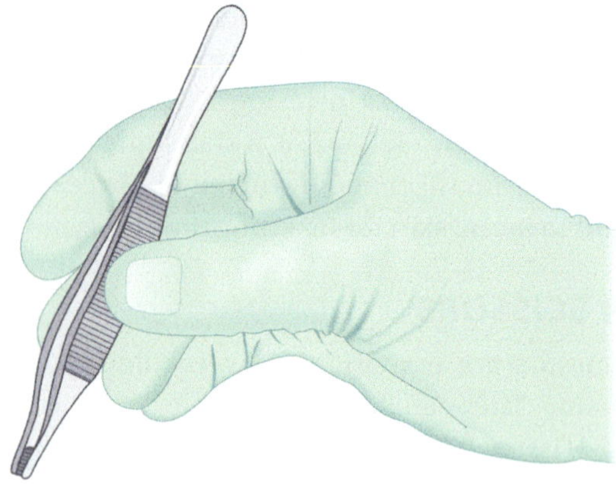

Fig. 8: Method of holding thumb forceps.

Babcock forceps are nontraumatic and are used for holding the gut, ureter, or bladder. Allis forceps have long blades with gaps between the blades. There are sharp teeth at the tip of the blades with grooves in between. When these forceps are locked, the tooth of one blade fits into the groove of the other blade and vice versa. These are used for holding tough structures such as skin, deep fascia, or aponeurosis. Lane's tissue forceps are heavy and traumatizing, with curved fenestrated blades. At the tip, there is a heavy tooth in one blade with a groove in the other blade. In the closed position, the tooth fits into the groove. They may be used for grasping a fibrosed salivary gland during excision or the breast tissue during mastectomy. They may also be used to encircle the spermatic cord around its curved fenestrated blade during hernia repair, or as a replacement of a lost towel clip.

ARTERY FORCEPS (HEMOSTATIC FORCEPS AND HEMOSTATS)

These were devised by the celebrated French surgeon, Ambroise Paré (1510–1590). His design was modified and improved by the introduction of a locking mechanism by Thomas Spencer Wells (1818–1897). Artery forceps are mainly used for holding bleeding vessels before they are occluded by a ligature or cauterized. They can also be used for dissection or for holding tough structures, such as fascia. They are pointed at one end, with rings at the ends of two shafts, linked with a hinge in the middle, and a ratchet to lock the blades.

Handling

Artery forceps and needle holders are held like surgical scissors **(Figs. 9 and 10)**. For locking the ratchet, handles are compressed. For unlocking, first lightly compress, and then separate the handles at a right angle to the hinge action. One should be able to lock and unlock them with either hand. For holding blood vessels, curved forceps are used with the concavity upward and the tips extending beyond the vessel. For ligating blood vessels which have been held by artery forceps, the assistant holds the forceps tip facing upward and visible, so that the surgeon can pass a ligature around the vessel. When the first half of the knot is being tied, the assistant gently releases and removes the artery forceps only at the verbal request of the surgeon, and not before.

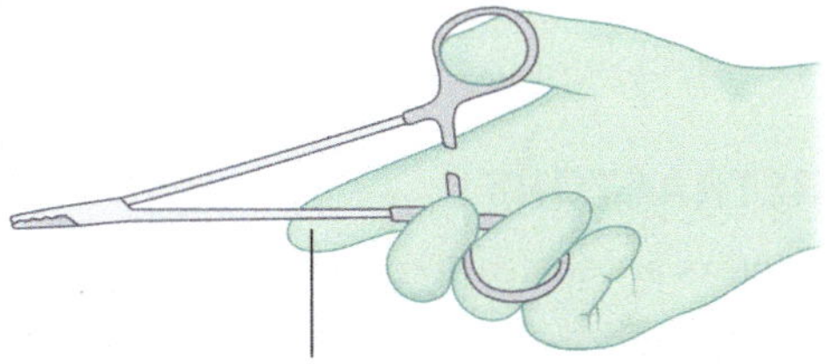

Fig. 9: Method of holding artery forceps.

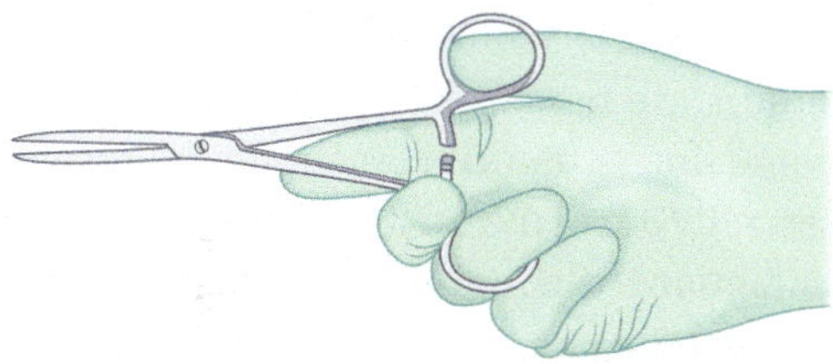

Fig. 10: Method of opening an artery forceps.

Artery forceps are available in different shapes and sizes. They can be either curved or straight. Small-sized artery forceps with fine tips are also known as Mosquito forceps. Other types include Kelly's, Spencer Well's, or Roberts. The Spencer Wells hemostatic forceps blades are usually half of the length of the shaft and have transverse serrations along the whole length of the blade with conical tips. In Kelly's clamps, the blades are short, and transverse serrations are present along the whole length.

NEEDLE HOLDERS

These are used for holding and driving needles through the tissue. They may also be called needle drivers. A needle holder is held in the same way as the surgical scissors. It can be differentiated from artery forceps by smaller, short blunt blades, criss-cross serrations, and a groove in the center of the blade for maintaining the orientation of the needle. A Mayo needle holder with a ratchet similar in design to that of artery forceps is commonly used. Plastic surgeons may use a smaller needle holder without a locking device and with a scissor at the tip. This type of needle holder was devised by Sir Harold Gilles, the famous British plastic surgeon.

Handling

Needle holders grip needles with especially designed jaws **(Fig. 11)**. Needles should be held at the junction of one-third and two-thirds of the way along the needle shaft from the suture material **(Fig. 12)**. Pronation and supination (backhand and forehand) are used to drive needle into the tissue. During a pronation/supination movement, the needle

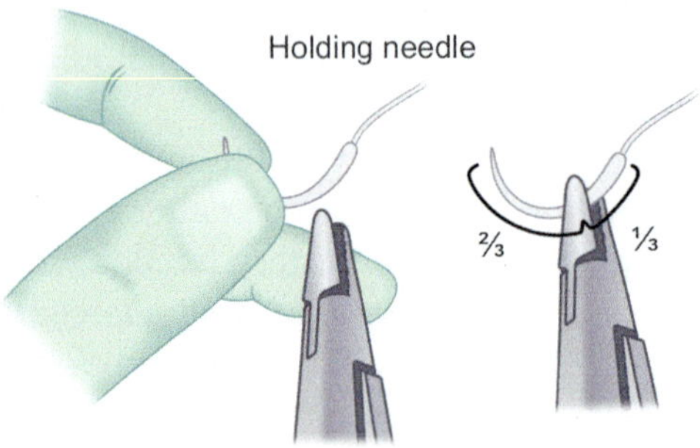

Fig. 11: Serrated jaw and smooth jaw needle holder.

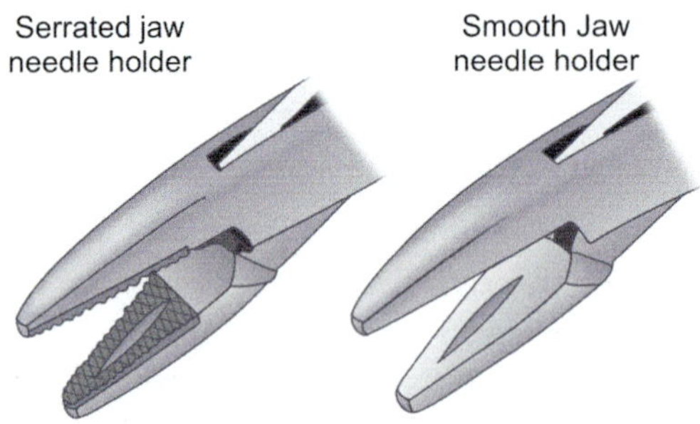

Fig. 12: Holding needle with needle holder at the junction of two-thirds and one-third from the tip.

holder rotates in its long axis and moves the needle in a curved plane through the tissue. A curved needle must be driven along its own curved shape through tissue and will bend if gripped incorrectly or driven in the wrong plane. Needles should be gripped at the tip of a needle holder, with a 90–105° angle with the shaft of the needle holder. The needlepoint should face the nondominant hand and point upward. When suturing in a deep cavity such as the pelvis, it is a good practice to use long needle holders in order to avoid hands blocking vision of the needle and tissues. While tying knots by hand, a needle holder with needle (mounted needle holder) may be kept on one side, in order to avoid a needle prick. Some surgeons palm the needle holder in the first interspace

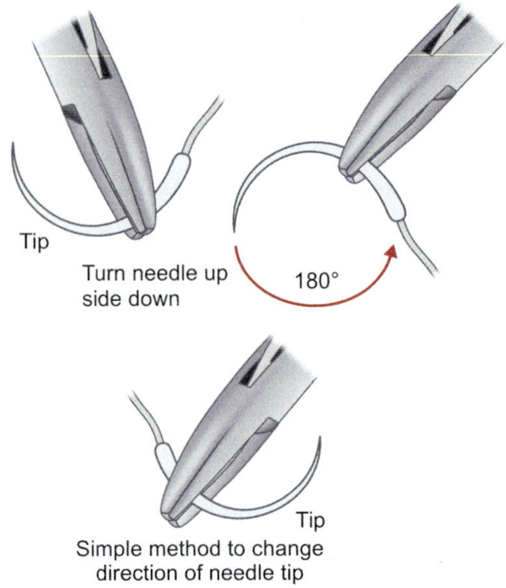

Fig. 13: A method to change direction of needle tip.

between thumb and second metacarpal, but this requires practice.

If it is essential to change the direction of a needle while stitching from right to left and vice versa, instead of taking out the needle from needle holder, turn the needle upside down inside the needle holder and then rotate the needle holder through 180° **(Fig. 13)**.

RETRACTORS

Retractors are instruments used to pull tissue aside to expose a surgical field. They are especially useful when working in a close cavity such as the pelvis or on a deeply placed organ such as the kidney or esophagus. Retractors are available in various sizes and shapes. Some are self-retaining, and others are handheld. The basic principle of retraction is that tissues should be displaced laterally out of the operative field. One should safeguard the underlying structure to be retracted against injury by putting a sponge or gauze beneath the retractor. An assistant

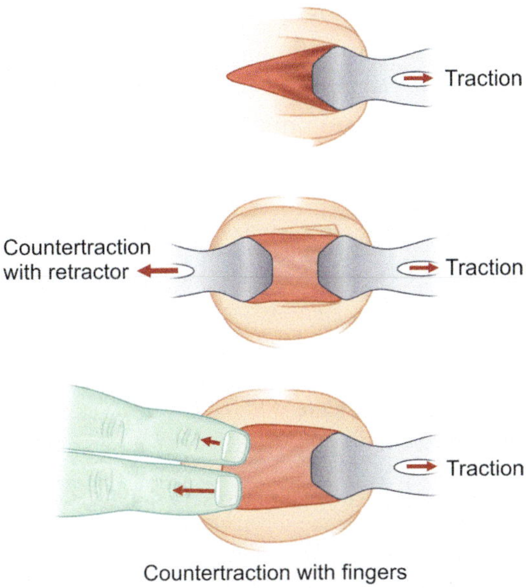

Fig. 14: Traction by retractor and countertraction either by retractor or by fingers.

who is retracting should be allowed to relax between surgical maneuvers in order to avoid fatigue and muscular cramps.

Retractors are used for traction, for countertraction, or for both **(Fig. 14)**. Traction is defined as pulling the tissue in one direction. Countertraction may be applied with another retractor or by hand, for example, using a Deaver's retractor to retract the liver, and hand to retract the duodenum and bile duct in displaying the cystic duct structures.

Retractors can be:

- Superficial retractors
- Deep retractors
- Self-retaining retractors.

These retractors are described in more details in the chapter of surgical instruments (Chapter 22).

Superficial Retractors

- *Langenbeck's retractor:* It has a long handle and small solid blade. It is commonly used for hernia surgery, open appendectomy, or in any superficial surgery to retract fascia or aponeurosis.
- *Czerny retractor:* It has thick small blade on one side and biflanged hook on the other side in an opposite direction. It is used during abdominal closure while performing hernia or open appendicectomy or during open technique for insertion of ports. Use of biflanged end is to retract the skin at the end of incision to facilitate closure of aponeurosis or deep fascia.

Deep Retractors

- *Morris retractor:* It is used for abdominal wall retraction.
- *Deaver's retractor:* It is used to retract liver, spleen, and other abdominal organs. It is an atraumatic retractor and has a broad gently curved blade. One needs four Deaver retractors for open cholecystectomy.
- *Doyen's retractor:* It is used during pelvic operations.

Principles of Retraction

- Retraction should be gentle.
- Injury to underlying structures should be avoided during retraction.
- During retraction of the abdominal wall, force should be directed laterally and upward.
- Retraction should be toward sky rather than laterally.

CLAMPS

Beside artery forceps which are used to permanently seal vessels, there are many other clamps with different uses in surgery.

Vascular clamps: For example, Bulldog clamp, Pott's arterial clamp, and Satinsky clamps. These are designed to occlude vessels temporarily without damaging them.

Intestinal clamps: These can be crushing or noncrushing. Crushing clamps are used during intestinal resection to control bleeding and leakage from the divided bowel and to create a clean edge for anastomosis. Noncrushing intestinal clamps may be used to hold a viscus, and to prevent intestinal spillage. They are not totally atraumatic and should be applied and locked up to one ratchet only.

KEY POINTS

- Proper handling of instruments is of paramount importance for optimum surgical outcome.
- Hold a scalpel like a pen if a small precise incision is planned.
- If a long incision on skin is planned, a scalpel may be held like a table knife.
- Number 3 BP handle accommodates size 10–15 surgical blades.
- Number 4 BP handle accommodates size 18–24 surgical blades.
- Scissors can be used for a variety of functions ranging from tissue dissection, raising skin flaps, and separating tissue planes.
- Hold scissors in a mid-pronated hand position with distal phalanx of thumb occupying the ring of the moving blade and distal phalanx of ring finger occupying the other ring. Ring should never go beyond the distal interphalangeal joint.
- In a needle holder, the needle should be held at the junction of two-thirds and one-third from the tip of needle.
- Never push a needle through the tissue, rather use a movement of supination and pronation of the hand to drive the needle through tissue along its own shape. If a knot is used, the hands should cross after one throw to lock it and make it safe.

CHAPTER 14

Drains in Surgery

Sudhir Kumar Jain, David L Stoker

"Drains never drain when they are really needed"

DEFINITION

A drain is a device used to prevent the accumulation of fluid in a cavity or closed space, whether this space is anatomical or created through surgical dissection. The fluids that may be drained include pus, blood, serum, urine, biliary or pancreatic secretions, intestinal contents, lymph, or air. Drains are used to continuously remove fluid from the body, as it is generally more beneficial for fluid to be outside rather than inside.

Determining the optimal timing for placing a drain after surgery remains somewhat subjective and varies among practitioners. For example, after cholecystectomy, some surgeons routinely place drains, while others do so selectively. In cases of uncertainty, it is often recommended to use a drain to ensure optimal management of fluid.

HISTORY OF SURGICAL DRAINS

The use of drains dates back to Hippocrates when metal tubes, glass tubes, and even bones were used to drain body fluids. Leonardo da Vinci observed the capillary action in small bore tubes, and this forms the basis of passive drain methods of the modern era. Heaton (1889) invented air vent suction drains or active drains.

Broad Functions of Drains

- To remove contents of body organs such as the urinary bladder by catheter or from the stomach by nasogastric tube
- To remove excessive secretions from cavities in the body, e.g., pleural cavity, peritoneal cavities, or to drain cerebral spinal fluid (CSF) from ventricles
- To remove excessive tissue fluid, serum, lymph, or blood after certain operations.

Indications

The following are indications for inserting drains—the list is not exhaustive, and some indications are relative:

- Drainage of pus
- After incision and drainage of any large abscess
- Drainage of empyema of thorax
- Drainage of empyema of gallbladder
- Drainage of infected pseudocyst of pancreas
- After surgery for diffuse or generalized peritonitis (controversial, but subphrenic and pelvis spaces may be at risk)
- Image-guided pigtail catheters can be inserted to drain many localized intra-abdominal collections or liver abscess.

When drains are employed for pus or in contaminated wounds, they should be kept in place for 5–7 days, so that a sinus track can become established. The purpose should be to keep the track open as long as it is needed to prevent reaccumulation of infected fluids inside the tissues. Premature removal of a drain can result in a deep-seated abscess.

Drainage of Blood

- Hemothorax
- After laparotomy for hemoperitoneum secondary to any etiology
- Drainage of scrotum after operation for large hydrocele
- Drainage of subcutaneous space following mastectomy, thyroid surgery or open surgery for large incisional hernias
- After liver surgery
- Radical excision of pelvic tumors.

Drainage of Intestinal Contents/Bile

- After anastomosis of intestinal viscus if there is increased risk of leak, e.g., in the malnourished or septic patient, or where blood supply is threatened. A drain may herald a leak, leading to early relaparotomy, or institution of early conservative primary management.
- After common bile duct (CBD) injuries during cholecystectomy
- After restorative surgery for bile duct strictures.

Drainage of Pancreatic Juice

- After pancreatic resection
- After pancreatic trauma

Drainage of Chyle

- Chylothorax
- Chylocele

Drainage of Urine

Surgery on the urinary tract where urinary tract has been opened and leak is likely to occur.

Drainage of Air

Intercostal tube drain is employed for pneumothorax. Common indications for inserting drain can be therapeutic or prophylactic.

Therapeutic Indications

- Tension pneumothorax
- Pericardial tamponade
- Solid organ abscess
- Intraperitoneal abscess
- Skin or subcutaneous abscess
- Hemothorax
- Empyema
- Pseudocyst of pancreas if it is infected.

Prophylactic Indications

- Post-thoracic surgery—cardiopulmonary or esophageal
- Postabdominal surgery (including urological procedures) if leak is suspected or likely to occur
- Postorthopedic joint surgery
- Head and neck surgery
- Any operation involving extensive skin dissection or creation of myocutaneous flaps, e.g., mastectomy, incisional hernia, and latissimus dorsi flap.

Palliative Indications

Drains can be used as a palliative measure to bypass a luminal obstruction. For example, in nasobiliary drainage (NBD) for patients with obstructive jaundice with or without sepsis. CBD stents are used to palliate jaundice in advanced malignancy.

Diagnostic Purposes

T-tube is placed after CBD exploration for diagnosis of retained CBD stones, by T-tube cholangiogram.

As Access Routes

For example, tubes are employed in percutaneous pyelolithotomy.

Monitoring Indications

Monitoring of urine output by urinary catheter or use of nasogastric tubes in subacute small bowel obstruction.

Classification of Drains

Based on mechanism of action: A drain can be passive or active. Passive drains act by the mechanism of capillary action, gravity, or the fluctuation of intracavity pressure. Examples of passive drains are the corrugated drain, Penrose drain, and sump drain. Passive drains are usually employed when the secretion is very viscid or thick and cannot pass through a tube.

Active drains are tubes, which drain by active suction. Suction used can be low continuous, low intermittent, or high suction. Examples of active drains are Redivac™ and Surgivac™. The advantage of these drains is that there is more reliable measurement of drain output. In a closed drainage system, there is minimal risk of wound infection. Skin excoriation around such closed systems should not occur.

Based on the nature of the drain: It can be a tube drain, sheet drain, or flat drain. They are described in the section here.

Based on their disposition: It can be open drain or closed drain.

Based on location: It can be external drain or internal drain. External drains are brought out through the body wall to outside. Internal drains are placed internally within the luminal organ to create passage or to connect two luminal organs. Double J stent in ureter, biliary stent in CBD, and ventricular-peritoneal shunt in hydrocephalus are examples of internal drains.

Based on property of material: The drain can be inert or irritant. The drains made up of irritant material such as latex, plastic, or red rubber excite fibrous tissue around drain, leading to track formation. Inert drain material such as PVC, silastic, and silicone do not provoke tissue fibrosis.

TYPES OF DRAINS (TABLE 1)

Tube Drains (Fig. 1)

Tube drains permit the formation of a closed drainage system, as they can be connected to bags or reservoirs. There are multiple holes at the end of the drain. Suction may be applied at the end of tube drains.

Sheet Drains (Figs. 2 and 3)

These consist of corrugated silicone material, or sheets forming parallel tubes (Yeates drain), in which fluid passes through and around the tubes. These drains are either exteriorized through a main wound or via a separate stab wound. They are fixed by either suture to the skin or passing a large safety pin through the drain at skin level. These drains are not used commonly in the present surgical era.

Gauze Packs and Ribbon Gauze Wicks (Figs. 4A and B)

Gauze packs are sheets of sterile cotton gauze placed on a raw surface where discharge is expected to occur over a wide area, e.g., in an abscess cavity or after the laying open of a fistulous tract. Gauze acts by capillary action, soaking up secretions. Packs may be soaked in saline with a lubricant such as liquid paraffin. Antiseptic agents such as betadine may also be used. Dry gauze packs are more

TABLE 1: Types of drains with their indications and mechanism of action.

Drain type	*Indications*	*Mechanism of action*
Penrose drain	Wound drainage, abscesses, and postoperative care	Provides passive drainage by gravity; drain is usually placed within the wound and allows fluids to seep out through capillary action
Jackson-Pratt (JP) drain	Postoperative fluid accumulation, such as seroma or hematoma and prevention of infection	Uses a suction mechanism to actively pull fluid out of the wound and into a collection reservoir; reduces the risk of fluid build-up and infection
Romovac drain	Postoperative drainage of blood, serous fluid, or other fluids; used in various surgeries	Similar to the JP drain but has a larger reservoir; also uses suction to actively draw fluids away from the wound
Blake drain	Postoperative drainage, especially for wounds with thicker or more viscous fluids	A type of closed-suction drain with a flat, perforated design that facilitates drainage of thicker fluids; helps in maintaining suction and reducing dead space
Chest tube	Drainage of pleural effusion, pneumothorax, hemothorax, or empyema	Inserted into the pleural cavity to remove air, fluid, or pus; uses gravity or suction to continuously remove fluids or gases from the chest cavity, promoting lung re-expansion
T-tube	Drainage of bile postcholecystectomy or common bile duct exploration	Inserted into the bile duct to facilitate bile drainage into the duodenum or collection bag; helps in preventing bile duct obstruction and allows for drainage of excess bile
Sump drain	Wound drainage with high risk of infection or complex fluid management	A double-lumen drain designed to reduce the risk of clogging and allows for both active suction and passive drainage; typically used in gastrointestinal surgery

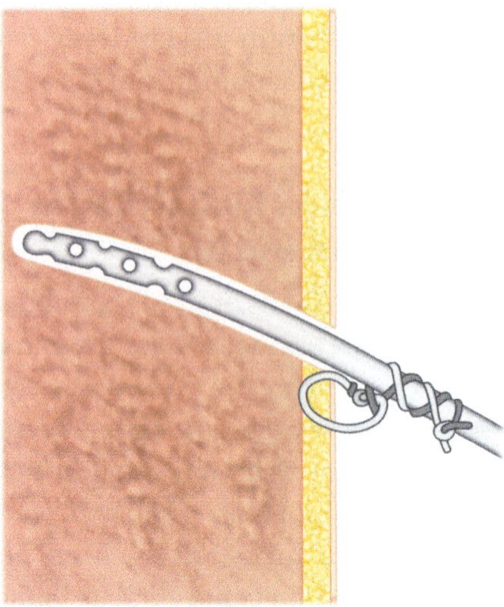

Fig. 1: Tube drain with multiple side holes.

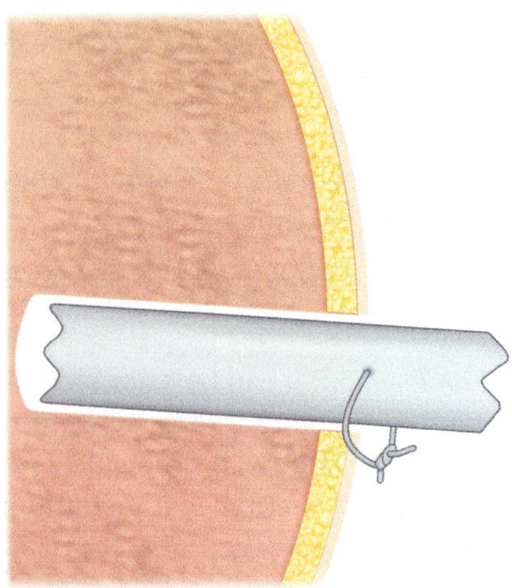

Fig. 2: Corrugated sheet drain.

effective but tend to adhere to raw areas and are difficult to remove. This may lead to pain and bleeding during removal. If a cavity is deep and discharge cannot be brought to the surface, it can be drained by a wick of folded gauze, which is passed down to the base of the cavity. To be fully effective, it should be moist. Sometimes wicks can be passed through a thin-walled latex tube, known as "cigarette drain". The latex tube prevents the wick becoming adherent to tissues **(Fig. 5)**.

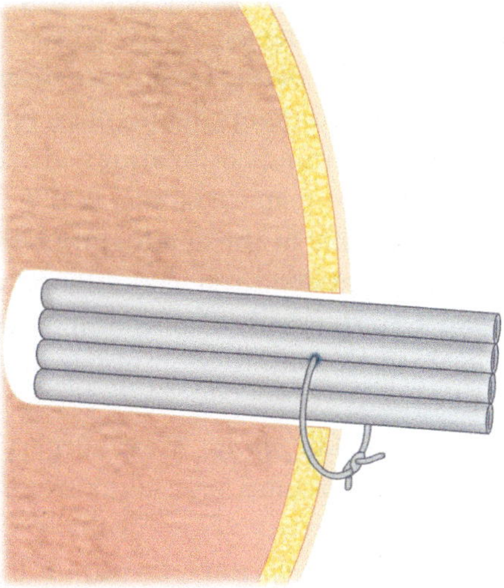

Fig. 3: Yeates drain.

Drain can be made of:

- *Latex rubber:* It is soft but excites a profound inflammatory reaction within 24 hours and renders them totally ineffective.
- *PVC:* This is much less reactive and more efficient. It is firm and more unyielding but tends to harden with prolonged use, especially when it comes in contact with bile.
- *Silicon:* This is the best material for drains because it is least reactive, most pliable, and does not become hardened with prolonged use.

TYPES OF DRAINAGE SYSTEMS

- *Open drainage:* In this system, Penrose drains, multitubular drains, or corrugated drains are used. The drain is taken out through the main operative wound or via a separate stab wound stitched to the skin

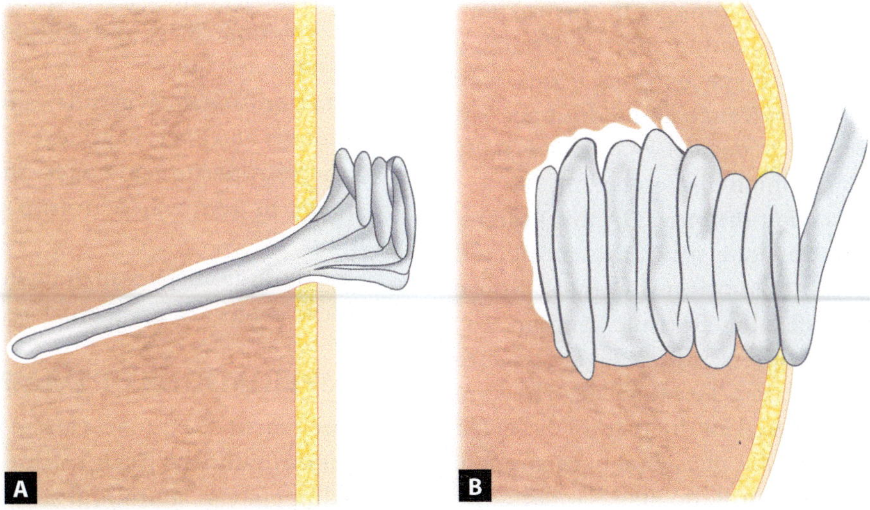

Figs. 4A and B: Wound being packed by a folded gauze piece (A) or A ribbon pack; (B) This is usually performed to drain a cavity.

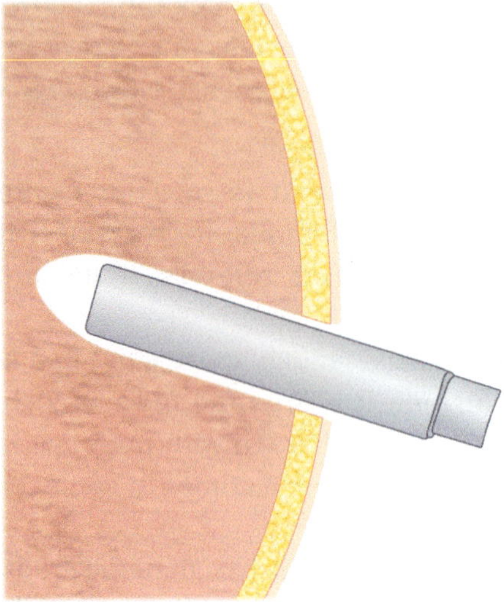

Fig. 5: "Cigarette" drain. This is formed by passing a folded gauze piece or a ribbon pack through a finger glove stalk or a thin-walled rubber tube.

or secured by a safety pin. This is then covered by a surgical dressing pad. This type of drain may increase the incidence of wound infection and if not managed effectively may disseminate infection to other patients in the surgical ward. The system is rarely used now.

- *Closed siphon drainage:* In this system, a tube drain is connected to a drainage bag. The drainage bag has a one-way valve at the entrance and a drainage tap at the opposite end. The tap allows daily emptying without disconnection.
- *Closed suction drainage:* In this system, firm polyethylene tubes are connected to portable suction devices. Some devices utilize low pressure vacuum, i.e., Romovac. Others utilize high pressure negative suction, i.e., Redivac. They are particularly used for drainage of dissected spaces, e.g., after incisional hernia repair. They should not be used inside the peritoneal cavity as they can cause injury to the gut due to negative suction.
- *Sump suction drainage*: These drainage systems also employ negative suction, but they have parallel air vents which prevent adjacent soft tissue from being sucked into the lumen. They are made of either silicon or PVC. They are useful in the management of small bowel fistula or pancreatic fistula.

Drains can be placed in the following anatomical spaces or planes:

- *Subcutaneous plane:* Drains are inserted below flaps to keep dead space empty of fluid. Common indications are after thyroid surgery, mastectomy, and ventral hernia repair. In these situations, there is significant dead space and blood may collect. In the neck, a collection of blood may lead to compression of the trachea and stridor.
- *Intramuscular plane:* After surgery for soft tissue sarcoma, e.g., compartmental excision.
- *After drainage of abscess:* A drain is put into the residual cavity preventing its premature closure and allowing the abscess cavity to heal from its base.
- In the pleural cavity to drain blood, pus, air, or infected fluid
- In the peritoneal cavity after surgery for peritonitis and after major resection
- In the retroperitoneal space after renal surgery or removal of retroperitoneal tumors
- In the retropubic space to drain urine after bladder surgery or open prostatectomy.

COMPLICATIONS OF DRAINS

- *Tissue reaction:* Fibrosis can be induced around a drain, which can lead to occlusion of a lumen, e.g., a urethral stricture may occur if a latex urinary catheter is left *in situ* for prolonged periods.

- *Source of infection:* There are increased chances of surgical site infection if a drain allows flow of content in reverse direction. It is advised to keep the drainage bag below the level of the wound at all times to prevent backflow and subsequent infection.
- *Retained foreign body:* A drain may break within a body cavity due to disintegration by proteolytic enzymes, trauma, or undue traction. This retained foreign body can act as a source of chronic pus discharge or can lead to an intra-abdominal collection.
- *Tissue necrosis:* The tip of a very hard or stiff drain may induce pressure necrosis and erosion of underlying viscera.
- *Drain site hernia:* There can be formation of hernia at the drain site.
- *Bleeding:* A rigid drain can erode into a blood vessel, leading to hemorrhage.

PRACTICAL TIPS FOR USE OF DRAINS

- The extended use of a drain after it has stopped draining offers no advantage.
- The correct drain should be selected depending upon indication.
- A drain should be placed centrally within a space to make it effective.
- After laparoscopic surgery, the use of surgical and nasogastric drains is likely to be less.
- The drain should not be used as a substitute for proper hemostasis or sound surgical technique.
- The drain should be protected from contamination, kinking, knotting, or blockage.
- External drains should be brought out from a separate stab wound and not from the main wound.

KEY POINTS

- A drain is a device to prevent collection of undesired or unwanted fluid in a cavity or a closed space.
- It can be used to drain pus, blood, intestinal contents, lymph, or air.
- Absolute indications for placing drains are tension pneumothorax, hemothorax, after pancreatic necrosectomy, and in a localized collection of pus.
- A drain itself can cause complications by erosion into viscera.
- Drains often reassure the surgeon rather than draining anything.
- Whenever in doubt about hemostasis always put a drain.

CHAPTER 15

Minimal Access Surgery

Raman Tanwar, Sudhir Kumar Jain, David L Stoker

"Conversion to open is just a continuation of laparoscopic procedure not a defeat of the surgeon"

DEFINITION

Minimal access surgery can be defined as the application of modern technology to minimize the trauma of surgical access, without compromising the exposure of the surgical site, or the safety of the patient.

INTRODUCTION

The historical development of laparoscopy dates back to 1901 when George Killing of Germany inserted a cystoscope into the abdomen of a living dog after creating a pneumoperitoneum using air. Wickman and Fitzpatrick in 1990 coined the term "minimally invasive surgery" in order to promote techniques with reduced operative trauma. Cuschieri in 1992 coined the term minimal access surgery (MAS), which in many regards is more accurate and descriptive. MAS is an amalgamation of surgical skills, surgical innovation, and technology advancement. The following techniques are included under the umbrella of MAS:

- Laparoscopic surgery including conventional laparoscopy with use of multiple ports
- Single-incision laparoscopic surgery (SILS)
- Hand-assisted laparoscopic surgery (HALS)
- Robotic assisted laparoscopic surgery
- Video-assisted thoracoscopy (VATS)
- Natural orifice transendoluminal surgery (NOTES)
- Endoluminal endoscopic surgery, e.g., surgery for early gastric carcinoma
- Arthroscopic surgery
- Minimal access thyroid surgery.

Minimal access surgery may not always be minimally invasive. For example, totally extraperitoneal (TEP) repair of groin hernia requires three 5–10 mm skin incisions, but also an extensive dissection in preperitoneal space.

In this chapter, the basics of conventional laparoscopic surgery will be discussed.

Laparoscopic surgery has following three main components:

1. Equipment for image production (a light source, the laparoscope or rod lens system, and a camera)
2. A method for the creation of a pneumoperitoneum (the insufflation of carbon dioxide gas to create space for operating)
3. Various sophisticated laparoscopic instruments

ADVANTAGES OF LAPAROSCOPIC SURGERY

In laparoscopy, abdominal wall retraction is provided by carbon dioxide (CO_2) pneumoperitoneum (8–15 mm Hg), which is gently and evenly applied to the abdominal musculature and diaphragm, in contrast to the localized pressure of a mechanical retractor. Incisions are small at 5–12 mm in comparison to open surgery, and therefore less painful.

The incidence of hypothermia and evaporative fluid loss during laparoscopic surgery is much less because there is no exposure of the abdominal contents to the atmosphere. There is a lower incidence of postoperative intestinal adhesions after laparoscopy due to minimal handling of gut. This results in less serosal tears, less adhesions, and a reduced incidence of postoperative paralytic ileus. In the past, there was a saying that "big surgeons make big incisions". A large incision, however, may be the cause of morbidity, increasing the likelihood of:

- Postoperative pain (both acute and chronic)
- Infection
- Bleeding
- Incisional hernia.

Any of these may prevent early ambulation and recovery. Delay in mobility may lead to deep vein thrombosis, pulmonary embolism, or pulmonary consolidation.

Causes of pain in open surgery include:

- Trauma of cutting muscles and other structures such as nerve, aponeurosis, or fascia
- Mechanical retractors, leading to localized bruising or ischemia to muscle or nerve caused by sustained pressure. A large incision is more painful than a small one.

All these are significantly less in laparoscopic surgery.

The following are absolute contraindications to laparoscopic surgery:

- Unwilling patient
- Untrained surgeon
- Untreated bleeding disorders
- Patient in shock.

Relative contraindications to laparoscopic surgery include:

- History of previous extensive abdominal surgery
- Known intra-abdominal adhesions
- Bowel obstruction
- Pregnancy.

BASIC LAPAROSCOPIC SKILLS

The following skills should be learned by the novice laparoscopic surgeon which are mentioned here.

Mechanical Limitations and Limited Degrees of Freedom of Instrument Movement

Currently available laparoscopic instruments offer only 4° of freedom of movement, i.e., rotation, up/down, left/right angulations; in/out movement for straight long instruments and 6° of movement for curved instruments. This limitation has been overcome by new instruments available for robotic surgery, which have 7° of freedom with better perception of the surgical field. In contrast, in open surgery, there are 360° of movement of instruments.

The limited degrees of freedom of movement make tissue handling with laparoscopic instruments more difficult. This is compounded by the fixed position of entry ports. Instrument changes during laparoscopic surgery are more laborious and distracting. Port sites should be planned very carefully, and an experienced team will have no difficulty in changing instruments.

Less efficient instruments: A typical laparoscopic instrument transmits the force of a surgeon's hand from its handle to tip in ratio of only 3:1 in contrast to 1:3 ratios with a hemostat. The surgeon's hand therefore works about six times as hard to complete the same grasping task with the laparoscopic instrument. This is rarely a problem and can be balanced by the fact that massively less retraction is required in awkward places.

Tactile feedback: There is a loss of direct tactile feedback because there is no direct contact of fingers with tissues. Indirect tactile feedback through instruments is markedly reduced due to the long length of instruments and because of friction between ports and instruments. This loss of indirect tactile feedback can lead to damage to tissue which has been grasped in an instrument, because the force which is being applied to grasped tissue is poorly appreciated by the surgeon's hand. This is true for a novice laparoscopic surgeon, and as the experience of the surgeon increases, this problem diminishes. Hand-assisted MAS does not have this drawback.

Dark room: Operating room lights are turned off during laparoscopic surgery, and the operating team works in reduced light. Dark operating rooms during laparoscopic surgery increase the risk of collision hazards and using the wrong instruments. This can be overcome by providing a separate head light over the instrument trolley.

More clutter: The amount of equipment, tubes, and cables is greater during laparoscopic surgery in comparison to open surgery. This creates a hazard for traffic movement. Multiple tubes and cables may create a jungle of connections in the operating field if not well organized. This may decrease the efficiency of instrument handling, positioning, and exchanges. In a well laid out modern theater, there are neatly laid cables to the laparoscopic stack **(Fig. 1)**, and the only extra cables to the patient are the light cable and video lead.

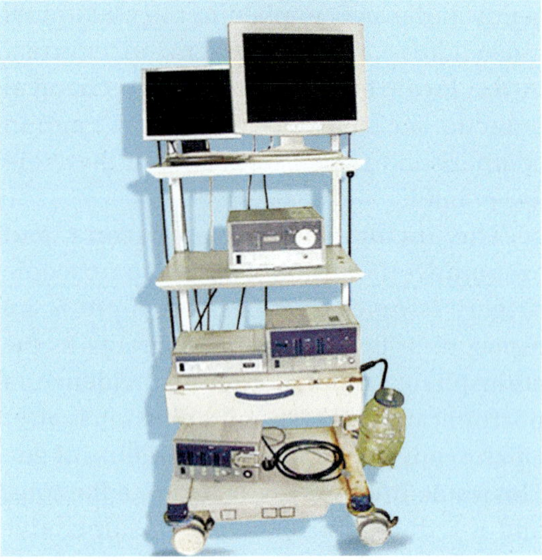

Fig. 1: Laparoscopic stack containing video monitor, camera processing unit, insufflator, and light source.

Tissue retrieval: Small port size limits the retrieval of solid or bulky organs, and sometimes a small separate incision needs to be made in order to remove organs, for example, colon. For solid organs, a morcellator can be used, or tissue can be broken up into small pieces by finger fracture. These methods may risk wound contamination or tumor cell implantation at port sites during retrieval. The risks are however low, and port site tumor recurrence should not occur if good surgical techniques are adhered to.

Skills to Overcome Visual Limitations

Two-dimensional imaging: Standard monitors in current use are two-dimensional imaging systems. The surgeon has to mentally reconstruct three-dimensional (3D) pictures from the two-dimensional output. This involves intense perceptual and mental processing, which continues throughout a laparoscopic procedure. Three-dimensional high-definition monitors are now available, but they add to the cost.

Limited view: There is a reduced field of vision, and there is a decrease in the sensory input from the periphery of the field. There can be incidental tissue injury, when the instruments move outside the field of view. Movement of instruments within the abdomen must take place under direct vision to avoid accidental injury. This limitation is partly counterbalanced by the fact that the view is greatly magnified, and instruments can move anywhere in the abdominal cavity with ease.

Decoupling of the Motor and Visual Spaces

The monitor should be placed in such a way that the visual axis formed between the surgeon's eyes and the monitor should be aligned with the hands and instruments. If they are not aligned, it leads to poor task performance.

Port placement ***(Fig. 2)****:* Proper port placement is extremely important for successful completion of a laparoscopic procedure. Manipulation angle, azimuth angle, and elevation angles guide the site for optimal port placement.

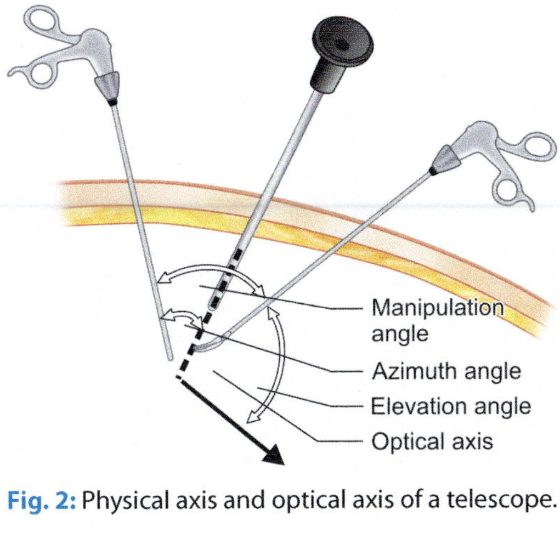

Fig. 2: Physical axis and optical axis of a telescope.

Manipulation Angle

This is the angle between the active and assisting instrument. Manipulation angle should be between 45° and 75° with the ideal angle being 60° for the efficient performance of intracorporeal knotting.

Azimuth Angle

This is the angle between either of the instruments and the optical axis of the endoscope. Better work efficiency is obtained with equal azimuth angles. Wide azimuth angles should be avoided as far as possible.

Elevation Angle

This is the angle between the instrument and horizontal plane. Ideally the elevation angle should be equal to the manipulation angle. Ports should be placed in such a way that the ratio of intracorporeal and extracorporeal length of instrument should be 2:1. Ports for instruments and endoscope should be placed in such a way that instrument and endoscope are aligned in the same direction. One should not operate against the camera, because the surgeon will be working with a mirror image, and manipulation can become difficult in that situation.

Monitor Location

The monitor should ideally be placed in front of the surgeon and below eye level range (0–45°, 25° ideal) in order to produce a gaze down view. Gaze down viewing permits sensory signals and motor control to have a closed spatial location and brings visual signals into correspondence with instrument manipulation. The design of laparoscopic stacks is such that the monitors are usually at eye level.

Principles of Camera Operation

The camera operator's role is crucial in laparoscopic surgery because the camera is the eye of the surgeon and he/she will only see those things that are shown by the camera. The camera operator actively takes part in the surgery.

Golden Rules for Camera Operation

- Keep the task in the center of the field, which has the best illumination and least image distortion, so that the surgeon sees the best quality image. Another reason for keeping in the center is that if the surgeon works in the periphery of the field, instrument movement may take place outside the displayed image and can accidentally damage adjacent structures.
- If the surgeon wants better resolution of the target area for doing fine work, e.g., dissection or picking up a fallen clip, advance the telescope toward the target area, which will increase the resolution but decrease the size of visual field. During insertion of instruments or knot tying, a wider visual field is required, and the laparoscope should be kept away from the target area. When the surgeon becomes more experienced, this may not be necessary.
- Avoid jerky movements because they hinder precise surgery.
- Keep the camera oriented at all times with a level horizon.
- Before starting the procedure, do a white balancing of the camera and focus the camera on a gauze swab for reference.
- During port insertion, keep the portion of the abdomen where the port will enter in the center of the monitor field at all times to avoid injury to intra-abdominal organs.
- During instrument insertion, the camera holder should guide the surgeon by showing a panoramic view for proper insertion of instruments. This becomes less important with a more experienced surgeon.

Selection of Laparoscope (Fig. 3)

Each endoscope has an optical axis and a physical axis. The optical axis is the axis passing through the center of the visual field of the laparoscope. The physical axis is the axis passing through the center of the endoscope. The endoscope can be 0°, 30°, or 45° depending on the angle between optical axis and physical axis. The 30° laparoscope is useful in pelvic surgery and for difficult cholecystectomy. The 45° laparoscope is used for bariatric surgery and for surgery around the esophageal hiatus. For common procedures, a 0° laparoscope is sufficient. Camera angles can be changed during a procedure by passing it through different ports, thus improving the field of vision.

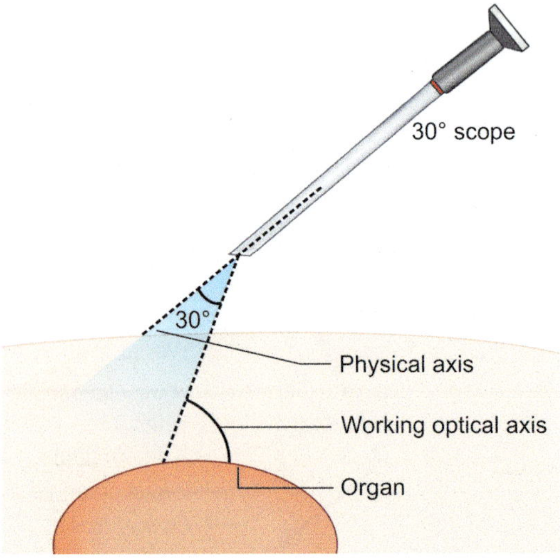

Fig. 3: Various axis of telescope.

CARE AND HANDLING OF TELESCOPES

The telescope is the most delicate laparoscopic instrument. It is also the most important and essential instrument which provides image and light through two distinct systems. A telescope must be handled with care from the start to the end of surgery, and also during the cleaning and sterilization process. All surfaces of a telescope should be inspected on a regular basis for any scratches or dents. The telescope should be carefully inspected before starting surgery to assess functional integrity. The eyepiece should be assessed to evaluate the clarity of image from the reflected light. The optical fibers surrounding the lens at the tip of the telescope should be checked by holding the light post toward a bright light. The presence of discolored or hazy image or black dots or shadowed areas indicates improper cleaning, a disinfectant residue, a cracked or broken lens, the presence of internal moisture, or external damage. While passing telescope through a metal port, it should be inserted gently into the lumen, so as not to break the lens. During the cleaning and disinfection process, the telescope should not be bent during handling, and heavy instruments should not be placed on top of it. Avoid placing the telescope near the edge of a sterile trolley or surgical field to prevent it from accidental dropping onto the floor. While transferring the telescope from one point to another, grip the ocular lens in the palm of the hand and never transfer by the shaft. Immediately after use, wash the surfaces of the telescope with a soft cloth or sponge using a neutral pH enzymatic solution and thoroughly rinse with distilled water to remove any residual cleaning solution.

BASIC REQUIREMENTS FOR LAPAROSCOPIC SURGERY

Important basic equipment for laparoscopic surgery includes:

- A rapid-flow insufflator
- A light source
- Video camera and camera cable **(Figs. 4 and 5)**
- A laparoscope
- At least one monitor but two (one behind the surgeon) are desirable and add comfort to the assistant

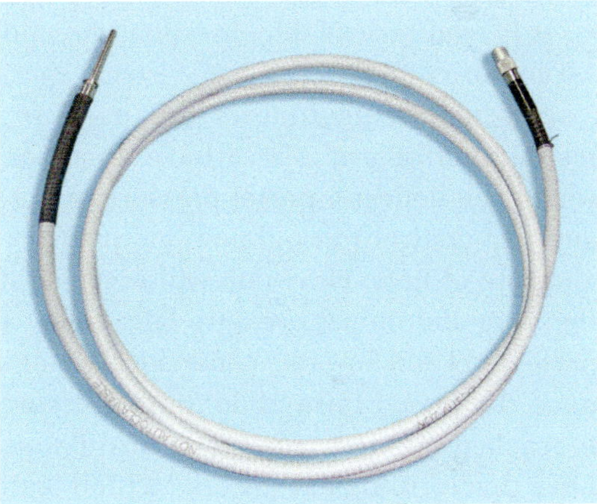

Fig. 4: Fluid-filled light cable.

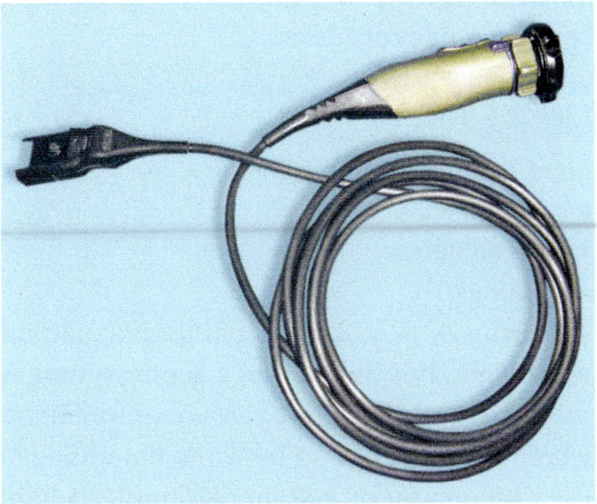

Fig. 5: Camera head.

- Electrosurgical unit
- Suction-irrigation machine
- Laparoscopic instruments and ports.

Rapid-Flow Insufflator

Carbon dioxide (CO_2) is used to create a pneumoperitoneum, creating a working space by distending the anterior and lateral abdominal walls. CO_2 is preferred because:

- It is an inert gas and does not support combustion.
- It is highly soluble, easily absorbed into the blood, and easily excreted by the lungs.
- It is readily available, inexpensive, and nontoxic.

Automatic insufflators are used for insufflation of gas. These have a sensor, which can deliver a preset pressure of CO_2 and can control intra-abdominal pressure and rate of flow. Flow rate will increase if the intra-abdominal pressure falls below a preset level and flow rate automatically stops once the preset intra-abdominal pressure is reached. Modern automatic insufflators have bacteriological filters, which can be incorporated along gas lines and can increase the temperature of the gas up to 37°C, to prevent hypothermia during long laparoscopic procedures.

Light Sources

Light sources commonly in use are:

- Xenon
- Metal halide
- Halogen

Both xenon and metal halide give natural white light, but the light of a xenon source is more natural. Halogen gives a yellow light, which is compensated by white balancing in the video camera system. All modern light sources have infrared filters. Commercially available xenon light sources can give an intensity varying from 150 to 300 lux. They have automatic intensity control which gives continuous optical illumination. Light from the source is carried to the laparoscope by a flexible light cable and down the laparoscope by a solid lens. Light cables are very delicate and should be handled with care.

Light cables can be:

- Glass fiber light cable
- Special fluid filled cable (*see* **Fig. 4**).

Glass fiber light cables are more flexible but less efficient than fluid light cables because of fiber mismatch at the source or fiber breakage. Glass fiber light cables can be autoclaved, but fluid-filled cables should not be autoclaved.

CARE OF LIGHT CABLES

The light cables are another important component of laparoscopic instrumentation. They transmit light from a light source on the stack to the telescope for onward transmission within the telescope to the operative field. Squeezing, stretching, or sharply bending the cable should be avoided. The light cable should be grasped by the connector piece when inserting or removing it from the light source. It should never be pulled directly when disconnecting it from the light source. One should be careful not to puncture the cable with towel clips, when fixing the cables to the surgical drape. The light source should not be turned on before connecting the light cable to the telescope as fire can be ignited on the surgical drape due to high temperature. Inspect the cable for broken fibers before each use. Inspect both ends of the cable to ensure they have a clean, reflective, polished surface. Wipe the fiber optic light cable gently to remove all blood and organic materials immediately after use, with a mild detergent.

Precautions to be taken during handling of light source and cable:

- The light source should not be shone directly into the eye when unplugged from the laparoscope, as the very high intensity of light can cause retinal damage.
- The ends of light cables can become very hot, with temperatures reaching up to 95°C, with the possibility of burns to anyone handling it.

To prevent injury, the light source should initially be set on its lowest level (10–25%) and should be switched off when laparoscope is not in use. Light sources should have a fan to prevent the temperature rising too high and also to increase the life of the expensive bulbs.

Video Cameras

The cameras used in laparoscopy are miniature cameras based on a charged couple device (CCD). Chip camera systems have two components:

1. The camera head attached to the laparoscope
2. The camera controller unit, which is located on an adjacent trolley which usually also holds the insufflator, and a monitor. The camera head consists of an objective lens and CCD chip. The lens focuses the image onto a CCD chip. The chip converts incoming photons into electronic charges and produces picture elements (pixels). This is possible because CCD chip is covered by a layer of light sensitive photoreceptors. The signal is then transmitted to the camera processing unit, where the image is generated for the monitor. There are two types of cameras, single chip and three chips. In the single-chip camera, only one chip processes all three primary colors. In three-chip cameras, there is a separate chip for each primary color, i.e., red, green, and blue. This improves image definition.

PHYSIOLOGY OF PNEUMOPERITONEUM

Carbon Dioxide

Carbon dioxide instilled into peritoneal cavity normally diffuses across the peritoneal surface into the venous circulation. After CO_2 is carried away by the venous system, it can be eliminated by the lungs or stored elsewhere in the body. The human body can store up to 120 L of CO_2, and bone is the largest potential long-term reservoir. Skeletal muscles and other potential visceral stores come into play if retention occurs for <1 hour. After storage, CO_2 is mainly eliminated by the lungs. Following a long laparoscopic procedure, it might take several hours for the accumulated CO_2 to be eliminated and for the body's acid base balance to be restored to normal. After laparoscopic surgery, oxygen should be administered to assist in elimination of CO_2.

Carbon dioxide is used for insufflation because it is colorless, noninflammable, nontoxic, readily soluble in blood, and easily expelled from the body through the lungs.

Effects of Carbon Dioxide

Direct local effects: These effects include decreased cardiac output, pulmonary hypertension, and systemic vasodilatation.

Centrally mediated effects: Hypercarbia leads to widespread sympathetic stimulation, resulting in tachycardia, vasoconstriction and increased central venous pressure, mean arterial pressure, pulmonary artery pressure, and pulmonary vascular resistance. CO_2 causes transient hypercapnia and respiratory acidosis which is made worse with an intra-abdominal pressure more than 12 mm Hg and a head down position. In healthy adults, this can be compensated and also can be avoided by controlled hyperventilation and increased respiratory oxygen concentration.

Volume Effects of Pneumoperitoneum

- Elevation of diaphragm and anterolateral abdominal wall
- Decreased venous return due to increased pressure on the inferior vena cava.

Physiological Effects of Elevation of Diaphragm

- Decreased functional residual capacity
- Increased ventilation-perfusion mismatch
- Increased intrapulmonary shunting
- Increased alveolar-arterial gradient of oxygen partial pressure.

These effects are overcome by increasing the mechanical ventilation rate and concentration of inspired oxygen.

Physiological Effects of Decreased Venous Return

- Initial increase in cardiac index followed by decrease in cardiac index (20–59%).
- Cardiac axis of the heart shifts causing electrocardiographic alteration
- 65% increase in systemic resistance
- 90% increase in pulmonary vascular resistance.

These effects are overcome by an adequate volume load.

Metabolic Changes after Pneumoperitoneum

- Four-fold increase of renin and aldosterone
- Release of vasopressin, adrenaline, and noradrenaline, leading to sympathomimetic response
- Renal vasoconstriction, leading to urinary sodium retention and temporary tubular renal dysfunction
- Hypothermia due to escape of water vapor along with gas leakage. Water vapor takes latent heat of vaporization along with it, causing heat loss. It is just like a wind blowing over the exposed abdominal contents. In prolonged procedure, core temperature can drop and hypothermia may result.

CREATING A SAFE PNEUMOPERITONEUM

Various methods of creating a safe pneumoperitoneum are:

- The closed method
- The open method
- Direct trocar insertion
- Optical trocar insertion.

The Closed Method

A Veress needle is used to create a pneumoperitoneum. The Veress needle is a hollow needle with a spring loaded blunt center core. The proximal end has a luer lock, which may be closed with a tap. The patency of the needle and spring loaded mechanism should be tested before using it.

The umbilicus is usually used for insertion of the Veress needle, but in very obese patients or in patients with a history of previous abdominal surgery, the midclavicular point in the subcostal region of left hypochondrium can be used provided spleen enlargement has been ruled out. This point is also known as Palmer's point. In both areas, the needle should be held like a pen and directed toward the pelvic cavity rather than vertically downward. Often, two "clicks" can be felt as the needle penetrates the abdominal wall, and the blunt trocar springs forward, firstly through muscle or linea alba, then again through peritoneum. It is necessary to ascertain the safe position of the needle in the peritoneal cavity following insertion. The following tests are performed to make sure the Veress needle is in a safe position.

- Attach a syringe to the Veress needle and aspirate. If intestinal contents or blood are aspirated, the needle should be withdrawn, as bowel or vascular injury may have occurred. In practice, this happens rarely.
- *The saline drop test:* A drop of saline put over the hub of the needle with the luer lock opened should be sucked inside the peritoneal cavity because of negative pressure. Saline should flow freely into the needle without difficulty.
- Initial slow insufflation of CO_2 at a rate of 1 L/min should produce an initial intra-abdominal pressure of 5–7 mm Hg. If the initial pressure reading is above 10 mm Hg, the needle may be lying in the preperitoneal space, mesentery, or omentum. Once a safe pneumoperitoneum has been created, the first port insertion is usually via the umbilicus, directed toward the coccyx, preferably with a retractable blade to minimize the possibility of visceral damage.

In a variation of this technique, the laparoscope can be placed down the center of a different sort of port (Optiview and Visiport), with a transparent blunt tip, enabling the operator to see the tissues splitting and the peritoneum opening *under vision.*

The Open Method (Fig. 6)

A vertical or horizontal 2 cm long infraumbilical incision is made. The incision is deepened down to the linea alba.

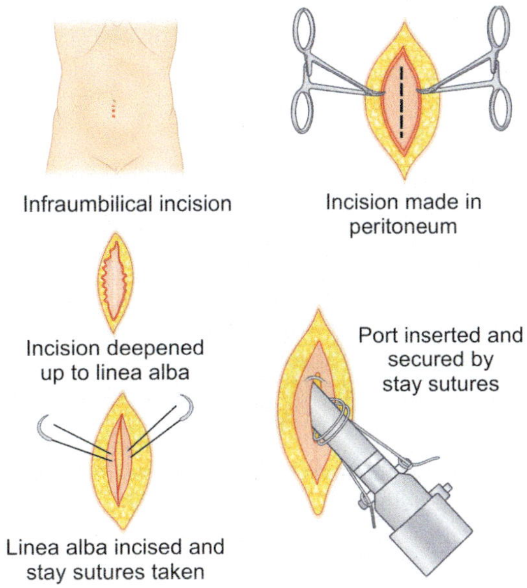

Fig. 6: Various steps for inserting first port by open method.

The linear alba is incised between stay sutures and peritoneum is exposed, and then incised for 1 cm *under vision.*

A finger is inserted inside peritoneal cavity to sweep away any adhesions, and a blunt tipped trocar is then inserted *under vision.* Stay sutures can be used to secure the port. Due to the size of the initial incision, gas leakage around the initial port can occur. A gas proof seal can be obtained by putting stitches around the port into skin over paraffin gauze, or a special port with occlusive balloons at the tip, known as a Hasson's cannula **(Fig. 7)**, can be used. The port has to be closed and repaired carefully at the end of the procedure, to prevent port site hernias developing.

The open method is now the most commonly used technique, as it has a lower incidence of bowel and vascular injury. It is not used universally, however, as the closed method is quicker and produces a smaller scar. The serious vascular injury rate for the

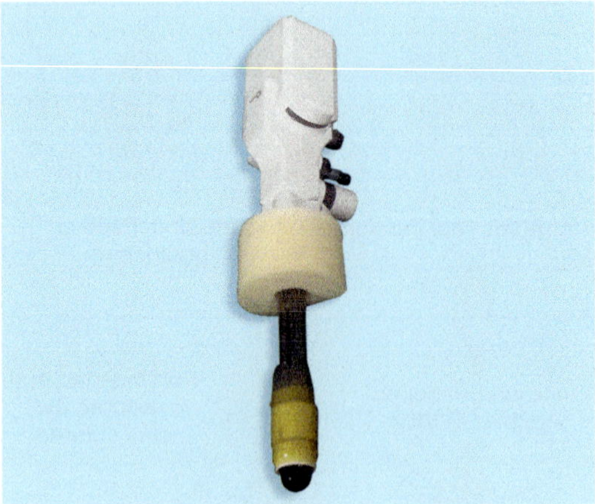

Fig. 7: Self-retaining Hasson port used in open method of pneumoperitoneum.

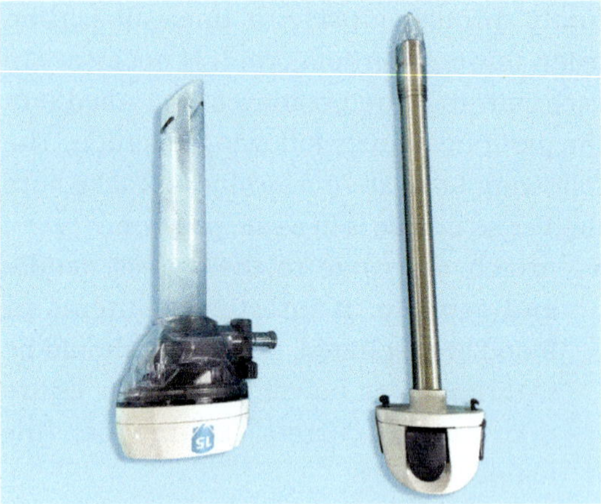

Fig. 8: Optical trocar.

closed technique is in the range of 1:1,000 insertions and practically nil by open technique.

Direct Trocar Insertion

This technique should be carried out only by experienced and skilled laparoscopic surgeons. The authors have not used this technique in their practice. It is a blind direct insertion which avoids the use of the Veress needle and a double blind puncture of the abdomen. In this technique, an adequate skin incision to avoid skin resistance during the sleeve insertion is given, and the periumbilical skin is lifted up using towel clamps on either side and a sharp trocar is used. The trocar must be held like a pen avoiding in this way to penetrate too deep. After the insertion of trocar, an explorative laparoscopy is carried out to check for any intra-abdominal injuries. This technique is mentioned just to condemn it and is not recommended.

Optical Trocar Insertion (Fig. 8)

These are hollow trocars either disposable or reusable in which telescope can be inserted. They are very useful in obese patients or in patients who underwent previous major abdominal surgery. Before insertion, a 0° telescope is inserted into the sheath and fixed. The use of this trocar allows entry into the peritoneal cavity under direct vision, layer by layer.

Summary of ergonomic physical recommendations for optimizing the working conditions in laparoscopic surgery:

- The foot pedal should be near the dominant foot and at the same level.
- Instrument handles should be at or slightly below elbow height.
- Shoulders should be relaxed, and arms should not be elevated.
- There should be proper choice of instrument handles and grasper configurations for each task.

KEY POINTS

- Minimal access surgery is not always minimally invasive.
- Proper selection of equipment and proper training is necessary before one embarks upon laparoscopic surgery.
- Proper placement of ports is the key to success of laparoscopic surgery.
- Safe creation of pneumoperitoneum is of paramount importance for starting of any laparoscopic procedure.
- Open method for creation of pneumoperitoneum is safer than closed method with minimal incidence of vascular injuries and a very low incidence of gut injuries.
- There are mechanical and visual limitations of laparoscopic surgery, which can be overcome by experience.
- If intracorporeal suturing is planned, the manipulation angle between active instrument and assisting instrument should be between 45° and 75°.

CHAPTER 16

Hemostasis

Sudhir Kumar Jain, David L Stoker

"An unexpected bleed during surgery is like a prey to a lion, which needs to be caught"

INTRODUCTION

The concept of hemostasis can be traced back to the primitive man's realization that uncontrolled bleeding can lead to death. Early Greeks and Romans used vegetables and minerals dressing to control bleeding. Surgeons in the early era avoided vessels in their incisions to avoid bleeding. Excessive bleeding is still a reality and sometimes nightmare for all surgeons. The ability to control bleeding is an essential surgical skill, which every surgeon must acquire. It is important during an episode of hemorrhage that the surgeon maintains his or her composure and controls bleeding without causing further damage to surrounding structures. One should always ask for a senior's help if one is not able to control the bleeding on his or her own. Galen (13 BC–200 AD) described several methods of controlling bleeding which are valid even today.

Drawbacks of excessive bleeding include:

- Systemic complications such as shock, clotting disorders, anemia, or impaired wound healing
- Retained blood in surgical field reduces visibility.
- Retained blood in wound provides culture media for bacteria, which can lead to break down of clots and red cells, leading to secondary bleeding.

TYPES OF BLEEDING

According to Source

- Arterial bleeding is brisk, bright red, pulsatile, and under high pressure.
- Venous bleeding is dark red, continuous, low pressure, nonpulsatile, and difficult to control in comparison to arterial bleeding.
- Capillary bleeding is constant slow ooze from a raw area. It can usually be controlled by pressure.

According to Time of Bleeding

- Primary hemorrhage occurs at the time of surgery or as a result of trauma. Bleeding may be excessive if there is an altered bleeding or clotting profile, e.g., liver disease, obstructive jaundice, malnutrition, hemophilia or if there is a disease involving arteries which prevents constriction of blood vessels, e.g., atherosclerosis.
- Reactionary hemorrhage occurs within 24 hours of an operation. It usually occurs from small blood vessels from raw surfaces or from a minor capsular laceration of the staple line of anastomosis. Reactionary bleeding is usually caused by a rise in arterial or venous pressure, leading to dislodgement of clots. This may be caused by pain, or excessive straining.

Reactionary hemorrhage can occur after laparoscopic surgery, when small blood vessels compressed by increased intra-abdominal pressure start bleeding when the pneumoperitoneum is desufflated. Careful hemostasis is of paramount importance to avoid this problem.

- Secondary hemorrhage usually occurs 7–10 days after surgery. It is usually due to an infection by organisms such as β-hemolytic *Streptococci* that cause dissolution of blood clots. Examples of secondary bleeding include bleeding from the tonsil bed after tonsillectomy, bleeding from an infected area after biliary surgery, or bleeding from infected vascular grafts. This type of hemorrhage may be secondary to autodigestion of blood clot following pancreatic surgery.

BLEEDING DURING SURGERY

During surgery, some bleeding is inevitable. Blood loss tends to be greater during long or complex procedures such as liver resection, esophageal resection, and major joint surgery. Every surgeon must acquire the skills necessary to firstly minimize blood loss, and secondly to control hemorrhage during surgery.

Prevention (Table 1)

- In certain diseases such as obstructive jaundice, malnutrition, chronic liver disease, and in hemophilia patients, there is an increased propensity to bleed. In these situations, the bleeding and clotting profiles should be brought to normal. In obstructive jaundice and chronic liver disease, intramuscular administration of 10 mg vitamin K often brings the prothrombin time to normal. In cases of emergency surgery, infusion of fresh-frozen plasma often replenishes the deficient clotting factors.
- If the patient is on oral anticoagulants, or heparin, these drugs should be stopped before surgery, and the coagulation profile should be brought back to normal. Aspirin and other antiplatelet drugs should ideally be stopped at least 5–7 days before surgery.
- Blood transfusion service protocols should be checked in order to decide if a blood sample is to be "Grouped and Saved", or if blood is to be cross-matched. The availability of cross-matched blood should be checked prior to surgery.
- The technique of hypotensive anesthesia may help minimize blood loss.
- During head and neck surgery, raising the head end of the table 15–20° reduces venous congestion and blood loss.
- While raising skin flaps during thyroid or breast surgery, blood loss can be reduced by infiltration of normal saline or normal saline mixed with adrenaline (1:200,000). Fluid raises the tissue pressure, renders tissue transparent, and opens up the plane of dissection. Adrenaline produces local vasoconstriction and reduces the blood loss intraoperatively.
- Revise the anatomy before starting any major surgery. This helps in identification of major blood vessels before they are injured.
- If you are operating upon blood vessels or major organs, control of inflow vessels often helps in reducing bleeding. Noncrushing vascular clamps can be applied across the pedicle of an organ, or the pedicle can be encircled with a tape prior to dissection.
- If operating upon huge vascular tumors, preoperative embolization of feeding vessels might reduce intraoperative

TABLE 1: Prevention strategy details.

Optimization of patient to reduce bleeding	
Address bleeding tendency in certain diseases	• For obstructive jaundice, chronic liver disease, and hemophilia, normalize bleeding and clotting profiles • Administer 10 mg of vitamin K intramuscularly for prothrombin time normalization • Infuse fresh-frozen plasma in emergency surgeries to replenish clotting factors
Manage anticoagulant and antiplatelet medications	• Stop oral anticoagulants and heparin before surgery and normalize coagulation profile • Discontinue aspirin and other antiplatelet drugs 5–7 days before surgery
Blood transfusion protocols	• Check protocols for "Grouped and Saved" or cross-matched blood • Ensure availability of cross-matched blood before surgery
Use hypotensive anesthesia	Employ hypotensive anesthesia to minimize blood loss
Positioning during head and neck surgery	Raise the head end of the table 15–20° to reduce venous congestion and blood loss
Techniques for skin flap surgery	• Use normal saline or saline mixed with adrenaline (1:200,000) for infiltration • Adrenaline aids in vasoconstriction and reduces intraoperative blood loss
Review anatomy before major surgery	Revise anatomy to identify major blood vessels and avoid injury
Control of inflow vessels	Apply noncrushing vascular clamps or encircle the pedicle with tape before dissection to control bleeding
Preoperative embolization for vascular tumors	• Consider preoperative embolization of feeding vessels • Perform surgery within 24–48 hours to avoid neovascularization
Use of tourniquet in limb surgery	• Contraindicated in chronic ischemia, impending gangrene, spreading cellulitis, or fractures • Elevate limb for 2–3 minutes before application • Apply pneumatic tourniquet over orthopedic wool • Optionally use Esmarch's bandage for exsanguination before tourniquet • Inflate tourniquet to 70–100 mm Hg above systolic pressure (200 mm Hg for arm and 300 mm Hg for leg) • Release tourniquet every 2 hours for at least 10 minutes before reapplying

bleeding, provided surgery is performed within 24-48 hours of embolization. After 48 hours, there is development of new blood vessels (neovascularization), which make surgery more difficult.

- The tourniquet is a commonly used method for reducing blood loss when operating upon limbs. It is contraindicated in the presence of chronic ischemia, impending gangrene, spreading cellulitis, and in the presence of fracture. Before applying a tourniquet, the limb is emptied of blood by elevating it for 2-3 minutes. A pneumatic tourniquet is applied on the proximal part of the limb over orthopedic wool. An Esmarch's bandage can be applied over the limb for more complete exsanguination, but it must be applied before applying the tourniquet. It is contraindicated in the presence of cellulitis. A tourniquet is applied around the upper arm or upper thigh over a thin layer of orthopedic wool and is inflated to 70–100 mm Hg above systolic pressure (200 mm Hg for arm and around 300 mm Hg for the leg). It should be released after every 2 hours for at least 10 minutes before reapplying it.

CONTROL OF HEMORRHAGE

- *Hemostasis by pressure:*
    - *Direct occlusion of hole in a vessel by finger tip* ***(Fig. 1)****:* If pressure is applied by a fingertip over a small cut on the vessel for 15–20 seconds, a small clot will form over the divided end of the vessel and prevent further bleeding. The smooth surface of a moist gloved finger is less likely to dislodge the clot when finger is removed. If gauze is applied to the bleeding wound, clot is more likely to get dislodged as it can get adherent to the gauze.
    - *Pressure against underlying bone* ***(Fig. 2)****:* If the incised skin wound happens to lie over bone, surgeon's hand can be placed on the external surface of that wound edge to compress the divided vessels against the firm underlying bone. Partial or serial release of that pressure will assist in identification of the open ends of any large vessel to be caught by artery forceps.
    - *Pressure with a knife or instrument tip* ***(Fig. 3)****:* The tip of the knife can be used to immediately compress the open lumen of the vessel, the moment it starts spurting during transaction by knife. The tip of the blade is quickly redirected to cover the cut vessel and to stop the bleeding until assistant

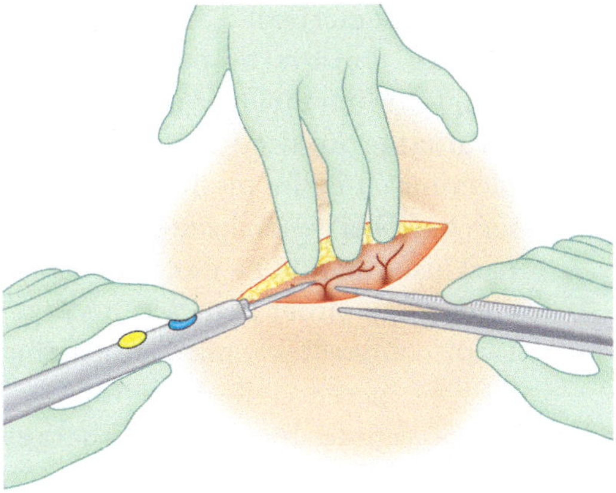

Fig. 2: Control of bleeding by pressure against bone.

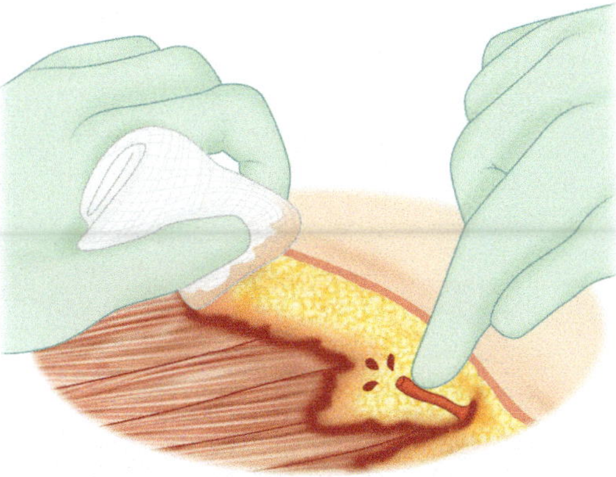

Fig. 1: Use of finger pressure directly over vessel to stop bleeding.

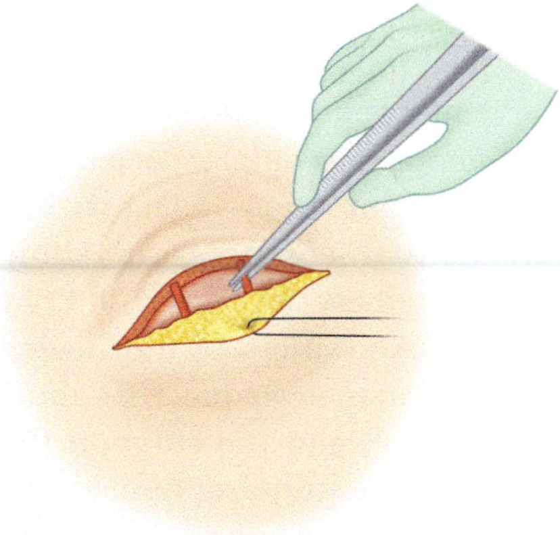

Fig. 3: Control of bleeding by pressure of instrument.

grasps the bleeding point with forceps and cauterizes it or ligates it. The tip of the suction cannula can also be used in a similar manner by the surgical assistant to momentarily compress and arrest a bleeding point.

- *Sponges* may be directly applied to a bleeding surface by the hand and fingers in order to arrest bleeding. If the bleeding occurs in a deep or narrow cavity where the hand cannot be put, a sponge mounted on a long-handled instrument can reach up to the bleeding point to compress it until the surgical team is ready to clamp, ligate, or cauterize it.
- *Manual pressure* by packing or by a metal retractor over a pack is an invaluable method for control of bleeding. It is the method of choice for control of generalized oozing. The pack used should be moistened with cold saline rather than warm saline. Warm compresses applied on bleeding surface increase the bleeding. Dry packs should be avoided as they cause tissue desiccation and tend to adhere to the newly formed clots. These fresh clots may be pulled free on removal of the dry pack. The packing should be immediately employed whenever there is a substantial bleeding, especially in a deep cavity or other inaccessible areas. Manual compression should be exerted over packs for 10–15 minutes observed strictly by the theater clock. This maneuver provides immediate control, and the surgeon then has time to prepare himself for any necessary further action. Packing alone may be sufficient for certain clinical situations, e.g., extensive liver injuries. It also provides an opportunity for the anesthetist to stabilize the patient. Manual pressure may occasionally be employed during laparoscopic surgery by using an atraumatic instrument or adjacent tissue over the bleeding area.

- *Ligature and sutures* are the mainstay to control bleeding from large vessels **(Figs. 4 and 5)**. Clips and simple ligatures are commonly used methods of securing hemostasis. Both absorbable and nonabsorbable material can be used to occlude divided vessels. Nonabsorbable materials are those which remain in the tissue for more than 60 days. These materials comprise of silk, cotton or metal clips, or vascular stapler. Absorbable material has some drawbacks of having less tensile strength and greater tissue reactivity. Absorbable materials also have poor handling qualities. However, in European countries where silk is no longer available, polyglactin 710 is commonly used for ligation of blood vessels. In Asian countries particularly in India, surgeons prefer to use free silk ties for this purpose. Silk has best handling qualities and knot setting accuracy. However, because of its multiple strands and associated large surface area, it produces more

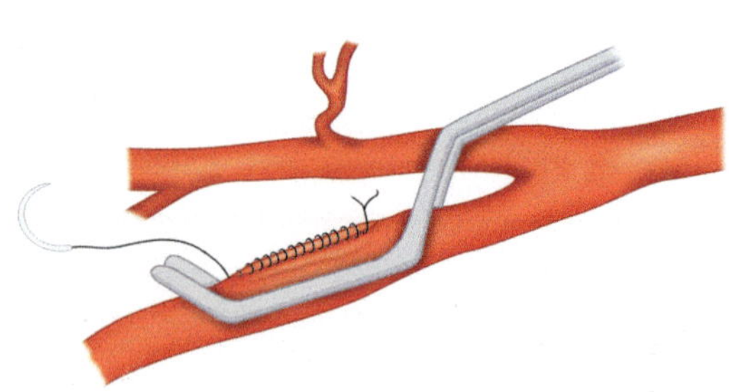

Fig. 4: Closure of large rent in an artery by continuous suture.

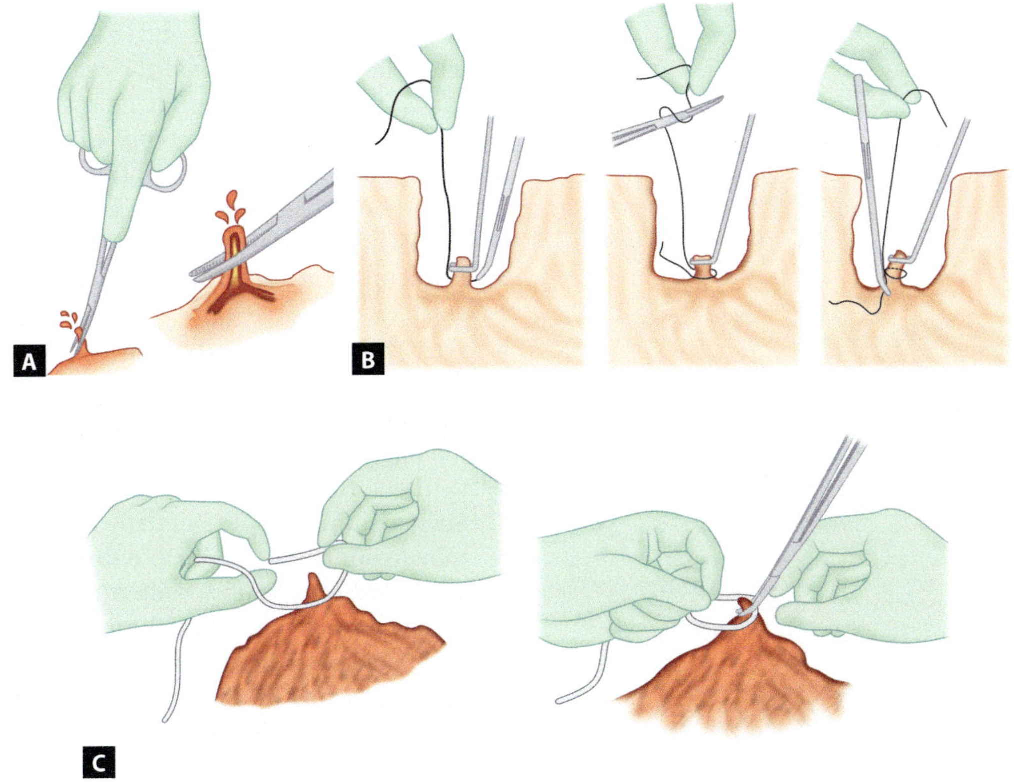

Figs. 5A to C: (A) Method of holding bleeding vessel by hemostasis; (B) Holding vessel in deep cavity; (C) Typing blood vessel.

fibrosis than monofilament sutures. While tying the vessel, the hands of the surgeon should not obstruct the view of the assistant surgeon, and the tip of the instrument which has clamped the vessel should be visible all the time to the assistant. Two-handed tie technique or tie on a clamp technique can be used for ligating clamped vessels. Tie on a clamp technique is used for tackling large vessels inside a deep cavity. Vessels of 2–5 mm in diameter can be occluded by clips or simple ligatures. While applying a clip, one should make sure that it surrounds the vessel completely. The clip should make an angle of 90° with the long axis of the vessel, which should then be divided 3–4 mm away from the clip or ligature, to prevent slippage. Clips and ligatures should not be too tightly applied, because it can lead to weakness of the vessel wall by the cheese-wire cutting effect, especially in cases of rigid, nonelastic arteries following atherosclerosis in older patients.

- *Suture of buried vessels* (***Fig. 6***)*:* Some vessels after division retract deeply into the tissue and cannot be easily clamped. In such cases, a figure of eight or running lashing suture can be placed so as to produce localized constriction of the cut surface along with the vessel.

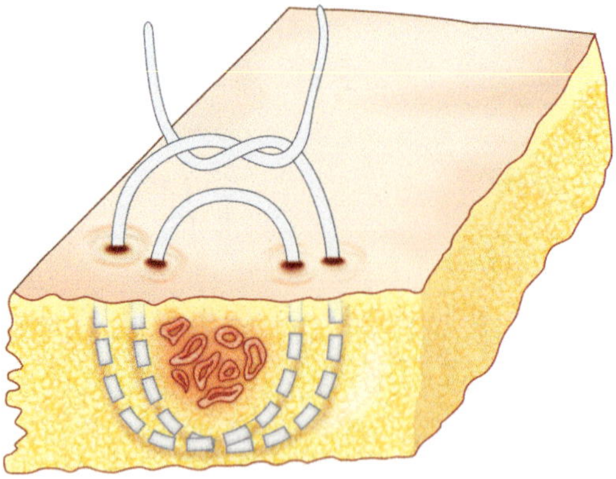

Fig. 6: Figure of eight sutures for control of deep-seated bleeding vessel.

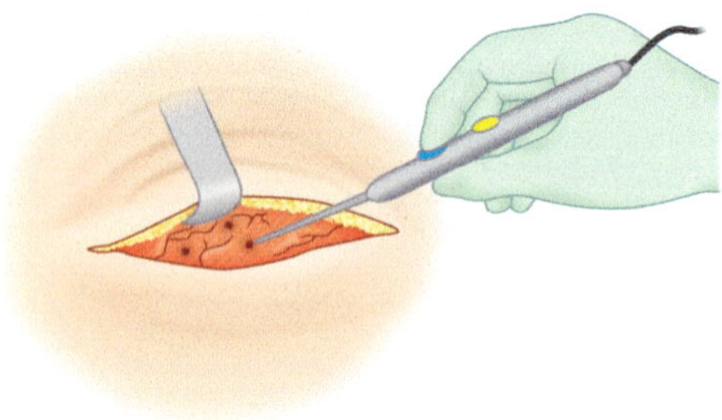

Fig. 7: Hemostasis by electrocautery.

- *Energized systems:* The following devices can be used for thermal coagulation and sealing of blood vessels:
  - Electrocoagulation
  - Ultrasonic sealing
  - Ligasure sealing
  - Photocoagulation.

  Electrocoagulation is safe for sealing of vessels up to 2 mm **(Fig. 7)**. Ultrasonic sealing is used for sealing of vessels up to 5 mm. Ultrasonic sealing uses sound waves not audible by the human ear, i.e., frequency >20,000 cycles/sec. They cause less tissue heating with reduced penetration. These machines generate waves between 20 and 60 kHz frequencies produced by a piezoelectric transducer. They can cut, coagulate, or separate tissue by high power density of around 100 W/sec and co-apt small vessels. The ligasure is used for sealing of vessels up to 7 mm in diameter. It provides a feedback loop that ensures complete sealing of the lumen before it breaks the flow of current. Photocoagulation uses an intense beam of light to produce denaturation and precipitation of proteins, leading to coagulation.
- *Transfixion and double ligature:* If an arterial stump continues to pulsate after simple ligature, this may indicate that the ligature is not safe and may slip due to the force of transmitted pulsation. Such a stump should be made safe by a transfixion stitch, in which either 2-0 or 3-0 Vicryl on a round-bodied needle is passed through the wall of the stump, and tied on one side, then encircling the stump, and tied firmly on the other side with a surgeon's knot. Transfixation prevents the displacement of ligature. Transfixation and double ligature are generally needed for vessels over 5 mm in diameter, such as the femoral artery, splenic artery, or renal artery. An experienced surgeon will often use a transfixion stitch on a large artery as a safety measure prior to division, during an elective procedure.
- *Suturing of stump:* Suturing of a proximal arterial stump is still occasionally performed, using a Prolene stitch to prevent hemorrhage.
- *Vascular stapler:* A vascular stapler can be used to provide a simple and safe way of dividing vascular pedicles during laparoscopic surgery. It may also be used in inaccessible areas during open surgery. The instrument fires three rows of vascular staples across the artery and then cuts between the two staple lines. Vascular cartridges are supplied in white

or gray color. It is quick and effective, but very expensive.

Things to do after control of hemorrhage:

- Do not close up immediately, but wait until the patient is stabilized, so that you can identify any other areas of bleeding, which may not have manifested then due to hypotension.
- One should wash out blood from body cavities with saline. Blood left inside a cavity can act as a nidus for bacterial proliferation, and the patient may also develop icterus in the postoperative period due to absorption of products of broken down hemoglobin.
- Before closure, always make sure that you have not caused damage to other vital structures, e.g., damage to the common bile duct while controlling bleeding from a cystic artery.

Hemostasis with Drugs

Vasoconstrictors such as epinephrine and norepinephrine are quiet valuable in reducing blood loss. They may be injected in skin and subcutaneous tissue before making an incision. They should be injected at least 5–10 minutes before starting surgery as smooth muscle constriction in vessel wall requires 6 minutes to appear. A concentration of 1:200,000 epinephrine in saline is used, and one can inject 40–50 mL of the solution into an average adult weighing 70 kg. Caution should be exercised in using regional injections within or close to the pedicles of flaps. Advice of anesthetist should be taken before injection of epinephrine. In long duration operations, the vasoconstrictor can be injected again after interval of 90 minutes.

Topical Hemostatic Agents

Generally, topical hemostatic agents are assigned to one of the five major groups:

1. Passive (i.e., mechanical) agents (e.g., oxidized regenerated cellulose and by wax derived from Bee)
2. Active agents (e.g., bovine thrombin, pooled human thrombin, and recombinant thrombin)
3. Flowables (e.g., bovine gelatin particles, human thrombin, porcine gelatin particles and with or without pooled human or recombinant thrombin)
4. Fibrin sealants (e.g., human plasma-derived fibrin sealants, the patient's own plasma combined with bovine collagen and thrombin, and the patient's own plasma used to create fibrinogen and thrombin)
5. Adhesives (e.g., skin sealants, synthetic tissue sealants, glutaraldehydes, and polyethylene glycol polymers).

Laparoscopic Prevention and Management of Active Hemorrhage

Preventive Steps

- Adopting sound surgical principles is of paramount importance. The surgeon should be well acquainted with the local anatomy of operating area. All structures should be visualized and identified prior to division.
- Avoid bluntly avulsing adhesions and adipose tissue; contained small vessels tend to retract into the divided tissue and are difficult to control.
- Safe application of energy to the area of the vascular structure to be divided, prior to its division, helps to prevent uncontrolled hemorrhage.
- If one is not sure about the vascularity of a structure to be divided, it is advisable to mechanically occlude it with a clip prior to its division or at least to have dissected free enough length to allow manual control if bleeding is observed after division.

MECHANICAL METHODS OF LAPAROSCOPIC HEMOSTASIS

- *Endoscopic clip appliers* **(Fig. 8)** were developed to facilitate ligation of small (2–5 mm) structures such as ducts and vessels. Metallic (titanium) clips are most often used. The common disposable clip appliers contain up to 20 clips and are available in a 10-mm diameter instrument or more recently a 5-mm instrument. High-quality reusable clip appliers available from several manufacturers allow the surgeon to considerably decrease costs, but these instruments have to be reloaded after each clip is fired. Clip application requires visualization of both sides of the clip to ensure adequate tissue length and to prevent inadvertent clipping of adjacent vital structures or tissues. There is theoretic risk of clip migration which has prompted the advent of absorbable clips usually made of polyglycolic acid polymers (Dexon or Vicryl). These clips have identical ligation properties but may pose less threat to adhesion formation or migration. Inadvertent mechanical ischemic necrosis can occur from metallic clips placed in close proximity to bile duct or bowel wall, resulting in stricture or perforation. These complications can be prevented by better visualization of the structures prior to placing the clip.
- *Linear stapling devices* **(Fig. 9)** are of vital use to prevent major hemostatic complications. Endoscopic linear cutters that deploy three parallel rows of hemostatic staples (staple height = 2.5 mm white cartridge) or (gray cartridge with staple height of 2 mm) are available to facilitate *hemostatic* division of large vessels like splenic artery or renal vessels or vascular tissue. With effective cutting lengths from 30 to 60 mm, larger vessels or highly vascularized tissues such as in the lung or bowel mesentery can be controlled and divided in one motion. Inspection of both sides of the device is mandatory prior to firing to avoid division of unintended structures and to ensure that the entire target tissue is within the active area as indicated in marks or numbers on the side of the device. Depending on the manufacturer, the shaft diameters of these linear cutters vary from 12 to 18 mm.

Appropriately large trocars must be strategically placed to allow opening of the

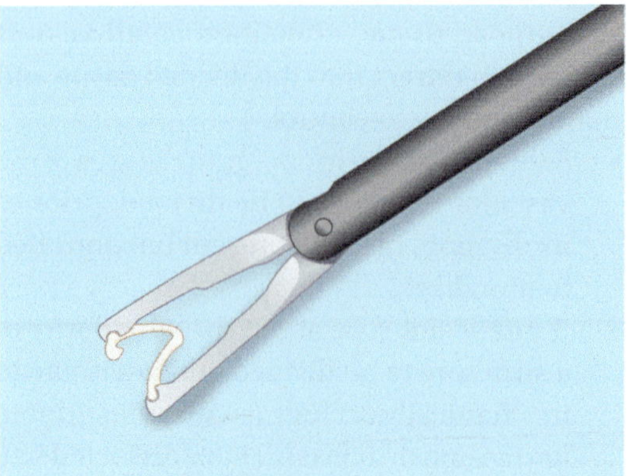

Fig. 8: Laparoscopic clip applicator.

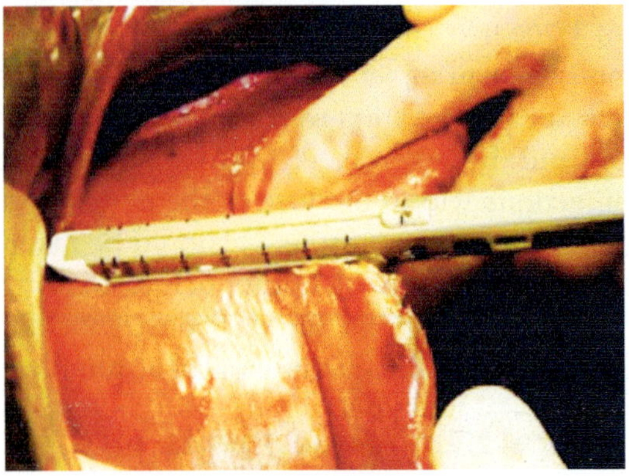

Fig. 9: Use of linear cutter with white cartridge to divide liver.

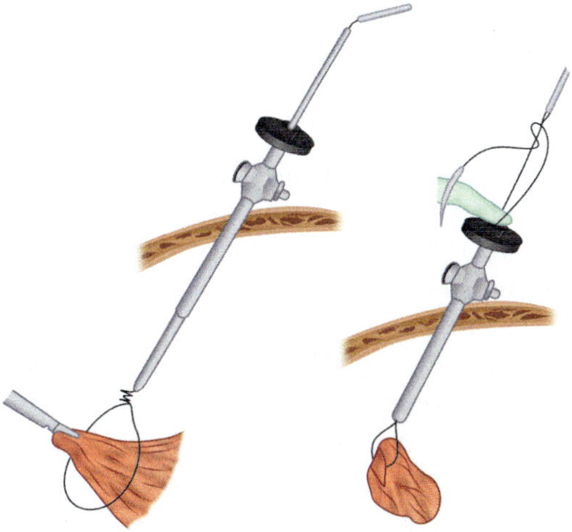

Fig. 10: Use of preformed knot used in cavity.

active portion of these instruments within the desired operative field.

- *Pretied suture loops* ***(Fig. 10)*** with slip knots have a limited use in *primary* hemostasis because the vessel or vascular pedicle must first be divided, grasped, and then encircled with the loop. This leaves a bleeding structure for a period of time while being encircled by the loop. However, the loops are extremely useful to secure bleeding vessels after transection. The bleeding structure is grasped and the field irrigated. An atraumatic grasper is passed through another port and passed through the loop of the suture ligature. The first grasper is then released, and the second grasper grasps the stump of the bleeding structure. The loop is snugged down over the shaft of the instrument, securing the bleeder.
- *Simple ligatures* need to be nothing more than a long suture (at least 40 inches) which is passed around a clearly dissected vessel. Care should be taken to employ an instrument which acts as a fulcrum and prevent "sawing" of the tissue as the ligature is being passed. If an intracorporeal knot is planned, the suture material should be fashioned about 6″ long (length of a scalpel handle is a convenient reference).
- *Suturing* in laparoscopic surgery has been used primarily for tissue approximation. When tissue approximation will result in hemostasis, suturing is a valuable adjunct. An obvious example is the use of figure-of-eight suture to secure a bleeding vessel.

Protocol Suggested to Control Active Bleeding during Laparoscopic Surgery

Even after the meticulous dissection and hemostatic techniques, one may occasionally encounter active bleeding, leading to panic decision of conversion to an open procedure. The following steps are suggested for the control of active hemorrhage. When bleeding is encountered and not easily controlled by electrocautery, the surgeon should:

- Visualize the bleeding source without moving any instrument that is providing retraction. Blind application of energy sources to the presumed bleeding point without proper identification should be avoided as it can be dangerous and can lead to injury to adjacent vital structures.
- Avoid the "reddening" or obscuration of visualized field which occurs when even small amount of blood obscures the laparoscope's view.
- Perform suction with a large-bore suction cannula (10 mm, if available) to avoid accumulation of blood. Irrigation, although might be helpful in identifying slow bleeding sites, should be avoided in active bleeding as it adds to blood/liquid pool and potentially can splatter onto the laparoscope and limit visualization.
- Application of a 5-mm atraumatic grasper to the bleeding point when

identified is useful. A maneuver for uncontrolled bleeding from the cystic artery may be useful. In this, the gallbladder infundibulum is grasped by the instrument through the right upper quadrant trocar to apply direct pressure over the actively bleeding area. This allows the surgeon to stop the bleeding temporarily by tamponade, aspirate blood from the field, clean the laparoscope, and place new instruments or trocars to control the cystic artery.

- If the vessel cannot be controlled under direct vision, the surgeon should convert to an open procedure.
- If the bleeding point is controlled with a grasper, the next step is to evaluate the trocar situation. Simply put, there must be enough trocars to control the bleeding and to introduce a clip applier or suture ligature. Most commonly, a clip will be used to control the bleeding. A trocar must be available that can accommodate a clip applier, without removing any instruments that are providing retraction. It is better to add a trocar than to compromise by moving instruments and risk losing control of the bleeder. The added port should be placed at least 15 cm away from the bleeding site in a vector that will allow torque-free clipping and at right angles to the laparoscope (so that the placement of a clip can be easily observed).
- Place a clip precisely on both sides of the atraumatic grasper with care not to create torque or displace the controlling grasper.
- Irrigate and evaluate. If it is not certain whether the clips are providing secure hemostasis or whether they have injured surrounding structures, the procedure should be converted to open exploration.

KEY POINTS

- Every surgeon must be able to control hemorrhage during surgery.
- In cases of unexpected bleeding, keep yourself cool and composed.
- Pack the bleeding area to buy time and organize yourself.
- Inform the anesthesiologist.
- Do not hesitate to ask for a senior's help if you are not confident.
- Wait for 10 minutes before removing the pack.
- After allowing sufficient time following packing, bleeding will often have reduced to a trickle to identify the bleeding point.
- If packing does not help, proximal and distal control of a vessel may be needed.
- If there is bleeding from a great vessel, suturing of a tear in the vessel may be required.

CHAPTER 17

Biopsy Techniques

MD Raihan, Sudhir Kumar Jain, David L Stoker

"Biopsy is like a mirror, which reflects the true nature of the disease"
"Properly performed biopsy lays the foundation stone for future surgical management"

INTRODUCTION

Biopsy is a process in which tissue is obtained for microscopic or other investigations. It is not analogous to fine-needle aspiration, which obtains only cells. Fine-needle aspiration is an alternative to biopsy but not a substitute, as there are many clinical situations in which there is no alternative to biopsy. Details of histological architecture and immunohistochemistry are only obtainable from biopsy specimens.

INDICATIONS FOR BIOPSY

- To confirm the diagnosis of malignancy, when there is strong clinical suspicion but repeated fine-needle aspiration is not conclusive or negative.
- In suspected cases of soft tissue sarcoma, lymphoma or follicular carcinoma of thyroid. In these cases, fine-needle aspiration cannot establish an exact diagnosis.
- To differentiate between primary malignancy and metastasis
- In cases of breast malignancy where determination hormonal receptor status is required.
- To differentiate between in situ carcinoma and invasive carcinoma
- Subtyping of malignancy for staging and prognostication
- In cases of testicular malignancy, if there are residual retroperitoneal masses post-radiotherapy or chemotherapy. Excision biopsy of residual masses is necessary to differentiate between residual malignancy and fibrosis.
- Tissue is mandatory if any disease requires investigation with electron microscopy, enzyme histochemistry, and immunohistochemistry.

Enzyme histochemistry is required:

- For diagnosis of myopathy
- For diagnosis of malabsorption and alactasia
- For Hirschsprung's disease

Immunohistochemistry is needed:

- For subtyping of lymphoreticular tumors
- For identification of germ cell tumors (placental alkaline phosphatase)
- Melanoma (by S-100, HMB45, and vimentin)
- Thyroid tumor (by thyroglobulin)
- Vascular tumor (endothelial marker, e.g., factor VIII)
- For identification of soft tissue tumors

The objective of a tissue biopsy is to obtain a tissue sample:

- From a lesion which is representative of the pathology
- With preserved tissue architecture

- Should include a portion of normal tissue for comparison.

RULES OF TISSUE BIOPSY

- In a large lesion, there can be areas of normal tissue in between lesions or lesion can be heterogeneous. To avoid sampling errors, one should take multiple biopsies from different places.
- In an ulcerated or fungating lesion, biopsy should not be taken from the center, because this will most probably show necrotic tissue. Always take a biopsy from the periphery of the lesion, including normal tissue with it.
- If it is surgically feasible and safe for the patient, always include the full thickness of the lesion in a biopsy to assess the depth of the lesion. This is especially important in staging of malignant melanoma.
- Deeply situated masses may be surrounded by compressed normal surrounding tissue, forming a pseudocapsule. One should make sure that the biopsy traverses through this normal tissue in to the actual site of pathology before obtaining tissue. Failure to do so might result in a false-negative report.
- Avoid handling biopsy tissue with crushing forceps or traumatic instruments, because this will lead to loss of tissue architecture, which is especially important in diagnosis of lymphoma.
- Do not use laser or the cryoprobe while obtaining a biopsy, as they destroy tissue.
- Do not use a morcellator for retrieving a solid organ after laparoscopic surgery, if you want a tissue diagnosis post-operatively.
- Orientation of the resected specimen is important, if you need information on tumor-free resected margins or staging. Orientation should be carried out in theater by pinning out, or labeling with colored sutures. This is of paramount importance in breast conservation surgery for cancer.

TYPES OF BIOPSY

- Open biopsy
- Percutaneous closed biopsy
- Endoscopic biopsy
- Laparoscopic biopsy

Open Biopsy

Open biopsy is usually performed for lesions in the skin and subcutaneous tissues. It is now unusual to open the abdomen or chest just for the sake of obtaining tissue.

Types of Open Biopsy

- *Shave biopsy:* A scalpel or razor is used to shave off a thin layer of the lesion parallel to the skin. Shave biopsies are simple to perform, need little training, and no sutures are required for closure. The lesion elevated above the skin or a pathology confined to the epidermis is most suitable for shave biopsies. Examples include seborrheic or actinic keratoses, skin tags, warts, and superficial basal or squamous cell carcinomas. Shave biopsies are contraindicated for pigmented lesions because if an unsuspected melanoma is partially removed, it cannot be properly staged.
- *Punch biopsy:* A small cylindrical punch is screwed in to the lesion through full thickness, and a cylinder of tissue is removed. Punch biopsy includes whole of epidermis/dermis and reaches up to subcutaneous fat. One to two stitches may be needed to close the wound. The punch is a good procedure for diagnostic skin biopsy or removing small lesions

and yields better cosmetic result than a shave biopsy. Punch biopsies yield a cone-shaped core of tissue with its widest diameter at the skin surface and narrowest at the biopsy base.

- *Incision biopsy:* Incision biopsy involves removal of a wedge of the lesion with adjacent normal tissue. Incision biopsy is used for large lesions prior to treatment.
- *Excision biopsy:* In this, entire lesion is excised with a surrounding rim of normal tissue. This is used for small lesions, which can be excised completely.

Biopsy of Skin Lesions

Biopsy of skin lesions can be in the form of punch biopsy, shave biopsy, or excision biopsy. Punch biopsy is indicated for flat or raised lesions (if melanoma is suspected). For pedunculated lesions, excision or shave biopsy is indicated. For a raised lesion, if melanoma is not suspected shave biopsy can suffice.

Biopsy of Oral Lesion

- *Excision biopsy:* Excision biopsy means removal of the whole of the lesion.

  Indications of excision biopsy are:
  - Should be employed with small lesions <1 cm
  - The lesion on clinical examination appears benign.
  - If complete excision with a margin of normal tissue is possible without mutilation
- *Incisional biopsy:* An incision biopsy is a biopsy that samples only a particular portion or representative part of a lesion. If a lesion is large or has different characteristics in various locations more than one area may need to be sampled. The hazardous location of lesions is another indication for incisional biopsy.

Indications for Biopsy in Oral Cavity Lesions

- Any lesion that persists for more than 2 weeks with no apparent etiologic basis
- Any inflammatory lesion that does not respond to local treatment after 10–14 days
- Persistent hyperkeratotic changes in surface tissues
- Any persistent tumescence, either visible or palpable beneath relatively normal tissue.

Characteristics of Oral Lesions that Raise the Suspicion of Malignancy

- *Erythroplasia:* The lesion which is totally red or has a speckled red appearance
- *Ulceration:* If the lesion is ulcerated or presents as an ulcer
- *Duration:* Any lesion which has persisted for more than 2 weeks
- *Growth rate:* If lesion exhibits rapid growth
- *Bleeding:* If lesion bleeds on gentle manipulation or touch
- *Induration:* If lesion and surrounding tissue are firm to the touch
- *Fixation:* If lesion feels attached to adjacent structures.

Percutaneous Closed Biopsy

- Image guided
- Blind

Image-guided percutaneous biopsy is the method of choice, usually reserved for deep seated inaccessible lesions. Image guidance can be through ultrasonography or CT, and with the help of either, it is usually feasible to find a safe path or window through which

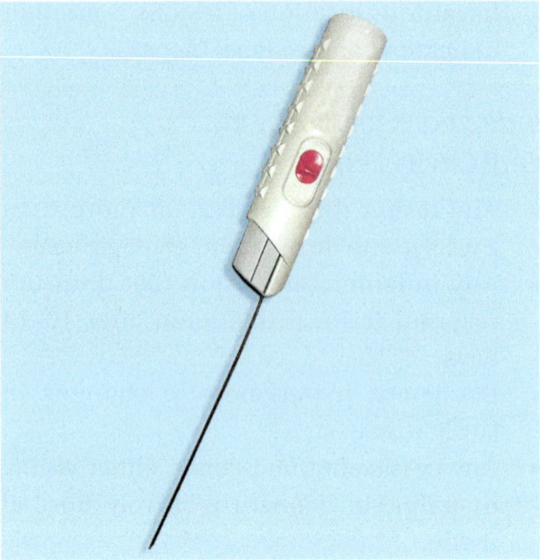

Fig. 1: Trucut needle.

the biopsy needle can pass into the region of interest.

Blind Biopsy

This can be used for superficial palpable lesions, kidney, liver, and prostate. Various types of needles may be used.

- Abraham's needle for pleural biopsy
- Menghini needle for liver biopsy
- Trucut needle
- Automatic, spring loaded modification of trucut needle **(Fig. 1)**
- High-speed drill biopsy for bone only.

Endoscopic Biopsy (Fig. 2)

This can be used in association with both rigid and flexible endoscopy. Varieties of biopsy forceps are available. Since these biopsy forceps remove a very small amount of tissue, multiple biopsies at different points may need to be taken.

Laparoscopic Biopsy

During diagnostic laparoscopy, biopsy can be taken from a suspicious area from liver, omentum, or mesenteric lymph node.

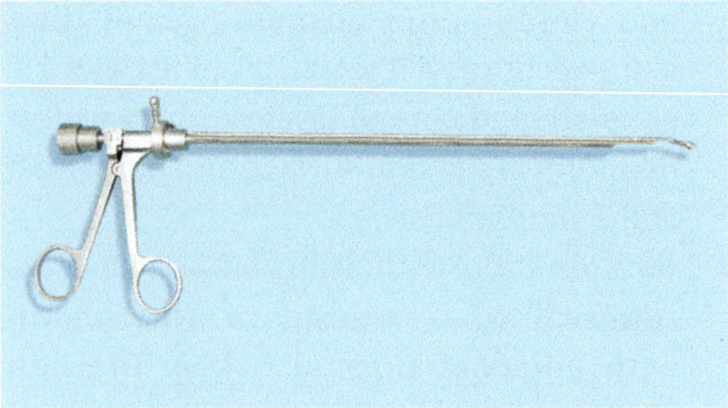

Fig. 2: Cystoscopic biopsy forceps.

POSTBIOPSY PROCEDURE

- A proper histology request form must be completed. Every specimen must be labeled correctly. The form must contain the patient's identification details, nature of specimen, clinical features, operative details, and presumptive diagnosis. Patient details on the request form should match with the label on the specimen jar or container. Pathologists will also need to know if the patient had neoadjuvant chemotherapy for a full pathological staging report.
- The specimen should be put in an appropriate fixative. Ten percent buffered formalin is suitable for most specimens.

FROZEN SECTION

This is a special technique in which tissue is sent fresh to the pathology department, where it is frozen to –25°C using either liquid nitrogen or CO_2. After freezing, the tissue is immediately sectioned using a microtome in a special chamber known as a cryostat. Cut frozen sections are stained with hemotoxylin and eosin for immediate reporting. There has to be good coordination between the surgical and pathology teams when using this technique. Frozen sections are more difficult to interpret than ordinary paraffin sections, and the services of an experienced pathologist are needed. It can be a highly accurate technique with false-negative rates of 0.5% and a false-positive rate of 0.1%.

Role of Frozen Section in Modern Day Clinical Practice

- To establish the benign or malignant nature of a lesion during surgery, in order to decide on the extent of a resection. An example of this would be the management of solitary nodular goiter with fine-needle aspiration report of follicular pathology. In this situation, the surgeon may perform a lobectomy and send it for frozen section. If the report is follicular carcinoma, he completes the procedure by doing a near total thyroidectomy. If the report is follicular adenoma, lobectomy itself is sufficient. However many times, it may not be possible to give definite opinion on frozen section, especially in follicular neoplasm of thyroid.
- To ensure that resected margins are tumor free in malignancy. One of the examples is breast conservation surgery, in which the surgeon can revise the resected margins if not tumor free.
- To establish that a biopsy contains sufficient material for diagnosis and is from a representative area in a difficult case.

Precautions to be taken during Special Situations

Biopsy of an impalpable breast lesion detected by breast screening:

- Preoperative X-ray localization and insertion of localizing needle under X-ray control, by the radiologist in a radiology suite is performed.
- Suspected lesion with localizing needle is removed.
- Removed specimen along with needle is X-rayed and compared with preoperative mammogram film.
- If image of removed specimen does not match with abnormality on mammogram, more tissue is removed.
- Boundaries of removed specimen are marked with dye.
- Removed specimen is sliced into serial 5 mm thickness sections on a special X-ray board and image again taken to determine which sections contain the exact lesion, which can then be further processed.

LYMPH NODE BIOPSY

Which lymph node should be removed?

- If there are involved lymph nodes in different anatomical areas, then choose an area which is more likely to be involved in the suspected pathology. For example, in a suspected case of Hodgkin's lymphoma with involvement of cervical, axillary and inguinal lymph node, biopsy from an axillary lymph node will be preferred to that of a cervical or inguinal one.
- If there are multiple lymph nodes in one anatomical group, then choose a lymph node which is least likely to be involved in nonspecific infection. Example is cervical lymphadenitis with involvement of submental, submandibular, and posterior cervical lymph nodes. In this clinical situation, biopsy from a posterior cervical group of lymph nodes is a more sensible choice because lymph nodes of submental and submandibular region are commonly involved in nonspecific infections of throat.
- Choose a lymph node for biopsy which does not overlie or underlie an important structure. Excision biopsy is preferred over incision biopsy.
- After biopsy, the lymph node is bisected to inspect for gross pathology, i.e., caseous material, stony hard lymph node, or

lymph node containing pus. On bisection, imprints are taken on glass slides and stained. One-half of the lymph node is sent in formalin for H and E staining. Remaining half is divided in to three parts. One piece is fixed in glutaraldehyde for electron microscopy. Another piece is snap frozen to –70°C for enzyme and immunohistochemistry. If infective pathology, e.g., tuberculosis is suspected, then remaining piece is kept in saline and stored at 4°C for microbiological examination.

VIRTUAL BIOPSY

Virtual biopsy refers to detection of tumor characteristics using a functional magnetic resonance imaging (MRI) or other imaging modalities to infer precise information regarding the size, extent, and nature of the lesion. Using virtual biopsy, the development of new vessels and the functional response to tumors can be studied. Brain lesions and colonic growths have been subjected to virtual biopsy with reliable results.

KEY POINTS

- In spite of advances in cytology techniques, biopsy techniques have a definite role.
- Taking a biopsy is a basic surgical skill which every surgeon must acquire.
- Tissue for biopsy must be taken from a representative area of pathology.
- Excision biopsy is preferable to incision biopsy.
- Avoid taking a biopsy from the center of an ulcerating tumor.
- Always include a portion of normal tissue while taking a biopsy from an ulcer.
- Core needle biopsy is a good alternative to incision biopsy.
- Always properly label biopsy specimens and give adequate details of clinical history and operative procedure to help the pathologist.
- Send a biopsy specimen in the proper solution.
- If planning for frozen sections inform the pathologist well in advance.

CHAPTER 18

Dissection Techniques

Sudhir Kumar Jain, Raman Tanwar

"Surgeon index finger is the best dissecting instrument"
"A good dissection is a hallmark for judging the quality of surgery"

DISSECTION

Dissection is an essential component for the successful completion of any surgical procedure. Quality of dissection is often judged as the hallmark of surgical competence. The technique of surgical dissection can be mastered by adopting sound surgical principles as well as by familiarity with surgical anatomy.

DEFINITION

Dissection is a Latin word derived from *dis* meaning apart and *secare* meaning to cut. It can be defined as "the exposure of a target organ or area by the process of separation of overlying tissue with hemostasis and preservation of surrounding essential or vital structures".

A good dissection requires not only a thorough knowledge of anatomy but also a good understanding of the pathology of the relevant area.

Components of dissection are as follows:

- Sensory component comprising visual and tactile elements
- Access component involving tissue manipulation and instrument maneuver. The end point of good dissection is exposure of the target structure so that the desired procedure can be performed upon it.

PREREQUISITE OF A GOOD DISSECTION

- Application of the right amount of stretch on the tissues (without trauma) before starting to dissect. This entirely depends upon tactile feedback which the surgeon acquires during the initial years of training. Tension or stretching of tissues in the correct direction helps in identification of attachments and natural planes of separation.
- Identification of proper tissue planes
- Economy of movement. Each and every action the surgeon takes should be productive and should help in achieving the desired objective. Unproductive actions increase the chances of complications and lead to fatigue. The surgeon should complete one step of the operation before proceeding to the next step.

MODES OF DISSECTION

Available modes of dissection are as follows:

- Blunt dissection
- Scissor dissection
- Scalpel dissection
- Ultrasonic dissection

- Dissection by electrocautery
- Hydrodissection by water under high pressure
- Dissection by laser.

Blunt Dissection

Blunt dissection is suitable in places where there is a good amount of loose areolar tissue, which can be separated by application of shear force. The safety of blunt dissection depends upon the sensitivity of tactile feedback to the surgeon's hands, which can differentiate between important structures, e.g., vessels or nerves and areolar tissue. Blunt dissection is especially useful in areas where anatomy is obscured.

Techniques of Blunt Dissection

Techniques are as follows:

- Separation or splitting of overlying tissue. This is especially useful while dissecting along tubular structures such as vessels, nerves, or ureter.
- Tearing or teasing
- Wiping
- Distraction
- Peeling.

Methods of Blunt Dissection

- *Fingertip dissection:* The tip of index finger allows living tissues to be opened without the need for excessive force. Fingertip dissection avoids heavy traction exerted by instruments. The use of heavy pressure can result in tearing of blood vessels, nerves and other structures with resultant heavy bleeding, loss of exposure, and delayed healing. Surgeon's index finger can safely open avascular layers of collagen bundles which have formed at the site of previous scarring and can readily dissect many lightly adherent normal tissue planes. A tearing or shearing action can be performed by a finger along the line of separation. The tip of the finger can be used to peel off a structure, e.g., separation of gallbladder from its bed during cholecystectomy. Sometimes blunt dissection is performed by gauze wrapped on a finger, e.g., dissection of a hernial sac from the cord structures during inguinal hernia repair. Finger fracture technique may be used for liver resection.
- *Sponge or gauze dissection:* If the density and adherence of tissue are significantly more than the tip of moist gloved finger, then fingertip dissection will not open the desired tissue planes. In these situations, if a moist gauze piece wrapped around surgeon's index finger is used, it will increase the coefficient of friction between the wound and fingertip and facilitate dissection. The movements of finger in this type of dissection comprises firm push and rotation of fingertips starting on the deeper or more fixed tissue which is followed by supination of hands and wrist so that mobile tissues get stripped and lifted away from deeper structures. Peeling action can also be performed by a pledget of gauze (Kuttner pledget) held in a pair of forceps to peel off fibrous tissue. During cholecystectomy, dissection in Calot's triangle is very often performed using this method. Peanut dissection is more effective when the gauze pledget is folded in half before clamping **(Fig. 1)**.
- Closed scissor tips can be used as blunt dissector. This technique is commonly used during lysis of adhesions during laparotomy. Blunt tipped scissors are excellent for opening tissue planes if the tissues are too dense for finger or sponge dissection but not so dense as

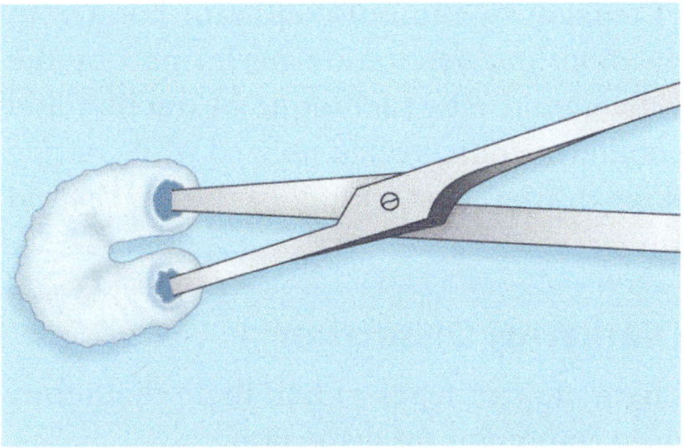

Fig. 1: Kuttner pledget for dissection.

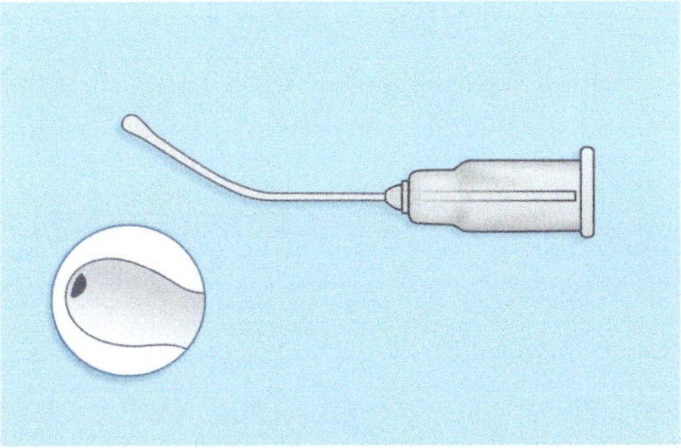

Fig. 2: Button hole or olive tip knife for dissection.

to require a scalpel. The technique of "spread, then look" is used for scissor dissection in which blades of closed tip scissor are first inserted in tissue planes then the blades of scissors are spread to open tissue planes, followed by division of any residual tough fascial bands. Scissor dissection is both safe and rapid in the hands of an experienced surgeon. Many small blood vessels get closed off and sealed the moment they are cut during scissor dissection due to shearing action of blades.

- Knife dissection is used when tissues are heavily scarred or very dense. Sharp edge of the knife is used for this dissection. Knife dissection should be performed under strict visual monitoring otherwise it can result in damage to important structures. A blunt or dull knife should never be used because it makes cutting uncertain and excessive pressure is needed to divide tissue. It will be difficult for surgeon to withdraw pressure immediately once desired depth of cutting has been reached resulting in damage to deeper tissues e.g., to gut while opening abdomen. Scalpel dissection is performed by applying a smooth horizontal stroke which delivers even pressure along the entire cutting edge. Small strokes with uneven pressure should be avoided as they result in greater tissue damage, enhanced bleeding, and increased operating time. Small strokes reflect uncertainty and indecisiveness in the mind of the operating surgeon. Special type of knives is also available for special situations. One such knife is olive tip or "button ended knife" **(Fig. 2)**, which can be inserted in a narrow space and used to make a lateral cut, e.g., lateral sphincterotomy in chronic anal fissure. Its rounded tip prevents any undesirable damage from the blade point, thus making insertion of knife into a pocket safe and easy. Iridotomy knife used by eye surgeons is an example of such type of knife. Freer knife has a rounded edge at its tip, and cutting is limited to that area only **(Fig. 3)**. It combines the features of

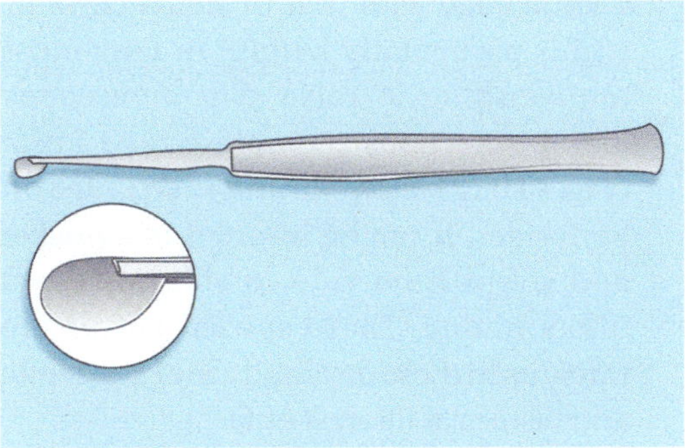

Fig. 3: Freer knife used for dissection.

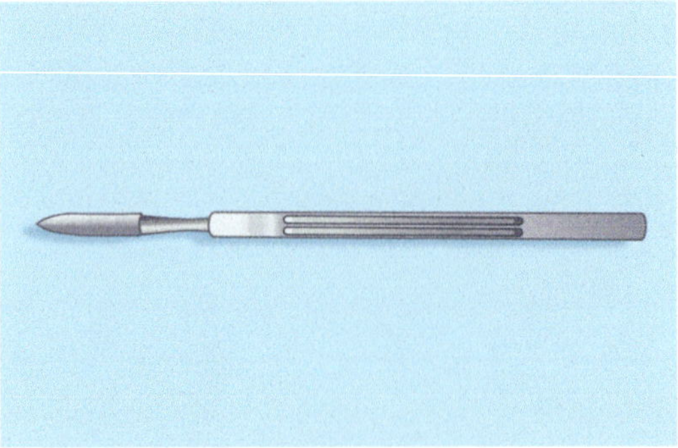

Fig. 4: Round tip knife for dissection.

a knife edge with that of sharp elevator and is particularly helpful in tangential undercutting to raise skin or mucous membrane flaps. Double-edged knife **(Fig. 4)** has a sharp tip and sharp edge on both sides. It can be inserted in a pocket and swept from side to side for rapid undermining. These special knives are rarely used these days and are of academic and historical interest only.

Splitting action is often performed by the pointed end of scissors to separate muscle fibers without cutting them, e.g., splitting of internal oblique/transversus abdominis muscle during appendicectomy.

- Right angle forceps or Maryland dissector is commonly used for blunt dissection behind vascular bundles. It can, however, split, peel off, or tear underlying structures and therefore needs to be used with care.
- Suction cannula is sometimes used as blunt dissection, especially during laparoscopic surgery, often in conjunction with hydro dissection.

Sharp Dissection

Sharp dissection involves division of tissues by cutting performed by scalpel or by scissors. Sharp dissection is a two-handed procedure and needs application of the desired amount of tension by the nondominant hand with division and separation performed by the active hand. The technique of traction and countertraction is often utilized while raising flaps during mastectomy or during thyroid surgery.

Diathermy Dissection

There are two types of handheld diathermy used commonly for dissection.

1. Handheld disposable diathermy probe with cutting and coagulation buttons. This is frequently used instead of scissors to divide tissues and coagulate small vessels simultaneously. It facilitates a bloodless field and has to be used carefully in the abdomen to avoid diathermy injury to bowel.
2. Monopolar and bipolar scissors. These are of the McIndoe variety and come in various lengths for superficial or deep dissection. They combine the dissecting properties of McIndoe scissors with the properties of the handheld diathermy probe. They are particularly useful during abdominal and neck dissections. The diathermy works from a foot pedal and can be used selectively for tissues such as peritoneum and serosa. They are useful for dividing adhesions. The bipolar scissors are safer to use, as adjacent tissues are not damaged by diathermy. This is because the current passes between the two scissors blades. These scissors have a limited life as they cannot be sharpened and have to be replaced after 20–30 uses.

Ultrasonic Dissection

Ultrasonic dissectors are of two types:

1. Low-power system
2. High-power system.

The low-power system (CUSA Selector) is used for liver surgery. These systems cleave water containing tissues by cavitation, leaving organized structures with low water content intact.

The high-power system, e.g., Autosonix and harmonic scalpel. This cleaves loose areolar tissue and blood vessels up to 3 mm diameter by fractional heating and performs coagulating and cutting action at the same time. It uses mechanical energy in the range of 55,000 cycles/sec and acts by disruption of hydrogen bonds and formation of a coagulum. It produces less heat in comparison to electrocautery and causes less collateral damage and tissue necrosis. The tip of the instrument remains very hot for several seconds after use, and caution needs to be taken to avoid it touching and burning adjacent tissues such as bowel or the surgeon's fingers. It also helps in simultaneous hemostasis by coapting large vessels.

High-Velocity Water Jet Dissection

This type of dissection disrupts friable, soft tissue but leaves ducts and blood vessels intact. It also has the effect of washing away adherent clot, which makes identification of anatomy much easier, e.g., in dissection of Calot's triangle during difficult laparoscopic cholecystectomy with dense adhesions in Calot's triangle.

Laser Dissection

A variety of lasers may be used in surgery for dissection. Laser light is used to heat a probe to white heat, e.g., a sapphire crystal. This very intense heat is highly efficient at cutting dense fibrous tissue and may help to produce an almost bloodless field. Lasers are very expensive and need strict protocols to avoid the hazards of eye exposure in theater. Training is required in their use in specialized situations. Types of lasers used include CO_2 laser, holmium laser, potassium titanyl phosphate (KTP) laser, Nd:YAG laser, and thulium laser. Holmium laser is being used these days for dissection in endourological procedures as in prostate removal for benign hyperplasia of prostate commonly known as holmium enucleation of prostate (HOLEP).

KEY POINTS

- Dissection is an essential component for successful completion of any surgical procedure.
- Quality of dissection is the hallmark of surgical competence.
- Good dissection requires application of the right amount of stretch, identification of tissue planes, and economy of movement.
- Dissection can be either sharp or blunt.
- Various devices such as diathermy, ultrasonic machine, or laser can be used for dissection.
- Blunt dissection is useful in places where there is plenty of areolar tissue and anatomy is obscured.
- Blunt dissection can be performed by finger, pledget of gauze held in a forceps, closed scissor tips, or by Maryland dissector.
- Sharp dissection involves division of tissues by cutting using scissors or scalpel.

CHAPTER 19

Surgical Diathermy: Principles and Precautions

Sudhir Kumar Jain, David L Stoker

"Beware of electrical current: It can burn you"

INTRODUCTION

Electrosurgical equipment is commonly referred as "Bovie" because Dr William T Bovie started electrosurgery and received his PhD for his work. William Bovie, along with neurosurgeon, Harvey W Cushing, MD, is credited with inventing the electrosurgical unit, which is known today as the "Bovie". The fact that whenever an electrical current passes through our body, it induces intense neuromuscular stimulation and alteration of cardiac rhythm was described by Michel Faraday. With the increase in the frequency of alternating current, neuromuscular stimulation decreases and disappears at 500,000 Hz (50 kHz). Electrical diathermy units work on the principle of converting normal-frequency alternating current (50 Hz) to high-frequency alternating current (50 kHz). Modern day electrosurgical units can produce currents in the range of 200–300 kHz. Neuromuscular stimulation does not occur at such high frequencies because the current changes direction so rapidly that ionic exchange at cellular level does not occur, and muscle is not stimulated. High-frequency alternating current, when concentrated on a small area, however, produces very high temperatures, capable of coagulating tissues. AJ McLean first detailed the histological analysis of animal tissue subjected to electrocautery. He also extensively analyzed principles regarding current density and heat transfer governing the effects of electric current on tissue.

DIFFERENCES BETWEEN ELECTROSURGERY AND ELECTROCAUTERY

These two terms are frequently confused and used interchangeably, but there are subtle differences between the two terms.

Electrocautery uses metal heated by electric current, which is applied to the target tissue in order to burn or coagulate the specific area of tissue. No current is passed through tissue but rather is applied directly onto the targeted area of treatment. In this technique, heat is passed through a resistant metal wire, which is used as an electrode. This electrode when hot is placed directly onto the treatment area destroying that specific tissue. This use of electricity is typically applied in superficial situations encountered by dermatologists, ophthalmologists, plastic surgeons, urologists, and related specialties. The electrocautery devices are usually compact, battery operated, and use physical heat to destroy the targeted tissues or cause a specific and desired effect, such as polypectomy. Electrocautery is only used for coagulation.

Electrosurgery uses electrical current which passes through tissue and the patient's body to achieve the desired result. An alternating current similar to that used to generate radio waves is used. The typical frequency is quite high, usually around 500,000 cycles/sec. This ensures that the current passes through patient tissue without causing neuromuscular contraction. The heat is generated at the point of resistance of the tissue to the electrical current. The various tools such as electrodes, blades, round balls, needles, and loop configurations can be used to apply the current. These instruments can be used to cut, coagulate, or even to fuse tissue. The electrosurgery devices are advanced radio-wave generators which pass modified electrical current through the target tissues to achieve the desired surgical effect.

USES OF DIATHERMY

- *Coagulation:* Three types of coagulation modes can be used:
  1. Soft coagulation is the safest for both open and laparoscopic surgery. In this mode, no electric arcs are generated between electrode and the tissue, as peak voltage is <200 V. In this mode, there is shrinkage and desiccation of tissue without charring.
  2. Forced coagulation uses electric arcs to achieve deep coagulation. Peak voltages of >500 V are utilized to obtain this. This is useful in areas with high vascularity.
  3. Spray coagulation, also known as fulguration, is a noncontact mode which uses intensely modulated high-frequency voltages (kV). A wider area of tissue is exposed to the current. Its main use is to control bleeding from an inaccessible vessel or to achieve hemostasis in a raw and bleeding area. The active electrode should not touch the patient's tissue during fulguration because in this mode the cell walls are destroyed through dehydration.

  For coagulation mode, current of *interrupted waveform of high voltage and low amplitude* is used. Cell walls contract using this mode due to protein denaturation and charring of cells.
- Cutting uses a current of *continuous waveform of high amplitude and low voltage*. There is rapid rise in temperature due to continuous wave form of current. Heat production resulting from a rapid rise of tissue temperature causes fragmentation of cells due to water evaporation.
- Blended mode, which can both cut and coagulate, amplitude, and voltage of current are equal.

MODES OF DIATHERMY

- Monopolar **(Fig. 1A)**
- Bipolar **(Fig. 1B)**

In monopolar diathermy, current passes from the generator via the active electrode **(Fig. 2)** through the patient and returns to the electrosurgical unit **(Fig. 3)** via a dispersive electrode (patient plate). In order to complete the circuit and to return the current to the electrosurgical unit, a patient plate is always required. This should be in good contact with the patient's skin over at least 300 cm^2 or more of area.

The amount of heat produced by electro-cautery depends upon:

- Current density
- Tissue resistance
- Time

Heat produced at the site of local application of cautery is governed by the modified Joule's law:

$$\text{Energy} = (\text{current/cross-sectional area})^2 \times \text{resistance} \times \text{time}$$

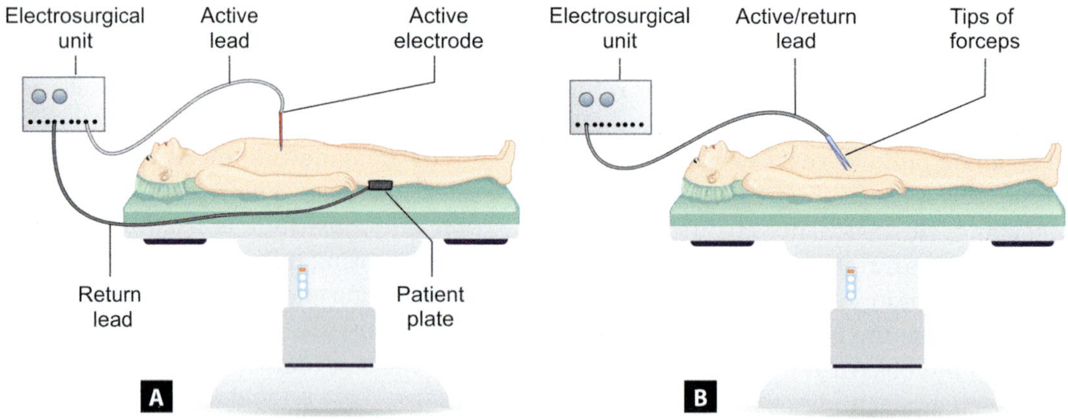

Figs. 1A and B: (A) Circuit of monopolar diathermy; (B) Bipolar diathermy.

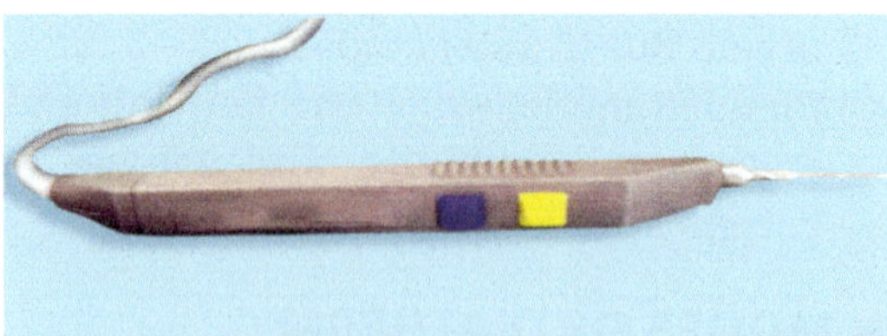

Fig. 2: Hand-operated electrocautery lead. Blue button for coagulation and yellow for cutting.

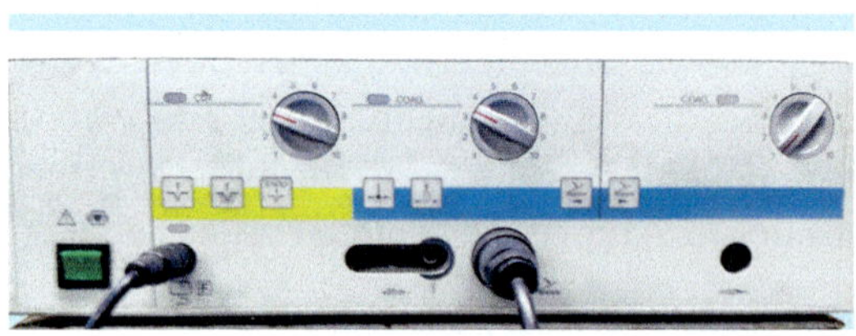

Fig. 3: Electrocautery machine.

In bipolar mode, current passes from the generator to one prong or arm of bipolar forceps (or scissors), then through the patient tissue caught between the forceps and returns back to generator through the second prong or arm. The current does not therefore pass through the patient's body, as the circuit is completed through the bipolar instrument. This mode does not require a patient plate.

USES OF BIPOLAR DIATHERMY

- When coagulation is required on a peripheral organ with a narrow pedicle, there is risk of channeling the current through the pedicle, leading to thrombosis of vessels and a deleterious effect on the organ's blood supply. It is, therefore, safer to use bipolar diathermy in this situation, e.g., circumcision.
- When pinpoint or microcoagulation is required, e.g., neurosurgery, ophthalmic surgery, or plastic surgery.
- When patient has a pacemaker in situ in order to avoid problems that may be caused by a unipolar current passing through the heart.

PRECAUTIONS WHEN USING DIATHERMY

- Equipment must be checked before use to ensure that it is in good working order. Regular check-up and maintenance of electrosurgery units should be performed to prevent injury to the patient and to theater personnel.
- The diathermy plate or return electrode should be of an appropriate size (300 cm^2 or more). The largest return electrode

appropriate to the patient helps to ensure that electrical energy is not concentrated enough to generate significant heat and cause a burn.

- The diathermy plate should be placed close to the operative site, and on the same side.
- The diathermy plate should be placed over a well-vascularized muscular area. Muscle is a better conductor of electricity, and good perfusion promotes electrical conductivity and dissipates heat.
- If the skin at the site where the plate is to be placed is hairy, it should be shaved, as hair prevents complete plate contact with the patient skin.
- The diathermy plate should not be placed over a bony prominence, scar tissue, skin over implanted metal prosthesis, or areas distal to tourniquets. Bone is not a good conductor of electricity. Tissue perfusion may not be adequate in scar tissue. The plate can become overheated if placed over an implanted metal prosthesis.
- The diathermy plate should have a uniform and good body contact to permit the uniform flow of current.
- There should not be any pooling of blood, body fluids, or irrigation fluid near the diathermy plate, as this may lead to loss of contact due to moisture.
- Patient's jewellery should be removed prior to transfer to the theater as metal jewellery presents a potential risk of burn from directed current.
- Contact of patient with grounded metal objects, e.g., intravenous (IV) stands, or anesthesia machine should be avoided as they may become an alternate pathway for current leak to ground and can lead to accidental burns.
- If there is a change in the position of the patient during surgery, the diathermy plate and wire should be reinspected to make sure that there is no tension on the plate, which can result in reduced plate contact.
- Alcohol-based solutions should be avoided for preoperative skin preparation because they may ignite and increase the risk of a thermal burn.
- The active diathermy electrode should be placed in an insulated quiver at all times when not in use.
- The active electrode should have a secure tip. A loose tip may cause a spark. Eschar which builds up on the tip prevents the electrode from working safely, and regular cleaning during a surgical procedure may be necessary.
- Electrosurgical smoke plume presents a potential biological and chemical hazard to both patients and staff. Smoke evacuation systems should be used for all procedures involving use of diathermy.
- Monopolar units should not be operated in the vicinity of an electrocardiogram electrode (minimum distance of 15 cm) as they may lead to monitor malfunction.
- Only the surgeon using the active electrode should activate the machine.
- One should be cautious while using diathermy inside bowel. This is because intestinal gas contains the inflammable gases such as hydrogen and methane, which are potentially explosive.
- Smoke plume generated from diathermy machine contains chemical by-products, e.g., toluene, benzene, hydrogen cyanide, and formaldehyde which are potent carcinogens. Inhalation of these smoke plumes should be avoided by use of inline filters, use of special smoke evacuation systems, or by use of improved surgical filtration masks.

PROCEDURE FOR STARTING A MONOPOLAR DIATHERMY MACHINE

As the safety of monopolar diathermy depends upon proper placement of the patient plate, and only few diathermy machines have patient plate monitoring systems, one should adhere to the following procedures during start-up:

- Place the patient plate on the patient at an appropriate place.
- Connect the return lead to the patient plate.
- Switch on diathermy machine, and plate continuity alarm will sound.
- Connect return electrode to the diathermy machine, so that continuity alarm is silenced.

HAZARDS OF SURGICAL DIATHERMY IN MINIMAL ACCESS SURGERY

Laparoscopic surgery has specific hazards in relation to electrocautery. These hazards arise due to the number of instruments and ports within the operative field.

The principal hazards are:

- *Insulation failure:* This is the most common cause of burns during minimal access surgery (MAS) and can be due to insulation failure, mechanical trauma, repeated sterilization of instruments, or manufacturing flaws. Defects in the tip of the instrument within the view of the laparoscope can cause injury to a nontarget area, e.g., liver during laparoscopic cholecystectomy. Insulation defects in the shaft of an instrument can cause undetectable injury to any bowel it comes in contact with. Insulation failure at the handle of the instrument can burn the surgeon or cause electric shock if the surgical glove is defective.

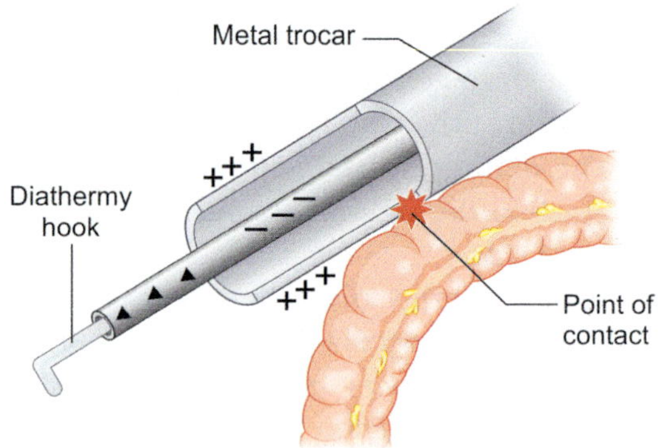

Fig. 4: Mechanism of capacitive coupling by diathermy.

- *Capacitive coupling* **(*Fig. 4*)**: This is a phenomenon where an electrical current in the instrument induces a current in a nearby conductor in spite of intact insulation due to electromagnetic induction. This is because current flowing through an instrument induces an alternating magnetic field around it.

  There is increased incidence of capacitive coupling with higher voltages. It is of clinical significance in the following situations:
  - Use of hybrid cannula, i.e., metal cannula within a plastic anchoring cannula
  - If an insulated electrode is passed through a metal port, there may be induction of current in the port.
  - If an electrode is passed through the working channel of the laparoscope, 70% of the current may be induced in the laparoscope.

  Induced current in a metal cannula or port may cause a diathermy burn if it touches bowel inadvertently.
- *Direct coupling:* If an activated electrode touches another metal instrument, there

will be direct transfer of current from the activated electrode to the metal instrument. Tissues which are in contact with the metal instrument may be injured. Situations where direct coupling can occur are:

- Touching of an active electrode to the laparoscope
- Touching of an active electrode to a metal clip or staple line

DIATHERMY AND PACEMAKERS

Diathermy currents can interfere with the working of pacemakers, which may be inhibited during diathermy activation, preventing cardiac pacing during cautery. A pacemaker may revert to a fixed rate of pacing during use of cautery and may require a magnet to reset it. If possible, the use of diathermy in a patient with a pacemaker should be avoided, and other sources of energy such as the ultrasonic scalpel should be used.

If it is mandatory to use diathermy in such patients, the following precautions should be taken:

- Use bipolar mode, avoiding the use of monopolar diathermy.
- If monopolar cautery is to be used, the patient plate should be sited in such a way that the current path does not pass through the heart or pacemaker.
- Monitor heart beat throughout the operation.
- A defibrillator should be available in case of dangerous arrhythmias.
- Cardiologist should be asked to check pacemaker function prior to surgery.
- Facilities for inserting a temporary pacemaker should be available.

KEY POINTS

- Diathermy uses high-frequency alternating current (>50 kHz) at which there is no neuromuscular stimulation.
- Whenever current gets concentrated in a small area heat is generated.
- One can use diathermy either for cutting or coagulation.
- Cutting diathermy uses a low voltage, high-frequency continuous waveform.
- Coagulation uses high voltage, low-frequency interrupted waveform.
- Bipolar diathermy is safer than monopolar diathermy because the current does not pass through the patient's body.
- Faulty position of patient's plate is the most common cause of a diathermy burn.
- Patient's plate must be fully in contact with the patient's body over a well-vascularized muscular mass with a minimum contact area of 300 cm^2.
- Avoid placing the return electrode over scars, bony prominences, or distal to a tourniquet.
- During laparoscopic surgery additional hazards of diathermy include direct coupling, insulation failure, and capacitive coupling.
- If possible, avoid monopolar diathermy in a patient with a pacemaker.

CHAPTER 20

Dressing and Wound Care

Sudhir Kumar Jain, Raman Tanwar

"Dress me elegantly so that I look good"

INTRODUCTION

The dressing of wounds is both an art and an important skill, which is sadly no longer thought to be a priority in many surgical curricula. A dressing can accelerate the healing process if properly applied but also has the potential to delay the same process. The surgeon must use the correct materials and should acquire knowledge of how and when to use them.

The ideal dressing should create and maintain a well hydrated wound environment. Some humidity beneath occlusive dressings increases the rate of epithelialization and promotes healing by creating a low oxygen tension. Modern day occlusive dressings increase cell proliferation and activity by maintaining an optimum level of wound exudate, containing vital proteins and cytokines produced in response to injury. Wound exudates facilitate autolytic debridement of the wound and promote healing.

Dressings should be properly secured under tension and should support the wound and give protection to it. The patient should not have discomfort or concern that a dressing may become dislodged unexpectedly during the postoperative period. Hairy areas of skin should be shaved off before applying adhesive tapes. Tincture Benzoin, if applied to surrounding skin before applying adhesive tapes, increases the tape's adhesiveness and also protects the skin. Surgeons should remember that patients quite often view their dressings as a reflection of the skill and care in their overall management.

The perfect dressing does not exist; however, if it did it would:

- Protect the wound from trauma
- Be impermeable to bacteria
- Allow oxygenation
- Retain moisture at the wound site while removing excess exudate
- Nonallergenic and nontoxic
- Not damage surrounding tissues
- Be free of particles and toxic wound contaminants
- Be removable without causing further trauma to wound
- Insulate the wound from thermal damage from outside
- Be economical
- Not require frequent changes
- Have long shelf life.

PURPOSE OF DRESSINGS

- *Wound protection:* Dressings serve the purpose of protecting the wound from external trauma or from the patient's own fingers. A simple absorbent gauze pad, well fixed with tape around the wound margin, often suffices for this. In areas of open wounds, gauze should be of fine mesh (30 μ) to avoid penetration of the gauze by granulation tissue. Removal of coarse meshed gauze after several days of application will cause renewed bleeding due to this granulation tissue ingrowth of budding capillaries. This will cause pain on removal of dressings **(Fig. 1)**.

- *Promotion of wound drainage:* Use of moist or wet dressings will promote wound drainage by ensuring that fluids do not get trapped inside the wound. Moisture prevents the formation of scabs and crusts, which usually occur if the wound is exposed to air. Liquid exudates are not thus blocked and will continue to escape into dressings in the postoperative period. This promotes normal mechanisms of wound healing by allowing drainage of harmful and necrotic material. Use of ointments or dressing material with ointment on wounds also reduces drying and crust formation. Ointments also prevent the dressing from adhering to the wound. Water-soluble ointments are preferred in comparison to oil-based ointments as oil molecules pool in wounds and act as foreign bodies, leading to slowing of wound healing.

Dressings Intended to Kill Bacteria

If the wound is expected to show a bacterial count of $>10^3$/g of tissue, a topical antibiotic ointment should be included in the dressing. Antibiotic ointment can be directly applied over the wound. Bacitracin is one such antibiotic which is well tolerated by living cells and seldom causes any tissue reaction. Neomycin or Furacin ointments may cause hypersensitivity reactions and should be used with caution.

Dressings to Splint the Wound

Many times dressings are applied to give rest to the body part during healing. Skin grafts require precise fixation and splinting during the first 7 days after surgery so that the graft can revascularize. Sudden displacement of the skin graft relative to the recipient bed during first few days will lead to disruption of revascularization from the graft bed, and the skin graft will fail to take up. Tie-on bolus dressing **(Fig. 2)** is one of the best

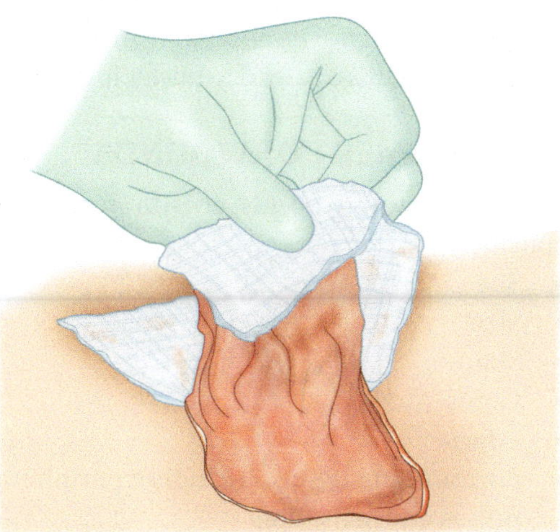

Fig. 1: Granulation tissue grows into coarse mesh and can cause renewed bleeding on removal.

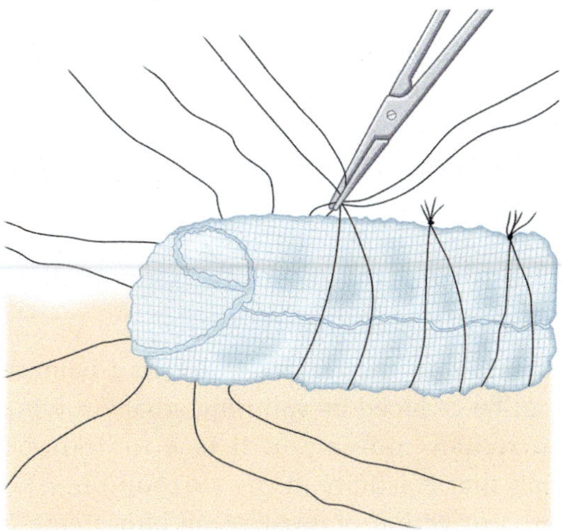

Fig. 2: Tie on bolus dressing.

methods to dress skin grafts. This technique is of paramount importance in areas where involuntary movement is bound to occur, e.g., eye lids, lips, fingers, and neck.

Splinting of One Structure to Protect Another Part

A dressing may also be used to position one part of the body so as to use that part to protect or splint another. An example of this is the use of a dressing to fix the upper eyelid in a closed position to protect the cornea from drying or injury in the postoperative period. To treat a fracture of the upper jaw, teeth in the nonfractured lower jaw are wired ("dressed") against those on both sides of the fracture in the upper jaw.

Splinting of Painful Joints or Muscles

When muscles or joints are inflamed as a result of trauma, immobilization by dressings may reduce discomfort and accelerate healing.

Dressings that Elevate a Body Part

Sometimes the function of the dressing is to simply elevate the part of the body above the heart to promote venous, capillary, or lymphatic return. The elevated part may be a lymphedematous or cellulitis limb. By elevating, the limb may benefit in the case of lymphedema, cellulitis, or deep venous thrombosis.

Dressings to Reduce Tension on Tissue in Healing Wounds

Tension on the tissues in healing wounds can be reduced by splinting adjacent joints to reduce movement. It is a well-known fact that elasticity of the surrounding skin or contraction of muscles on either side of a wound may work against the healing of the wound. These forces may even produce wound separation or dehiscence.

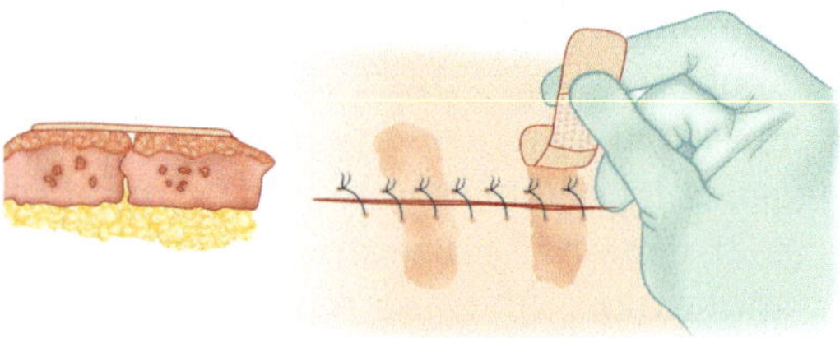

Fig. 3: Use of adhesive tapes to reduce tension on wounds.

External dressings or support may reduce such tension and reduce the chances retarding wound healing. The following methods are used as antitension dressings:

- *Adhesive skin tapes* ***(Fig. 3)****:* Adhesive skin tapes are the most commonly used method for antitension dressing. These tapes can be porous, impermeable, rigid, or elastic. Porous tapes have the advantage that they permit drainage of serum and blood through pores. Tapes are used commonly to support a row of interrupted skin sutures, e.g., in thyroid surgery.
- *Elastic strip:* Elastic strip can expand to some extent if there is edema of the tissues in wound after 2–3 days. Elastic tapes should not be applied with excessive tension as this can lead to blister formation.

ASSESSMENT OF WOUNDS

When assessing wounds, it is important to consider:

- Site
- Size
- Shape
- Depth
- Edges
- Surrounding tissues including peripheral pulses and sensation
- Base-slough, eschar, necrotic tissue, and granulation tissue

- Malignant change in a chronic ulcer (Marjolin's ulcer).

Microbiology swabs should be sent regularly. The presence of pathological organisms does not necessitate antibiotic treatment unless there is cellulitis or systemic sepsis. Regular dressing changes and debridement prevent bacterial counts from rising.

Necrotic Tissue

Necrotic tissue is devitalized or dead tissue. It is important to debride necrotic tissue to prevent infection and enhance healing.

Slough

Slough is a mixture of dead cells, fibrin, serous exudates, white blood cells, and bacteria. Sloughed wounds correspond to the proliferative stage of wound healing, and it is important to encourage formation of granulation tissue. Large quantities of exudates can macerate surrounding tissues. If large volumes of exudate are present, then an absorbent dressing is required. If the wound is dry, a dressing that retains moisture should be used.

Granulation Tissue

Granulation tissue is very vascular, resulting in a bright red color. Dressings should be chosen according to the amount of exudates. Overgranulation prevents epithelialization and healing of the wound. It appears as prominent, friable pink tissue overgrowing the edge of the wound. It can be treated by application of a silver nitrate pencil.

Epithelialization

Epithelial cells within the basal layer duplicate and migrate across a wound. A low-adherence dressing should be used to avoid damage to these tissues. Dressing changes should be kept to a minimum, although it is important not to allow penetration of fluids through a dressing as this increases the risk of infection.

Exudates

Exudate contains leukocytes, enzymes, growth factors, and cytokines, all of which are vital in wound healing. There is evidence to suggest that keeping a wound moist with exudate encourages healing.

Principles of Wound Care

When treating any wound, it is necessary to consider:

- Nutrition status
- Pressure care
- Management of primary cause
- Drain sepsis/debride wound
- Treatment of cellulitis
- Cleaning the wound
- Promotion of healing
- Regular review by same group of individuals/team
- Documentation of progress.

Methods of Debridement

Autolytic

Autolytic debridement uses the body's ability to dissolve dead tissue. Dressings are used to enhance water retention in the wound, which traps enzymes, growth factors, and other factors involved in healing.

Surgical

Debridement of necrotic tissues can be carried out in the ward during dressing changes. This should not be painful provided there is minimal inflammation of the surrounding tissues. More extensive debridement may require regional or general anesthesia and must be performed in a theater.

Biological

Larval therapy involves the application of sterile larvae to the wound, where they selectively digest necrotic tissue.

Enzymatic

A pharmacologically developed version of collagenase has been developed that can aid digestion of necrotic tissue.

Mechanical

Mechanical debridement involves the application of saline soaked gauze to the wound. It is allowed to dry and is then removed the next day, removing with it the superficial layers of tissue.

TYPES OF DRESSING

Low Adherence

Low-adherent dressings are economical and widely available. They allow exudates to pass through into a secondary dressing while maintaining a moist wound bed. They are manufactured in different forms such as tulles, which are open weave cloth soaked in soft paraffin or chlorhexidine. Tulles may also be textiles, or plastic films, and may be multilayered or perforated. They do not adhere at the wound bed and are particularly useful for patients with sensitive or fragile skin. Adherent dressings allow easy removal without damaging the wound or surrounding tissues. Examples of this type of dressing are Jelonet or Mepitel.

Semipermeable

These dressings are permeable to gas and water vapor but not to fluids or bacteria. The moisture and vapor transmission rate of such dressings depend on the brand, and it is through this mechanism that the dressing creates a moist wound environment. These dressings are used in clean, dry wounds or in wounds with minimal exudates. They are made of sheets of polyurethane coated with hypoallergenic acrylic adhesive and are primarily used as a transparent primary wound cover. They are flexible and are ideal for wounds on "difficult" anatomical sites—for example, over joints. They are not suitable for wounds with large amounts of exudate and may result in maceration of the skin surrounding the wound bed if they are used injudiciously. Examples include Bioclusive, Mefilm, OpSite, OpSite Plus, and Tegaderm. Opsite spray is a transparent film dressing spray, which is permeable to gas and water vapor, but water resistant. It is used on areas where a dressing is unlikely to adhere, e.g., flexible areas such as fingers or scalp.

Foam

Foam dressings are manufactured as either a polyurethane or silicone foam. They transmit water vapor and oxygen and provide thermal insulation to the wound bed. Polyurethane foams consist of two or three layers, including a hydrophilic wound contact surface, which can absorb large volumes of exudate preventing leakage onto surrounding skin. There is usually a hydrophobic or semipermeable backing. Allevyn and Lyofoam are examples of this class. Polyurethane foam dressings are also available as a cavity dressing—small chips of hydrophilic polyurethane foam enclosed in a membrane of perforated polymeric film, giving a loosely filled bag. Silicone foams consist of a polymer of silicone elastomer derived from two liquids, which, when mixed together, form a foam while expanding to fit the wound shape forming a soft open-cell foam dressing. The major advantage of foam is the ability to contain exudate. In addition, silicone foam dressings protect the area around the wound from further damage.

Hydrocolloid

Sodium carboxymethyl cellulose, gelatin, pectin, elastomers, and adhesives are bonded to a carrier of semipermeable film or a foam sheet to produce a flat, occlusive adhesive dressing that forms a gel on the wound surface, promoting moist wound healing. Cross-linkage of the materials used influences the viscosity of the gel under the dressing. This gel, which may be yellow and malodorous, may be mistaken for infection by the uninformed. Hydrocolloids are virtually impermeable to water vapor and air and can be used to rehydrate dry necrotic eschar and promote autolytic debridement. They are reported to reduce wound pain, and their barrier properties allow the patient to bath or shower and continue with normal daily activities without disturbing or risking contamination of the wound. Caution should be exercised when using hydrocolloids for wounds that require frequent inspection—for example, for diabetic foot ulcers. Hydrocolloid fibers are now available in the form of hydrophilic, nonwoven flat sheets, referred to as hydrofiber dressings. On contact with exudate, fibers are converted from a dry dressing to a soft coherent gel sheet, making them suitable for wounds with a large amount of exudate. Hydrocolloids contain gel forming agents and form a gel on contact with exudate. They are used for absorbing mild-to-moderate amounts of exudate and promoting autolysis. They are initially impermeable to exudate and bacteria. However, as the gelling process occurs, they become increasingly permeable to exudate. Aquacel, Tegasorb, and Granuflex are examples of this class.

Hydrogel

Hydrogels comprise of a matrix of insoluble polymers with up to 96% water content enabling them to release water molecules to the wound surface and hence maintain a moist environment at the wound bed. The hydrogels have also the ability to absorb a degree of wound exudate, the amount varying between different brands. They transfer water vapor and oxygen, but their bacterial and fluid permeability is dependent on the type of secondary dressing used. Hydrogels promote wound debridement by rehydration of nonviable tissue, thus facilitating the process of natural autolysis. Amorphous hydrogels are the most commonly used and are thick, viscous gels. Hydrogels are considered to be a standard form of management for necrotic wounds with slough. They are not indicated in wounds with high levels of exudate or if there is evidence of gangrenous tissue, which should be kept dry to reduce the risk of infection. They are water or glycerine-based products and therefore are gel-like in consistency. They are used in cavities to promote autolysis of tissues in necrotic wounds. In dry wounds, they are used to provide a moist environment; however, they can macerate surrounding normal tissue. These dressings are not used for exudative wounds as they exhibit poor absorption of exudate. They are nonadherent. Examples include Aquaform, Intrasite, GranuGel, Nu-Gel, Purilon, and Sterigel.

Antimicrobial

Silver, in either ionic or nanocrystalline form, has been used as an antimicrobial agent particularly in the treatment of burns (in the form of silver sulfadiazine cream). The recent introduction of dressings impregnated with silver has widened its use for many other wound types, e.g., colonized or infected. Iodine which has the ability to lower the microbiological load in chronic wounds is mainly in one of two formats: (1) As povidone-iodine (polyvinylpyrrolidone-iodine complex), an iodophor (a compound of iodine linked to a nonionic surfactant), which is produced as impregnated tulle; and (2) as cadexomer iodine (a three-dimensional starch lattice containing 0.9% iodine). Cadexomer iodine has good absorptive properties: 1 g of cadexomer iodine can absorb up to 7 mL of fluid. As fluid is absorbed, iodine is slowly released, reducing the bacterial load and also debriding the wound of debris. This mode of action facilitates the delivery of iodine over a prolonged period of time, thus, in theory, maintaining a constant level of iodine in the wound bed. It should be used with caution in patients with a thyroid disease because of possibility systemic absorption of iodine. The thyroid function should be monitored in patients who are treated with iodine dressings. Metronidazole gel is often used for the control of odor caused by anaerobic bacteria. This is particularly useful in the management of fungating malignant wounds. It may be used alone or as an adjunct to other dressings. Antimicrobial aims to reduce bacterial load. However, if a wound is overtly infected, they will not convert it to a clean wound.

Capillary

Capillary dressings consist of a sandwich foam dressing that is highly absorbent and is therefore used for wounds with large amounts of exudate. These dressings damage dry wounds.

Alginate

Alginates are natural products derived from calcium and sodium salts of alginic acid seen in a family of brown seaweed (Phaeophyceae). They are broadly of two types: one containing 100% calcium alginate, and the other a combination of calcium with sodium alginate, usually in a ratio of 80:20. Alginates contain high contents of mannuronic acid or guluronic acid, the content of each determining the amount of exudate absorbed and the shape the dressing will retain. Alginates form a hydrophilic gel as a result of the exchange of sodium ions in wound fluid for calcium ions in the dressing as they partly dissolve on contact with wound fluid. Alginates high in mannuronic acid (as seen in Kaltostat) can be washed off the wound easily with saline, but those with high in guluronic acid (such as Sorbsan) tend to retain their basic structure and should be removed from the wound bed in one piece. They can absorb fluid 15–20 times of their weight, making them suitable for highly exuding wounds. They are contraindicated on wounds with little or no exudate as they will adhere to the healing wound surface, causing pain and damaging healthy tissue on removal. They are useful for dressing cavities. A secondary covering dressing is required. Examples include Algisite, Kaltostat, SeaSorb, Sorbsan, Tegagen, and Urgosorb.

Gauze

It is used as a secondary dressing, often on top of low adherence/hydrocolloid dressings to absorb exudates. It is also used on top of semipermeable dressings to provide pressure, reducing the risk of hematoma formation. They should not be applied directly to the wound as they will stick, damaging tissue when removed.

Waterproof

Waterproof dressings are permeable to gas but not to water vapor, fluids, or bacteria. Therefore, they maintain a moist wound environment and so can lead to maceration. They are used over surgical wounds where there is a high risk of infection due to wound position (for example, over a laparotomy wound next to a stoma). Elastoplast is a waterproof dressing.

Vacuum-assisted Closure Device

The vacuum-assisted closure (VAC) pump applies low negative pressure to draw excess fluid from the wound, promote granulation tissue, aid wound contraction, and reduce bacterial counts. A polyurethane foam dressing is cut to size and applied to the wound. The suction device is embedded within this and an adhesive, impermeable drape covers the wound and overlaps normal skin. The setup allows equal pressure to be applied across the whole wound. The evacuation tube is connected to an external canister in which the fluid is collected. These devices can be used on an outpatient basis but can also be effective in large wounds such as laparostomy.

Examples of Dressings in Various Common Clinical Scenarios

Necrotic Wound—Pressure Sore

The dead tissue in necrotic wounds loses moisture rapidly and so often becomes hard and dry to touch. In order for healing to occur, this hard dead tissue must first be removed, either by surgical debridement, or by rehydrating the tissue, thereby promoting autolysis. Typically a hydrogel, such as Intrasite, is applied to the necrotic areas. A barrier cream is used on the edges to prevent maceration of the surrounding tissue. The area is then covered with a semipermeable dressing and reinspected every 24 hours.

Sloughy Wound—Ulcer

The presence of a thick layer of slough predisposes to wound infection. Therefore, slough should be removed to promote healing, either by mechanical, biological, or surgical debridement. Typically a hydrocolloid dressing is applied to promote autolysis and absorb exudates. For highly exudative wounds, an alginate may be used. Gauze is then applied as a secondary dressing.

Granulation Tissue

For granulating wounds, a low-adherence dressing is used to prevent damage to the delicate tissue. A secondary dressing such as hydrocolloid/alginate is used to absorb exudates. Gauze is then applied to absorb any excess exudate.

Unwanted Effects of Dressings

Maceration of the skin surrounding a wound may occur if a less absorptive dressing is used on a heavily discharging wound. If the dressing is highly absorptive, then more frequent dressing changes may be required.

The skin surrounding a wound with large amount of discharge may be further protected through the use of emollients or the application of barrier films. The use of a highly absorptive dressing on a dry wound may lead to disruption of healthy tissue on the wound surface and cause pain when removed. Allergic reactions are known to occur. If allergic reaction occurs, the dressing should be avoided, and the allergy should be treated with potent topical steroids. Tapes used to keep dressings in place are common causes of allergy.

KEY POINTS

- Dressing is both an art and skill.
- Properly chosen dressing accelerates healing.
- Ideal dressing should protect wound from trauma and infection, be nonallergic, allow oxygenation of the wound and should retain moisture.
- A variety of dressings are available, and one should choose according to the requirement of the wound.

CHAPTER 21

Basics of Staplers and Lasers in Surgery

Mrunal Bharat Kshirsagar, Sudhir Kumar Jain

"Technology is not a substitute for fine surgical skills"

INTRODUCTION

Stapling devices have become increasingly prevalent and efficient in soft tissue surgery, promising improved patient outcomes by reducing complications and surgery duration. The primary focus is on identifying and assessing the most commonly used and innovative stapling devices, such as linear, linear cutting, circular, and powered staplers. Additionally, it explores the emerging field of bioabsorbable staples, examining the materials used and their applications in surgery. To enhance understanding, the information gathered is presented in tables, highlighting key parameters for each stapling device. This thorough research on stapling devices aims to assist healthcare practitioners and researchers in making well-informed decisions when selecting the most suitable instrument for specific surgical procedures.

This chapter discusses surgical staplers, which are utilized internally during surgeries to deliver staples to tissues within the body. These staplers are used for various purposes, including removing portions of organs, cutting through and sealing organs, and creating connections between structures. Modern surgical staplers are typically disposable and have a predetermined maximum number of firing actions. They utilize cartridges and other associated products for surgical stapling. The staples used today have a rectangular cross-section and take on a "B" shape when compressed against the anvil of the stapler. This design minimizes the risk of ischemia by allowing blood to flow through them to the tissue edges, promoting adequate vascularization and supporting wound healing.

There are three primary types of stapling devices commonly employed in both open and laparoscopic surgery: linear, linear cutting, and circular. Linear instruments form a straight staple line and may or may not incorporate a blade, while circular instruments have staples arranged in a circular pattern and always include a blade. The increasing adoption of laparoscopy and robotic surgery has led to the development of stapling devices tailored for endoscopic techniques. Linear and circular stapling devices are predominantly used in gastrointestinal procedures such as complex gastrectomies, bariatric treatments, and colorectal oncological resections.

HISTORY

The history of surgical staplers began nearly a century ago with Hümér Hültl, a Hungarian physician often hailed as the "father of

TABLE 1: History of surgical staplers.

Year	*Development/event*
1959	Publication of pivotal article on surgical stapling
1907	Frenchman Jean-Nel pioneers use of metal staples
1908	Hungarian surgeon Humer Halti constructs first stapler
1921	Surgeon Aladar Petz presents improved stapler model
1945	Soviet engineer Vasiliy Gudov designs first vascular stapler
1951	Establishment of scientific research institute in Moscow
1967	Introduction of first American surgical stapler (TA)
Late 50s to early 60s	Western surgeons introduced to surgical staplers
1983	Soviet production of surgical staplers declines

(TA: transverse anastomosis)

surgical staples". In 1908, he developed the first-ever prototype, weighing approximately 8 pounds. This early model required extensive time for assembly and loading, making the dispensing process arduous and cumbersome for physicians. The most significant technological advancements enhancing stapler performance emerged prominently from the 1970s onward **(Table 1)**.

PROPERTIES OF STAPLES

Properties of staples are mentioned in **Figs. 1A to C**.

DIFFERENT TYPES OF STAPLERS

Depending on Material

Tables 2 and 3 show the different types of material-based staplers.

Based upon the staple architecture/design:

Linear Stapler

This device is a surgical device with control buttons on the handle to prevent accidental firing. It typically features a retention pin or lever for manual or automatic actuation. The device includes buttons for aligning the cartridge, positioning tissue, and opening jaws for tissue release and reloading after the operation **(Fig. 2)**.

Linear Cutting Stapler

This device features a sliding knob for activation, aligning and firing the blade simultaneously with stapling. The cutting line is intentionally shorter for safety. A release button disengages the cartridge after firing, and a safety tag covers the blade to prevent accidental firing during reloading **(Fig. 3)**.

Linear Endo Stapler

This device has an articulating end effector attached through a rotating locking system. After correct alignment, the handle is pushed to close jaws over tissue. A side button unlocks the firing mechanism, and continuous handle pressure delivers staples while the blade moves forward, gradually compressing and cutting the tissue **(Fig. 4)**.

Circular Stapler

This device consists of a detachable anvil and a handling part with a trocar for the cartridge, cutting element, rotary knob for jaw control, and an operating handle. The process involves opening the rotary knob to extract the anvil, detaching it for tissue insertion, and then assembling it with the cartridge by rotating the knob until an indicator confirms sufficient tissue compression **(Fig. 5)**.

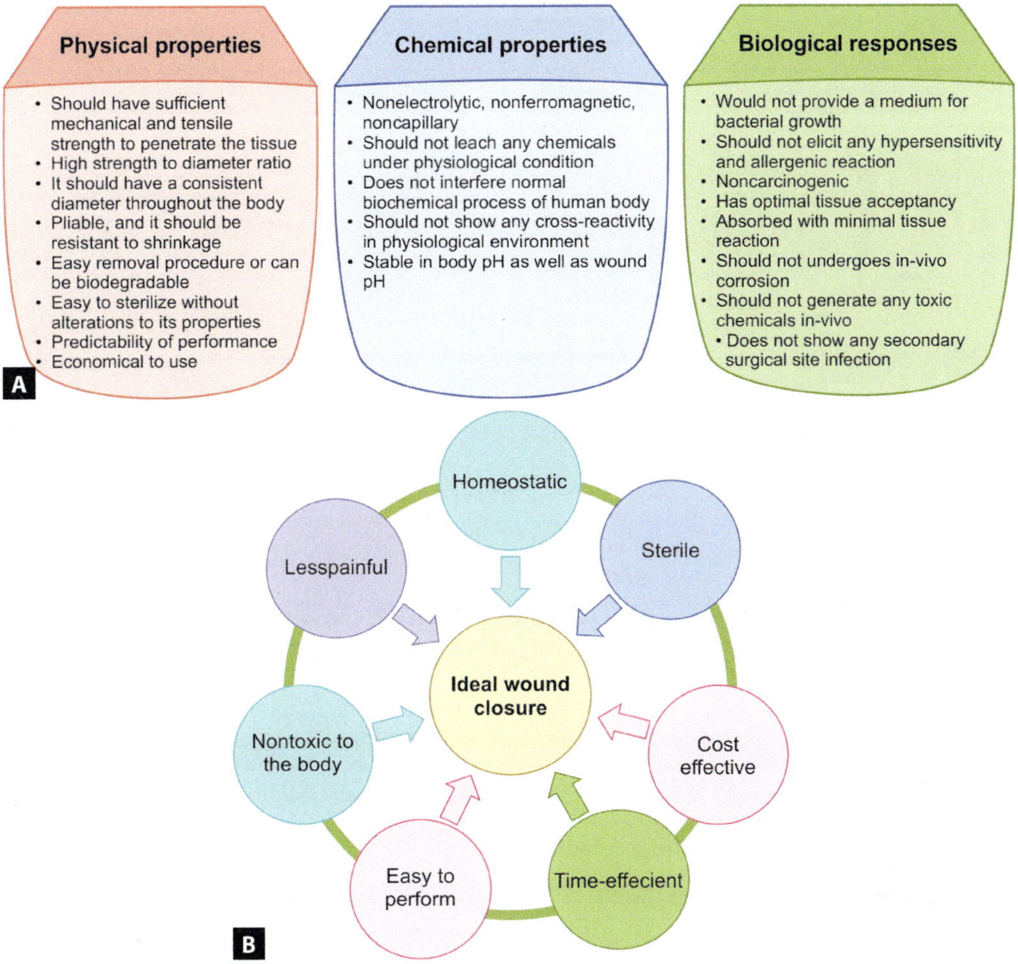

Figs. 1A and B

Powered Stapler

This device features battery-driven actuation, eliminating manual control. The firing mechanism is powered by a battery, operating an electromechanical system that controls the cutting element and the cartridge **(Fig. 6)** **(Table 4)**.

DIMENSIONS OF COMMONLY AVAILABLE CARTRIDGES IN STAPLER (TABLE 5)

LASER is an acronym that stands for *Light Amplification by Stimulated Emission of Radiation.* Albert Einstein published the theoretical basis for the laser in 1917. It was only in 1960 that the first functioning laser was constructed by Theodore Maiman in California, using a ruby crystal to produce laser light. Laser is a light made up of monochromatic (one color or wavelength), coherent, parallel photons moving in the same direction, which potentiates the amount of energy carried by it compared to white light. The wavelength and power output of the laser determine its application in terms of cutting, vaporizing, or sealing

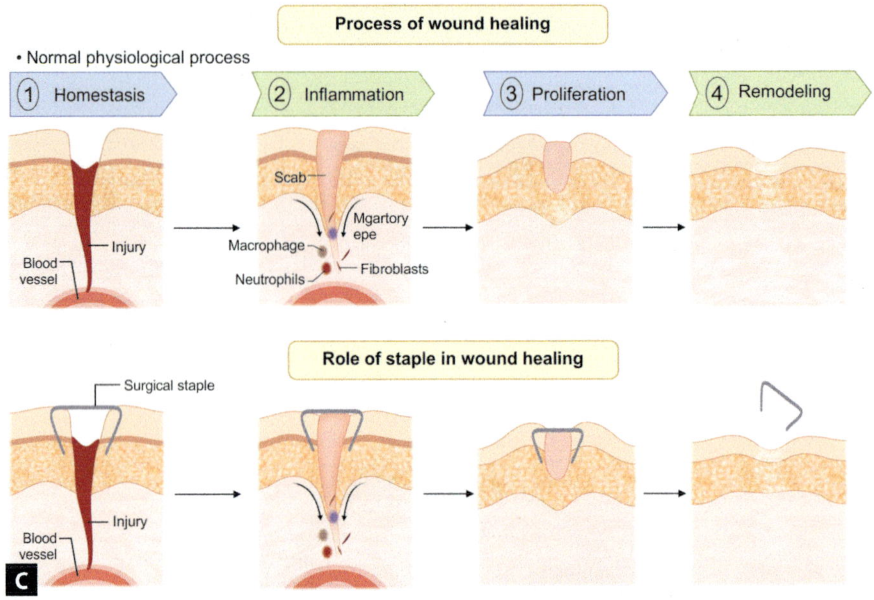

Figs. 1A to C: (A) Some ideal characteristics of surgical staples; (B) Common gold standards of the ideal wound closure system; (C) Pathophysiological role of surgical staples in the wound healing process.

TABLE 2: Some Mg-based wound closing materials with their applications.

Sl. No.	*Material (Mg-based)*	*Application in wound closing*	*Proved in the model*
1.	Mg with high purity	As wire, sheets, and tubes	Human, guinea pig, and rabbit
2.	Pure Mg, mix. of eq. part: Mg/Al, Mg/Cd, and Mg/Zn Seelig	As clips, wires, as a ligature in the anastomosis	Dogs
3.	AZ91E Mg alloy coated with graphene oxide nanoparticles-polythreonine	As staple in gastrectomy application	In vitro proven no. of reported deaths
4.	Mg–2.5 wt%, Nd–1 wt% Y, and FAsorbMg™	As a staple in intestinal anastomosis	Pig
5.	High-purity Mg	As a staple in the gastric anastomosis	Pig
6.	Mg–Cd	Screws, rod-plate	Humans

tissues. These three properties of laser light, i.e., monochromaticity, in directionality and coherence make them more hazardous than ordinary light, as laser light can deposit focused energy within a small area. The device produces a beam of coherent light with a specific wavelength in the infrared, visible, or ultraviolet regions of the electromagnetic spectrum. The aim of this chapter is to outline the basic fundamentals of laser and the precautions which should be observed during its use.

TABLE 3: Comparisons of different potential materials concerning some critical aspects for staple application.

Parameters	***Mg based***	***Zn based***	***Polymer based***
Mechanical features:			
Fabricated alloys or composites	Pure Mg, $MgNd_2$, Mg/Al, Mg/Cd, Mg/Zn	Zn–5Ge, Zn-Fe, Zn–1Cu-0.1Ti, Zn-Mg	PLA, PGA, PLGA, polyglactin, polydioxanone, polyglytone, and polyglyconate
Yield strength	80–220 MPa	<150–290 MPa	*Bulk:* 10–75 MPa (varies with polymer types)
Ultimate tensile strength	200–550 MPa	150–386 MPa	224–1,380 MPa (for suturing purpose)
Young's modulus	45 GPa	For pure Zn-94 GPa, for Zn-alloys-100–110 GPa	0.4–7 GPa
% of elongation	5–30%	1–20.5%	42–144%
Biodegradability/biocompatibility characteristics:			
Maximum consumption level (daily)	375–450 mg	6.5–10 mg	–
Presence of trace elements	Yes	Yes	No
Adverse events/side effects	–	This leads to copper deficiency	Adverse tissue reaction such as inflammation and aneurysm
In vivo corrosion behavior:			
Corrosion process/ pathway	Site-specific or localized	Site-specific or localized	Enzymatic or hydrolysis
Rate of corrosion	0.25–0.38 mm/year	0.05–0.1 mm/year	1->24 months
Production of gaseous component	Hydrogen gas production	No	No

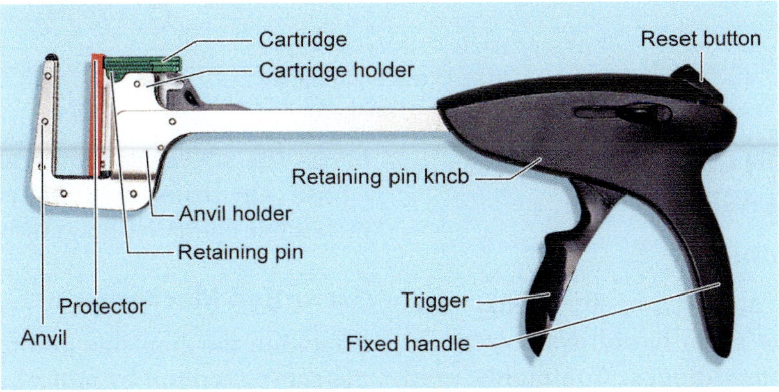

Fig. 2: Linear stapler.

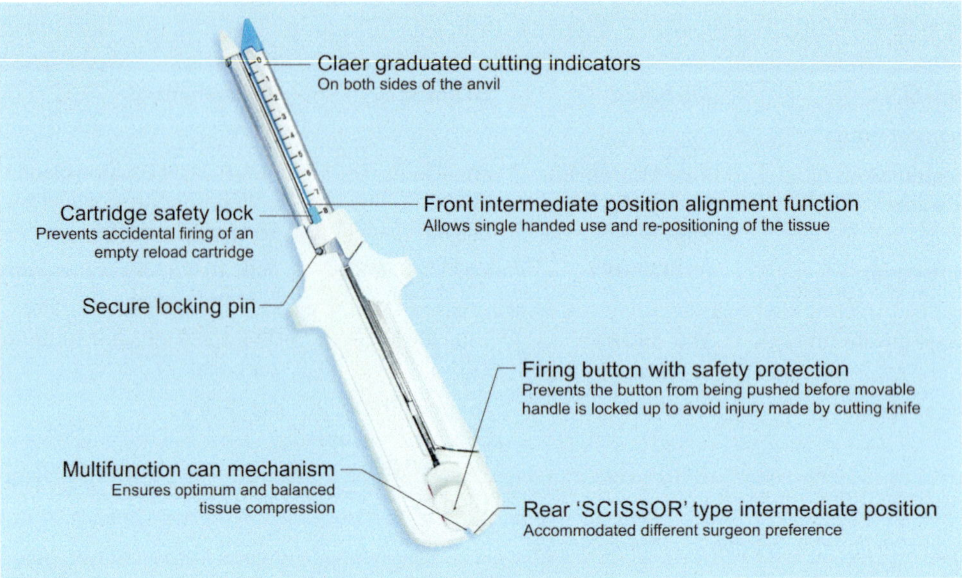

Fig. 3: Linear cutting stapler.

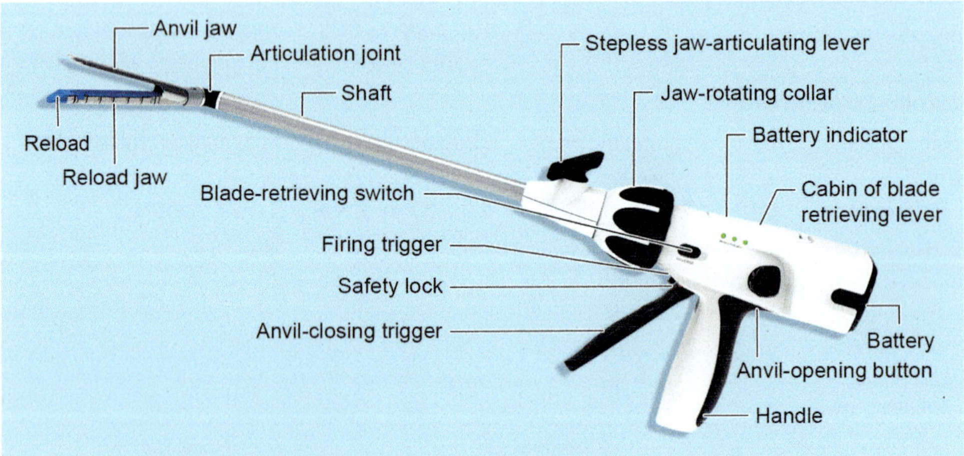

Fig. 4: Linear endo stapler.

COMMON COMPONENTS OF ALL LASERS

Active Medium

The active media may be solid state, tunable solid state, liquid dyes, gases, or semiconductors/diodes. Commonly used media are Ruby, Nd:YAG, CO_2, or helium/neon. The active medium contains atoms whose electrons may be excited to a metastable energy level by an energy source.

Excitation Mechanism

Excitation mechanisms pump energy into the active medium by optical, electrical, or chemical methods.

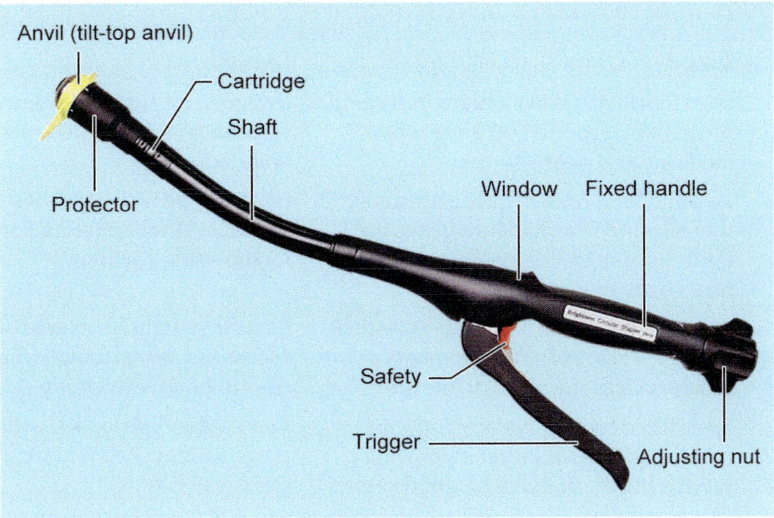

Fig. 5: Circular stapler.

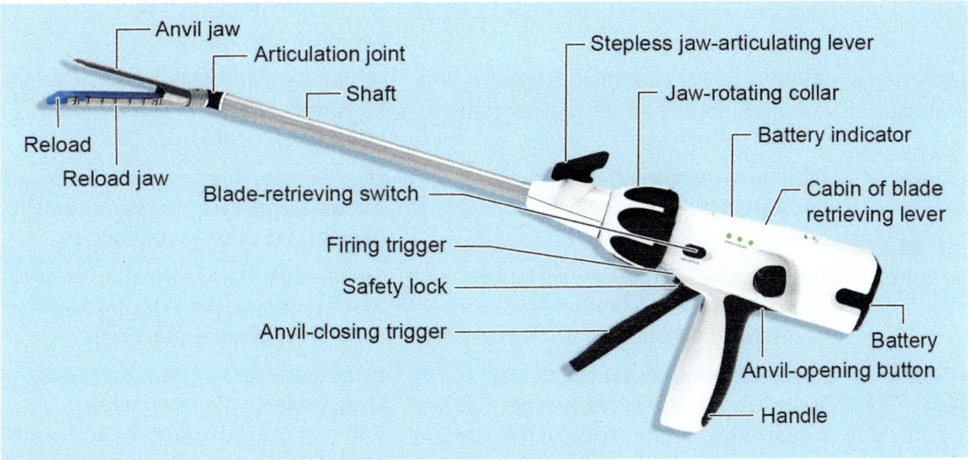

Fig. 6: Powered stapler.

High Reflectance Mirror

This is a mirror which essentially reflects 100% of the laser light.

Partially Transmissive Mirror

This is a mirror which reflects less than 100% of the laser light and transmits the remainder.

The earliest use of laser in medical treatment dates back to 1961 when the first solid state (Nd:YAG) and gaseous state (based on helium and neon) lasers were developed. Consequently, argon and the carbon dioxide lasers were developed within a span of 2 more years. Coumarin and Ruby lasers were some of the earlier lasers to be used in

TABLE 4: Types of staplers and their features and uses.

Stapler type	*Uses*	*Features*
Skin staplers	Used for closing skin incisions in surgical procedures, especially in emergency medicine and plastic surgery	Designed for superficial skin closure. Disposable, single-use devices with small, fine staples
Linear staplers	Versatile tools used in gastrointestinal, thoracic, and abdominal surgeries for creating straight-line staples and cutting tissue simultaneously	Linear shape with a row of staples. Available in various sizes. Some allow for multiple firing actions
Circular staplers	Crucial in colorectal and gastrointestinal surgeries for joining two segments of tissue, such as the colon or intestines	Circular, doughnut-shaped design for secure tissue anastomosis. Commonly used in bowel resections
Endo GIA staplers	Specialized tools for laparoscopic and minimally invasive surgeries, providing precise closure of tissue or blood vessels	Compatible with laparoscopic access ports. Various shaft lengths and staple sizes available
Thoraco-abdominal staplers	Used in thoracic and abdominal surgeries, reaching deep tissues and creating secure staples in challenging locations	Long, slender shaft for deep tissue access. Some models have articulating heads for better maneuverability
Hemorrhoidal staplers	Used in treating hemorrhoids by stapling and removing excess hemorrhoidal tissue	Rectal or anal access design for precise placement of staples. Effective in treating hemorrhoidal disease
Multifunctional surgical staplers	Versatile devices combining stapling and cutting functions for general surgeries	Single-use or reusable options. Designed for abdominal, thoracic, and gastro-intestinal surgeries
Reloadable staplers	Commonly used in open surgeries, reloadable for multiple uses	Durable, reusable design compatible with various staple cartridge sizes. Used in general and colorectal surgeries
Linear cutter staplers	Designed for creating linear staples and cutting tissue, commonly used in gastrointestinal and bariatric surgeries	Straight-line staple formation for precise tissue cutting. Used in gastric bypass surgery and bowel resections
Skin Closure Staplers	Specialized devices for plastic and reconstructive surgeries, precisely closing incisions in delicate areas such as the face	Fine staples for cosmetic purposes. Disposable, single-use devices. Commonly used in facelifts and eyelid surgery
Vascular staplers	Used in cardiovascular and vascular surgeries for creating secure anastomoses between blood vessels	Delicate, fine staples for vascular tissues. Commonly used in CABG and vascular reconstruction
Powered surgical staplers	Advanced devices using electrical or mechanical power for stapling, reducing manual effort during surgeries	Enhanced control and precision. Commonly used in laparoscopic, thoracic, and gastrointestinal surgeries
Curved staplers	Designed for minimally invasive surgeries, allowing access and stapling in tight spaces	Curved shaft for improved access. Precise tissue stapling and cutting. Commonly used in bariatric and colorectal procedures

(CABG: coronary artery bypass grafting; GIA: gastrointestinal anastomosis)

TABLE 5: Color, open, and closed height of the cartridges used in stapler.

Color	Rows	Tissue type	Open staple height	Closed staple height
Gray	6	Mesentery	2.0 mm	0.75 mm
White	6	Vascular	2.5 mm	1.0 mm
Blue	6	Standard	3.5 mm	1.5 mm
Gold	6	Standard/thick	3.8 mm	1.8 mm
Green	6	Thick	4.1 mm	2.0 mm

medicine and have been replaced in the modern era by more efficient and flexible lasers with higher peak power.

Lasers exert their effect in various ways depending on their unique properties. Of these the photothermal and photoablative effects are the most commonly exploited properties in the field of surgery. When used in delicate areas such as blood vessels or mucosa, the laser can cause ablation of tissue, which can be precisely controlled. This is often referred to as the photoablative effect. Lasers can also exert a photothermal effect, which can be exploited for coagulation and vaporization of stones as commonly used in the genitourinary system. Stones can also be broken by using the photomechanical effect of laser, which has been incorporated in intracorporeal intraluminal laser systems. Another important property is the photodynamic or photochemical effect wherein preferentially larger amounts of laser energy is focused on tissues which uptake photochemical substances. Such tissues include tumors. Short duration pulse lasers can also exert a photoacoustic effect which can be used for management of stones.

Lasers can be used in various modes:

- *Continuous mode:* In this mode, the laser is produced and directed continuously with a low-power output varying from 1,000 to 5,000 W.
- *Pulsed mode:* In the pulsed mode, short duration peaks of laser are directed at a 100fold higher power.
- *Q switch mode:* Excited photons are directed suddenly producing a very high-power output.

MEDICAL LASERS

Medical lasers may be operated in continuous wave or pulsed wave modes. The continuous wave laser's output is measured in watts, and for pulsed lasers, the output is measured in joules. Irradiance, or power density, refers to laser power per unit area (W/cm^2). Energy density (fluence) is irradiance multiplied by exposure time (J/cm^2). The interaction between the laser beam and the tissue is determined by the wavelength, power density, and exposure time. It is the monochromatic nature of laser light that is responsible for its selective effect on biological tissues. When the light comes into contact with the tissues, it can be transmitted, scattered, reflected, or absorbed. The laser light has to be absorbed by the tissue in order to exert biological effects. Examples of the main absorbing components in tissues are:

- *Water:* Absorbs infrared light
- *Hemoglobin:* Absorbs visible light, especially green
- *Melanin:* Absorbs visible and ultraviolet light.

The wavelength also determines the depth of penetration. As the wavelength decreases toward the ultraviolet spectrum, more scattering occurs, which limits the depth of penetration within the tissues. Hence, the argon laser is used for retinal surgery and portwine birthmarks. The Nd:YAG laser operates at the near infrared spectrum, which has a greater depth of penetration and is, therefore, used for the cutting and coagulation of tissue.

LASER AND TISSUE INTERACTION

A number of specific interactions can occur when laser light is delivered to tissue or any surface. If laser light is transmitted through material, there will no or very little absorption resulting in little or no thermal effect. A laser that is not transmitted through tissue is absorbed, resulting in heat energy production and thermal damage to tissues. Medical lasers work on principle of selective absorption, which targets a particular wavelength to a particular tissue or site such as hemoglobin in a blood vessel. So, by selecting a particular wavelength which is preferentially absorbed by a specific tissue, that structure can be targeted and leaving surrounding structures unaffected. Depending upon the rate of energy absorption, thermal energy (if rate of absorption is slow), or a shock wave (if rate of absorption is fast) is produced. The shock wave will result in explosive mechanical disruption. The amount of thermal energy produced depends upon length of exposure to the target structure. Hence by selecting a particular wavelength, fluence, and pulse duration, selective destruction of a particular target by laser is possible. This phenomenon is known as selective photothermolysis. Oxyhemoglobin absorbs light primarily in ultraviolet, green, and yellow regions of the spectrum. Melanin absorbs light in ultraviolet, infrared, and visible regions. In between 630 and 1100 nm melanin absorption is more than hemoglobin absorption, and penetration is deeper. Water and collagen absorb light in the region of infrared region.

Argon Beam Laser

The argon beam laser was developed in 1962 as a gaseous state laser and has been widely used for its photocoagulative ability. The laser breaks down the covalent bonds in protein molecules (photodissociation), resulting in nonthermal ablation.

Argon beam laser has a commonly used wavelength of 488 nm and falls in the blue green spectrum of light. Argon is rapidly absorbed by pigment such as melanin and hemoglobin, making it a suitable candidate for controlling bleeding. The argon plasma beam electrocoagulation system is used widely as an important method of coagulation, especially in dealing with vascular organs. Directed through an endoscope, this system can help ablate early cancers of the gastrointestinal tract and manage acute bleeding from the airways and the gut.

Argon gas, being inert and nontoxic, is the ideal gas for passing electrosurgical current. When current is introduced to a beam of argon laser, there is rapid ionization of the particles. This ionization takes place at much faster speeds than room air and can act as an effective surgical cautery by forming a link between the cautery and the tissue for transfer of energy.

Nd:YAG Laser

The wavelength of this laser is 1,064 nm and produces light in the infrared region. Since the wavelength in this region is invisible, a visible aiming beam is required to target tissues. The active medium in this laser is solid state and uses a crystal which is made up of the rare trivalent element neodymium (Nd) with yttrium aluminium garnet (YAG) ($Y_3Al_5O_{12}$). Nd:YAG laser took a long time to make its way into medical equipment. This laser has been used in various modes depending upon the characteristics needed. The high-power continuous wave operation is used in heavy duty cutting and exploits the thermal lensing phenomenon. The high-intensity Q-switched operation is more commonly employed in surgical lasers where high-power laser is fired in pulses. The Nd:YAG laser can also be used in single-mode operation.

Nd:YAG laser has a deep penetration of 5–6 mm from the point of contact. It offers excellent hemostasis and causes tumor ablation by coagulative necrosis. This laser has found application in most fields of surgery including ophthalmic surgery, management of endobronchial and other endoluminal tumors, skin lesions, ablation of thyroid, in management of stone disease, and prostate growth. It is commonly employed at a setting of 20–30 W.

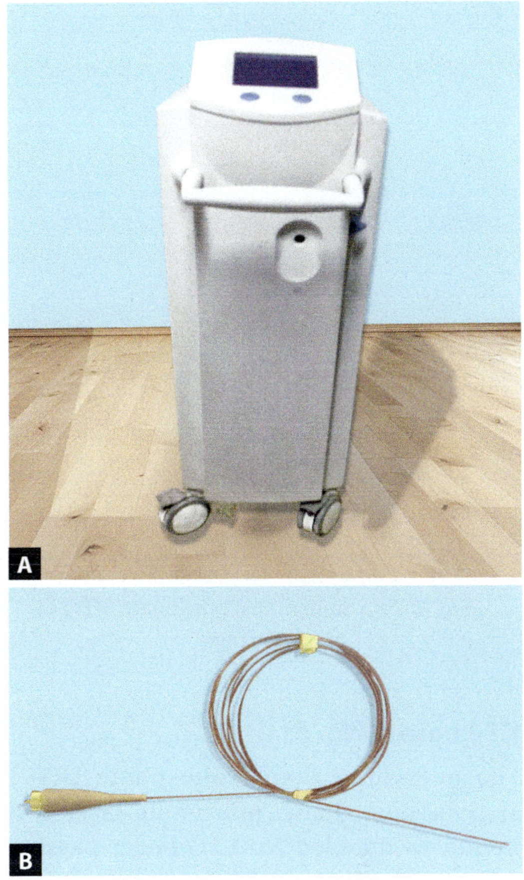

Figs. 7A and B: (A) Holmium laser machine; (B) Fiber of holmium laser.

Ho:YAG Laser (Figs. 7A and B)

The active medium of the Ho:YAG crystal laser is made up of aluminum, yttrium, and garnet doped with holmium. Holmium-based lasers have found their existence and application in surgical fields in recent times. This laser has a wavelength of 2,100 nm, positioning it in the near infrared spectrum of light. It is also a solid-state laser with minimal penetration in tissue, up to a distance of 0.5 mm. It is very well absorbed in water, making it relatively safer to use. In the Q-switched mode, the laser is used with pulse duration of 250–350 μs and a setting of 0.6–1.2 J at 8–10 Hz, which allows precise cutting and tumor ablation.

The laser is widely employed for procedures such as dacrorhinocystostomy and lithotripsy. The higher margin of safety has made this laser extremely popular among urologists, and its use is employed in vaporizing stones, cutting through strictures and ablating prostatic and bladder tissue. *There is a clinical concern regarding production of cyanide as a by-product of uric acid stone lithotripsy, but the risk is still undetermined and should be taken while using holmium laser for uric acid stones.*

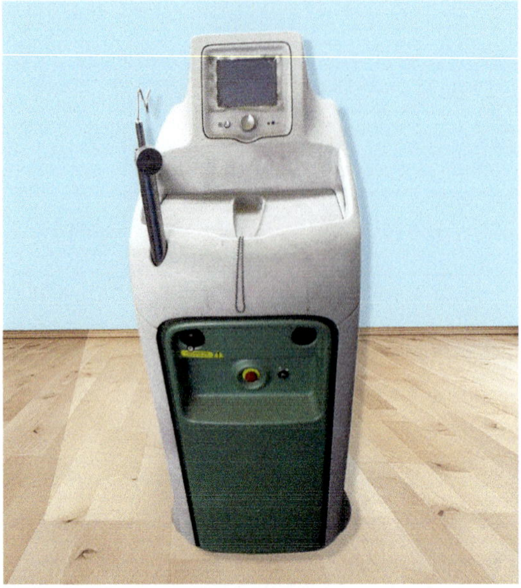

Fig. 8: Potassium titanyl phosphate (KTP) laser machine.

KTP Laser (Fig. 8)

The potassium titanyl phosphate (KTP) or potassium titanyl phosphate laser is a frequency doubled Nd:YAG beam passing through a KTP crystal. With a wavelength of 532 nm, this laser falls in the visible spectrum and emits green light. The light emitted by the KTP laser is absorbed mainly by hemoglobin, which is protective for the surrounding tissue due to vascular selectivity of this laser. KTP laser causes photo selective vaporization and desiccation of tissue and has been used in treating endoluminal growths, skin lesions, hypertrophy of the prostate, and ocular surgery. These lasers have a greater depth of penetration.

Diode Laser

The diode laser is produced by a pn type *(Comment—this needs explaining)* of linear array which provides flexibility and portability of use. It employs a small crystal over which substances such as indium gallium nitride or aluminum gallium arsenide are doped *(Comment—I think this means a thin layer added, but again doping needs to be explained)*. These lasers are, therefore, small and have found uses in various fields. Common wavelengths range from 300 to 3,000 nm depending upon the crystal used and the substance doped on the crystal. Diode lasers have a high gain, signifying that they are more efficient compared to other lasers. They can be used in continuous mode as well as in the pulsed mode. Diode lasers have been used for cosmetic surgery, superficial skin tumors, and early stage endoluminal lesions. Also, they are used in otorhinolaryngology, urology, and endovascular surgery.

Carbon Dioxide Laser

The carbon dioxide laser is a 10,600 nm laser that falls in the far infrared spectrum and requires visible aiming by a diode laser. It can be used in both continuous and short pulse mode and is considered the gold standard for ablative resurfacing. It can be used in several different gas combinations of CO_2 with helium and nitrogen. It provides more control over the depth of penetration and can be absorbed by both the intracellular and extracellular water to produce vaporization. The CO_2 laser is one of the earliest gaseous state lasers to be produced and is a major workhorse in dermatological resurfacing surgery.

Thulium Laser

The thulium laser is a continuous wave laser with a wavelength of 2,130 nm. The wavelength is similar to the holmium laser and is near the peak absorption of water, making it a good laser for enucleation of tissue. The depth of penetration is 0.25 nm owing to its slightly shorter wavelength. When used in high power of 50–100 W, it can act as a bleeding-free cutting tool, especially for the prostate due to its continuous nature.

Here are some of the various applications for laser in surgery:

- Resurfacing skin and management of keloids and hypertrophic scars
- Managementofcutaneousvascularlesions such as telangiectasias, hemangiomas, and venous malformations, various lakes, and angiomas
- Cosmetic applications such as resurfacing, dermatosis, photoepilation, pigmentation, and hypopigmentation
- Management of malignant and benign skin tumors and inflammatory conditions
- Management of varicose veins in the form of intravenous laser therapy (IVLT)
- Ophthalmic surgery of the cornea, uvea, vitreoretinal, and more
- Urological applications such as management of stones, benign prostatic hyperplasia (BPH), and strictures
- Coagulation in surgery of solid vascular viscera
- Photodynamic therapy
- Orthopedic arthroscopic surgery, meniscal surgery, disc compression, etc.
- Pulmonary and thoracic surgery
- Endoluminal management of polyps, varices, and strictures in gastroenterology

TYPES OF LASER HAZARD

- *Eye:* Acute exposure of the eye to lasers can lead to corneal or retinal burns. Chronic exposure to excessive levels may cause corneal injury, cataracts, or retinal injury.
- *Skin:* Acute exposure to high levels may cause skin burns, while carcinogenesis may occur for ultraviolet wavelengths (290–320 nm).
- *Chemical:* Some lasers require hazardous or toxic substances to operate (i.e., chemical dye and exciter lasers).
- *Electrical:* Most lasers utilize high voltages that can be lethal.
- *Fire:* The solvents used in dye lasers are flammable. High-voltage pulse or flash lamps may cause ignition. Flammable materials may be ignited by direct beams or specular reflections from high-power continuous wave (CW) infrared lasers.

Lasers and Eyes

Laser light in the visible to near infrared spectrum (i.e., 400–1,400 nm) can cause damage to the retina, resulting in scotoma (blind spot in the fovea). This wave band is also known as the "retinal hazard region". Laser light in the ultraviolet (290–400 nm) or far infrared (1400–10,600 nm) spectrum can cause damage to the cornea and/or to the lens. Photoacoustic retinal damage may be associated with an audible "pop" at the time of exposure. Visual disorientation due to retinal damage may not be apparent to the operator until considerable thermal damage has occurred.

Symptoms of Laser Eye Injuries

- Exposure to the invisible *carbon dioxide laser* beam (10,600 nm) can be detected by a burning pain at the site of exposure on the cornea or sclera.
- Exposure to a visible laser beam can be detected by a bright color flash of the emitted wavelength and an afterimage of its complementary color (e.g., a green 532 nm laser light would produce a green flash followed by a red afterimage). *The site of damage depends on the wavelength of the incident or reflected laser beam:* When the retina is affected, there may be difficulty in detecting blue or green color secondary

to cone damage, and pigmentation of the retina may be detected. Exposure to the *Q-switched Nd:YAG laser* beam (1,064 nm) is especially hazardous and may initially go undetected because the beam is invisible, and the retina lacks pain sensory nerves.

SKIN HAZARDS

Exposure of the skin to high-power laser beams can cause burns. Under 5 W, the heat produced from lasers will cause a flinch reflex, which is a sensation similar to touching any hot object in which one tends to pull one's hand away or drop an object before any major damage occurs. These burns can be quite painful as the affected skin can be cooked and forms a hard lesion that takes considerable time to heal.

Ultraviolet laser wavelengths may also lead to skin carcinogenesis.

Chemical Hazards

Some materials used in lasers [i.e., excimer *(Comment—this has not been mentioned before—what is it?)*, dye, and chemical lasers] may be hazardous and/or contain toxic substances. In addition, laserinduced reactions can release hazardous particulate and gaseous products.

Electrical Hazards

Lethal electrical hazards may be present in all lasers, particularly in highpower laser systems.

Secondary Hazards

- Cryogenic coolant hazards
- Excessive noise from very high energy lasers
- Explosions from faulty optical pumps and lamps
- Fire hazards.

LASER SAFETY STANDARDS AND HAZARD CLASSIFICATION

- Lasers are classified by hazard potential based upon their optical emissions, and necessary control measures are determined by these classifications. In this manner, unnecessary restrictions are not placed on the use of many lasers which are engineered to assure safety.
- In the United States, laser classifications are based on American National Standards Institute (ANSI).

AMERICAN NATIONAL STANDARDS INSTITUTE CLASSIFICATIONS

- *Class 1* denotes laser or laser systems that do not pose a hazard under normal operating conditions.
- *Class 2* denotes lowpower visible lasers or laser systems, which do not normally present a hazard but may present some potential for hazard if viewed directly for extended periods of time.
- *Class 3a* denotes some lasers or laser systems having a *caution* label that normally would not injure the eye if viewed for only momentary periods (within the aversion response period) with the unaided eye but may present a greater hazard if viewed using collecting optics. Some Class 3a lasers have *danger* labels and are capable of exceeding permissible exposure levels. If operated with care, Class 3a lasers pose a low risk of injury.
- *Class 3b* denotes lasers or laser systems that can produce a hazard if viewed directly. Normally, Class 3b lasers will not produce a hazardous diffuse reflection.
- *Class 4* denotes lasers or laser systems that produce a hazard not only from reflections

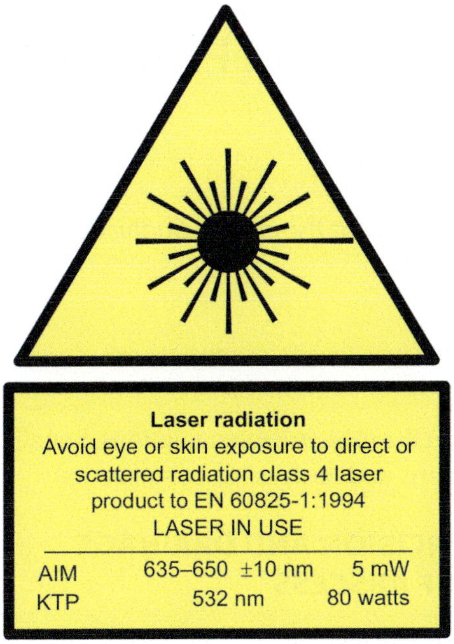

Fig.9: Display warning regarding laser safety precautions.

but may also carry significant skin and fire hazards.

General precautions while using lasers:

- Notification in the area where laser is used in the form of warning labels or signboards **(Fig. 9)**
- Safety goggles must be worn at all times to prevent ocular trauma.
- Keep the tip of the optical fiber visible at all times.
- Keep the laser in standby mode whenever the fiber is outside the patient's body or is not visible during that part of the procedure.
- Gentle handling of the optical fiber is necessary to prevent accidental breakage of the fiber within the scope, to prevent injury to both the patient and the scope.

LASER PROTECTIVE EYEWEAR REQUIREMENTS

- Laser protective eyewear should be worn by all personnel within the nominal hazard zone (NHZ) of Class 3b and Class 4 lasers where exposures above the maximum permissible exposure (MPE) could occur.
- Optical density of the laser protective eyewear at each laser wavelength should be notified by the laser safety officer (LSO).
- All laser protective eyewear should be clearly labeled with the optical density and the wavelength for which protection is afforded. This is especially important in areas where multiple lasers are housed.
- Laser protective eyewear should be inspected for damage prior to use.

KEY POINTS

- Lasers are commonly used in surgery.
- All persons using lasers should read the standard operating procedure (SOP) of that particular laser before using it.
- Laser operating areas should be clearly demarcated.
- All persons entering that area should use an appropriate eye protection device.
- There should be a laser safety officer to give appropriate training to the staff and to maintain the laser machine.

CHAPTER 22

Basic Surgical Procedures

Mrunal Bharat Kshirsagar, Sudhir Kumar Jain

"Mastering basic surgeries lay down good foundation for advance operations"

INTRODUCTION

Basic surgical procedures included in this chapter are:

- Incision and drainage of abscess
- Circumcision
- Intercostal chest tube drainage
- Hydrocele repair
- Open appendectomy
- Laparoscopic appendicectomy
- Open hernia repair
- Cholecystectomy
- Laparoscopic cholecystectomy.

Surgical procedures are an activity requiring careful preoperative work-up and dedicated postoperative monitoring. The preoperative work-up includes the following:

- Informed consent
- Marking the site to be operated
- Investigations for fitness of patient for anesthesia
- Specific investigations pertaining to that surgery.

INFORMED CONSENT

Informed consent is the consent given by the patient to undergo a treatment after being fully educated about the advantages and potential harm by the procedure. It should be specific for procedure, in the patient's language, taken by a surgeon competent to perform procedure. The patient must be explained about the other treatment options, benefits of surgery, and its possible complications.

INCISION AND DRAINAGE OF ABSCESS

Indications

General indication: All abscesses secondary to cellulitis and skin infections, which are not responding to oral/intravenous antibiotic coverage, generally require incision and drainage.

Steps of Procedure

1. *Preoperative preparations:*
    a. *Consent:* Obtain patient consent and mark the procedure site.
    b. *Antibiotics:* Consider if cellulitis is present.
    c. *Anesthesia:* Local or general anesthesia may be used.
2. *Positioning and theater setup:*
    a. Ensure optimal exposure of the abscess.
    b. Wear eye protection and have diathermy ready for hemostasis.
    c. Prepare skin for sterile field creation and appropriate draping.
    d. Conduct World Health Organization (WHO) knife check and inform the anesthetist before starting.

3. *Procedure:*
    a. Create a sterile field around the procedure area.
    b. Incise over the most fluctuant point of the abscess.
    c. Take pus swab for microscopy, culture, and sensitivity.
    d. Deroof the abscess, break loculations, curette the cavity, and irrigate with saline for hemostasis.
    e. Pack with normal saline and betadine soaked gauge dressing material.
    f. Apply gauze dressing ± surgipad.
4. *Postoperative care:*
    a. Patients can usually eat, drink, and go home the same day.
    b. No routine follow-up is necessary; wound care is managed by district or practice nurses until healing by secondary intention.
    c. Consider completing antibiotics if cellulitis was present.
5. *Postoperative complications:*
    a. Bleeding
    b. Infection
    c. Residual collection
6. *Tips and tricks:*
    a. Make a sufficient incision for effective drainage and easier packing by nurses.
    b. Always wear eye protection to avoid exposure to projectile pus.

DRAINAGE OF BREAST ABSCESS

Breast abscess, an acute, painful condition which may lead to breast destruction, is a surgical emergency and may discourage breastfeeding. Breast abscess usually results from bacterial mastitis caused by ascending infection by *Staphylococcus aureus*. Drainage or percutaneous needle aspiration is performed if:

- There is no response to antibiotics in 48 hours.
- There is persistence of an area of tense in duration after completely emptying the breast.
- Patient is presenting with area on the breast that is erythematous, warm, and fluctuant. Operation is performed under general anesthesia, but in case of small abscess, local anesthesia can be used.
- Patient lies supine, and part is cleaned draped.
- The incision is placed directly over abscess cavity in a radial direction. The abscess cavity is drained using a long sinus forceps.
- All loculi inside abscess cavity should be broken with the tip of sinus forceps or finger, to prevent any recurrence and to achieve complete drainage.
- Some large abscess can be drained through periareolar incision. Drain is placed in the abscess cavity in such cases and brought out through inframammary fold. Periareolar incision gives better cosmetic result and minimizes scarring. Drain is kept in place by fixing it by safety pin and removed only when drainage subsides.
- Large abscess cavity on the posterior aspect breast can be drained through an incision in the inframammary fold and a catheter is placed in abscess cavity.
- The cavity is thoroughly irrigated with saline and peroxide.
- The abscess cavity is loosely packed with ribbon gauze.
- A drain may be left in the dependent portion for drainage of abscess cavity.
- If the patient presents with extensive erythema of overlying skin, biopsy of the skin should be taken to exclude inflammatory breast cancer.

INTERCOSTAL CHEST TUBE DRAINAGE

Indications

- Empyema
- Hemothorax
- Pneumothorax involving more than 10% of the cavity
- Tension pneumothorax
- Recurrent pneumothorax after repeated aspiration
- Hydrothorax
- Surgeries with pleural violation

After taking an informed consent, the patient is made to lie in a supine position with the limb on the affected side in overhead abduction. The procedure is performed under local anesthesia.

Steps

1. Part is cleaned and draped.
2. The site for insertion is marked by counting the intercostal spaces from the sternal angle downward.
3. The site of insertion is marked in the triangle of safety which is bound by the lateral border of pectoralis major, the mid axillary line, and the upper border of the fifth rib.
4. Local anesthetic agent is infiltrated and allowed to act.
5. A transverse incision is made along the Langer's line in the site marked just above the lower rib of the intercostal space.
6. Incision is developed in layers using artery forceps. Muscles encountered are split till the pleura is reached.
7. The pleura is punctured using a hemostat under vision. Resistance is encountered on puncturing the pleura.
8. A finger is then introduced in the pleural cavity, and any loculus is broken.
9. A chest tube is introduced through the incision and directed toward the paravertebral gutter.
10. The chest tube is connected to an underwater seal bag, and the movement of fluid column is ensured.
11. Purse string sutures are applied after ensuring the adequate depth and position of the chest tube. A drain fixing suture is also employed to safeguard the chest tube.
12. A sterile dressing is applied around the chest tube, which secures the drain in position.
13. Patient is given clamping instructions and sent for a postdrainage chest radiograph.

CIRCUMCISION

Indications

- Phimosis
- Recurrent balanitis
- Balanitis xerotica obliterans
- Bowen's disease
- *Condyloma acuminata*
- Penile carcinoma confined to prepuce
- Paraphimosis
- Preputial trauma
- Social or religious
- Penile lymphedema.

Circumcision is contraindicated in defects of the penis or meatus and in bleeding disorders.

The procedure is performed under local anesthesia as an office procedure. It is also sometimes performed under general anesthesia.

Steps

1. Prepuce is completely retracted, and the glans is thoroughly cleaned.

2. A clean cut incision with a knife is made through the outer surface of the prepuce at the coronal sulcus down to the Buck's fascia.
3. A second incision is made 5 mm proximal to the coronal sulcus.
4. Hemostasis is secured, and the frenular artery is secured with a figure of 8 sutures.
5. The two layers are held together with the help of forceps.
6. Interrupted sutures of 3-0 chromic catgut are used to approximate the two incisions.
7. Soft paraffin gauze dressing is applied.

HYDROCELE REPAIR

Indications

- Large hydrocele causing difficulty in carrying out daily activities
- Hydrocele associated with symptoms of pain
- Difficulty in urination due to burying of penis in the hydrocele
- Concern with body image
- Hydrocele secondary to suspected malignancy
- Hydrocele prone to repeated trauma.

Surgery for hydrocele can be performed by either the inguinal or the scrotal approach. Scrotal approach is useful in benign hydrocele and is the most common approach utilized.

Steps

1. A vertical or transverse incision is made and developed up to the tunica vaginalis.
2. Blunt dissection is performed between the hydrocele sac and the incised layers of the scrotum.
3. Opening is made in the anterior wall of the parietal layer of the tunica, and the fluid is sucked out.
4. The opening in the tunica is extended both upward and downward.
5. If the sac is too large, a part of it is excised and hemostasis secured along the cut margins.
6. The sac is everted, and margins of the tunica are sutured using an absorbable catgut suture.
7. The suturing of the cut margins should be loose enough to permit a finger between the margin and cord structures.
8. The testis is returned back to the scrotum, and the scrotal wall is stitched in layers.
9. Alternative to the eversion of the sac is plication of the sac or the Lord's procedure wherein the hanging curtain of tunica after incision is plicated along the mediastinum of the testis using vicryl sutures. 8–10 sutures are applied all around the testis after which the complete unit is reposited back into the scrotum.
10. If bleeding is suspected or in cases of very large hydroceles where extensive blunt dissection is done, a corrugated drain may be placed through a separate stab incision.
11. Scrotal bandage is applied with mild compression to prevent the formation of hematoma and infection.

APPENDECTOMY

Appendicectomy is the most commonly performed emergency surgical operation around the world.

Indications

- Acute appendicitis is the most common indication for removing the appendix
- Interval appendicectomy, 6 weeks after the conservative management of appendicular lump

- Patients with recurrent attacks of subacute appendicitis previously known as chronic appendicitis in whom other causes of pain has been ruled out.
- Mucocele of appendix if detected during abdominal exploration for unrelated pathology.
- Diverticula containing appendix if detected during course of some other operation
- Appendix which is found to contain appendicoliths should be removed because of high chances of future appendicitis in these patients.
- Intussusception of the appendix
- Appendicectomy is part of Lord's procedure for intestinal malrotation.
- Appendicectomy should be carried out if appendix is found to be congested after reduction if ileocolic intussusception.
- Carcinoid tumor of appendix if <2 cm, not involving the base, cecal wall, or lymph nodes.
- Appendicectomy to facilitate appendicostomy may be used for intraoperative colonic lavage in the presence of obstruction.

Preoperative Preparation and Anesthesia

A preoperative dose of broad-spectrum antibiotic is administered to all patients to cover aerobic and anaerobic organisms; it should be continued if there is significant peritonitis. Spinal anesthesia or general anesthesia is employed.

Position of the Patient

Patient lies supine. Abdomen should be palpated after induction of anesthesia. If appendicular mass is found in right iliac fossa, it is advisable to postpone the surgery in favor of conservative management.

Following incisions can be employed for appendicectomy:

- Grid iron incision
- Transverse skin crease incision (Lanz, Rockey Davis, or Fowler Weir-Mitchell incision)
- Lower midline
- Rutherford Morrison incision employs cutting of internal oblique and transversus muscle fibers in the line of gridiron skin incision. This is usually done in difficult cases, i.e., retrocecal position of appendix.

Gridiron incision was first described by McArthur is at right angle to Mc-Burney point along one-third of the way on line drawn from anterior superior iliac spine to the umbilicus. Lower midline incision is used if diagnosis is in doubt or if there are features of peritonitis.

- After skin and subcutaneous tissue incision external oblique is divided in the line of skin incision.
- Fibers of internal oblique and transversus abdominis are split to expose peritoneum which is opened.
- Incision can be extended medially either by retraction of rectus muscle or by its division.
- After opening abdomen medial end of the wound is elevated by retractor.
- A finger is placed inside the peritoneal cavity to identify and deliver the appendix.
- If the appendix is not felt in this manner, the cecum is held by a moist gauze and delivered in to the wound by gradual and gentle side to side motion. Appendix is identified by following one the tenia of the cecum.
- A finger is used to hook around the appendix to deliver it in the wound. A Babcock tissue holding forceps is applied around appendix to hold it without crushing.

- Mesoappendix along with appendicular artery is divided between clamps and ligated till the base of the appendix is clear.
- Once the junction of appendicular base with cecum has been identified, appendix is crushed with straight clamp about 3–5 mm away from cecum and is reapplied 3–5 mm away from initial site of crushing.
- The perceived advantages of crushing the base of appendix are following:
    - The serosa becomes rough, and the chances of slipping of ligature become less.
    - Crushing inverts the mucosa.
    - Crushing blocks the lymphatics, thus decreasing the chances of retrograde transmission of infection when appendix is being transected.
- The base of the appendix is doubly ligated with 2-0 absorbable suture (chromic catgut or polyglactin) the crushed site.
- Appendix is divided between ligature and clamp.
- Exposed mucosa of appendicular stump is cauterized by a spirit swab more often as surgical ritual without any evidence of benefit behind this practice.
- Removed appendix along with clamp and scalpel used to transect the appendix is discarded in a separate kidney tray to minimize contamination.
- Inversion of the appendicular stump is justified only if the base of the appendix is inflamed and cannot be crushed, or there is edema of the appendicular base and there is a fear that ligature may slip.
- Closure of wound peritoneal lavage is done with warm saline.
- It is not necessary to drain the peritoneal cavity in case of nonperforated appendix. However, if there is a localized appendicular abscess or frank purulent fluid right iliac fossa can be drained through a separate stab incision.
- Wound is closed in layers. Internal oblique and transversus muscles are approximated by interrupted absorbable 1-0 suture. External oblique is closed by continuous suture.

LAPAROSCOPIC APPENDECTOMY

- Patient is placed supine with the left arm tucked in at the side and a mild Trendelenburg position.
- Three ports are placed namely a 10 mm infraumbilical midline port through vertical incision for insufflation and for telescope, 15 mm suprapubic port in midline, and another 10 mm port is placed in left lower quadrant **(Fig. 1)**.
- A pneumoperitoneum is established using open technique.
- Abdominal cavity is inspected, and right colon and cecum are identified.
- Teniae coli can be traced toward the cecum and base of appendix.
- Atraumatic bowel-grasping forceps are used to elevate the cecum and terminal ileum into the operative field.

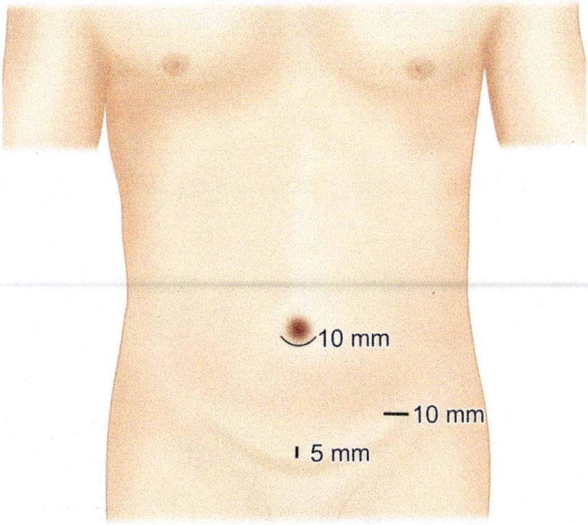

Fig. 1: Port placement for laparoscopic appendicectomy.

- The appendix is brought toward the surgeon and held by Babcock forceps **(Fig. 2)**.
- Curved dissecting scissors are used to free the lateral and inferior peritoneal attachments of the appendix.
- The appendix is mobilized with electrocautery or harmonic scalpel and appendiceal artery isolated at the base of the appendix with an angled dissecting forceps and controlled with either surgical clips or harmonic scalpel **(Figs. 3 and 4)**.
- Dissection of the mesoappendix is continued until the base of the appendix, and its junction with the cecum is freed from any adhesions or peritoneal attachments **(Fig. 4)**.
- Three pretied laparoscopic ligature made of 0 chromic catgut or synthetic sutures are applied, two near the junction with the cecum and a third placed on the proximal portion of the appendix **(Fig. 2)**.
- The appendix is divided, leaving the two ligatures on the cecum intact **(Fig. 5)**.
- Specimen is placed in an endobag and removed either through umbilical or suprapubic port.
- Ports are closed in layer after removing all instruments and ports under vision.

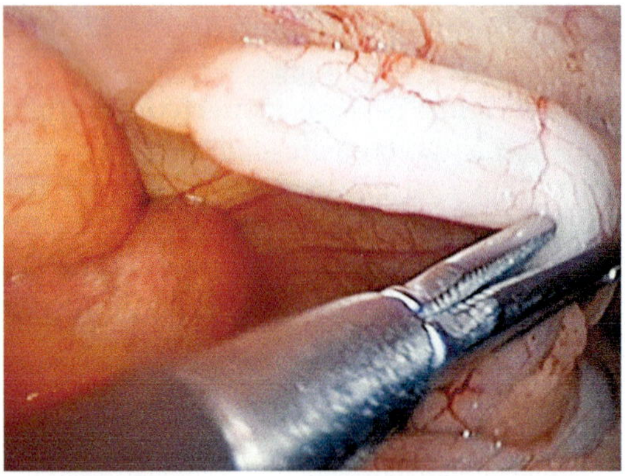

Fig. 2: Appendix being held by endograsper.

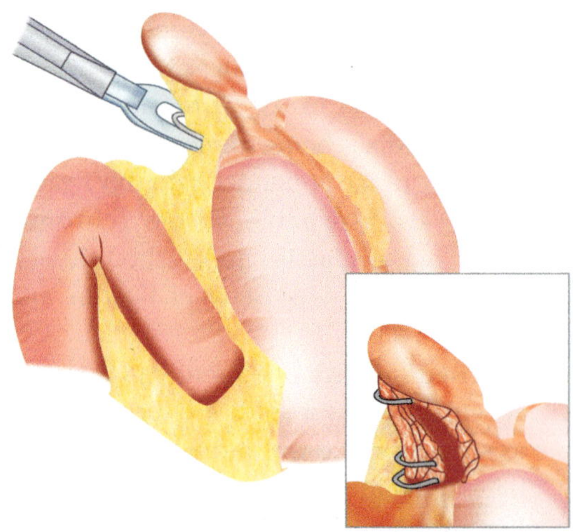

Fig. 4: Clipping of the appendicular artery.

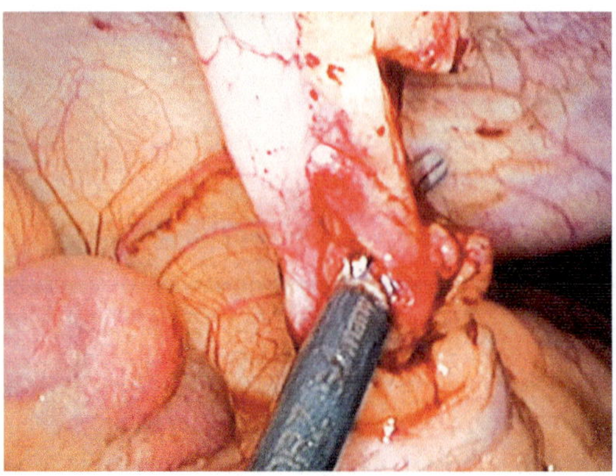

Fig. 3: Mesoappendix being isolated.

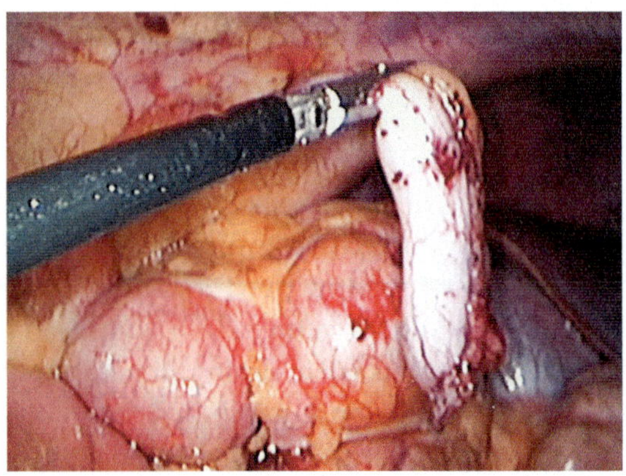

Fig. 5: Appendicectomy completed.

LIVER RESECTION

Indications

- *Primary malignant tumors:*
  - Hepatocellular carcinoma (HCC)
  - Cholangiocarcinoma
- *Secondary malignant tumors (metastases):* Most commonly from colorectal cancer
- *Benign tumors:*
  - Hepatic adenoma (with risk of malignant transformation)
  - Hemangioma (especially if causing mass effect)
- *Other conditions*:
  - Biliary stones
  - Congenital choledochal cysts
  - Infectious hydatid cysts.

Steps of Procedure

1. *Preoperative preparation:*
   a. Confirm absence of extrahepatic disease with staging laparoscopy.
   b. Assess cardiopulmonary fitness.
   c. Check bilirubin, prothrombin time (PT), and platelet count.
   d. Consider preoperative interventions based on laboratory findings.
   e. Cross-match blood products and prepare tumor markers [Ca19.9, carcinoembryonic antigen (CEA), and alpha-fetoprotein (AFP)].
2. *Positioning and theater setup:*
   a. Surgeon on patient's right, assistant, and scrub nurse on the left
   b. Urinary catheterization and administration of induction antibiotics.
   c. Patient positioned supine with arms extended

Steps of Surgery

1. Make an incision (reverse L or rooftop) based on surgical preference.
2. Fully mobilize the liver by dividing ligaments and posterior attachments.
3. Ligate caudate veins (for right-sided resections) and secure hepatic vein.
4. Ligature of right hepatic artery and portal vein aids in identifying Cantlie's line and reduces blood loss.
5. Secure left portal triad if needed, considering intrahepatic left hepatic vein.
6. Mark resection line using intraoperative ultrasound.
7. Prepare for Pringle maneuver if required, and then transect parenchyma using appropriate dissectors.
8. Manage biliary and vascular structures with ties, clips, or staples.
9. Ensure hemostasis and inspect resection margin for leaks or bleeding.

Postoperative Care and Instructions

- Monitor hemoglobin, bilirubin, PT, and platelet count.
- Administer fresh-frozen plasma (FFP) as needed based on PT levels.
- Consider further interventions for biliary issues.
- Provide proton pump inhibitors and heparin for peptic ulcer prophylaxis and deep vein thrombosis (DVT) prophylaxis, respectively, depending on patient's condition.

Postoperative Complications

- *Bleeding:* Requires urgent intervention to control bleeding sources
- *Bile leak:* Managed with conservative measures or endoscopic procedures if necessary
- *Liver failure:* Requires comprehensive management with supportive care and potentially interventional radiology procedures.

Tips and Tricks

- Preoperatively optimize liver function and hemodynamics to minimize complications.
- Consider advanced techniques such as laparoscopic or robotic approaches to reduce surgical morbidity, especially for anterior and lateral liver resections.

Left Hemicolectomy Indications

- Neoplastic lesions involving the descending colon or sigmoid colon
- Complex, symptomatic diverticular disease

Steps of Procedure

1. *Preparation:*
   a. Bowel preparation one night prior to day of surgery.
   b. Administer thromboembolism prophylaxis.
   c. Give prophylactic antibiotics after anesthesia induction.
   d. Insert urethral catheter after anesthesia.
2. *Position:*
   a. Position the patient in Lloyd-Davies position.
   b. Make a lower midline incision extending above the umbilicus.
3. *Procedure:*
   a. Conduct WHO checklist.
   b. Assess resectability of tumor, presence of liver metastases, peritoneal deposits, and synchronous tumors.
   c. Protect small bowel with wet packs and tilt the table to the right.
   d. Retract sigmoid colon to the right and medially.
   e. Have assistant retract lower left abdominal wall.
   f. Use diathermy to divide peritoneum lateral to sigmoid and descending colon.
   g. Separate mesentery from retroperitoneum, protecting structures such as gonadal vessels and ureter.
   h. Lift descending colon off Gerota's fascia and separate greater omentum from transverse colon.
   i. Extend incision along left paracolic gutter toward splenic flexure.
   j. For splenic flexure tumors, divide gastrocolic omentum and remove with specimen.
   k. Mobilize splenic flexure cautiously to avoid spleen damage.
   l. Lift sigmoid colon and divide peritoneum on right side from inferior mesenteric artery origin to sacral promontory.
   m. Identify and ligate inferior mesenteric artery and vein carefully.
   n. Divide transverse mesocolon and marginal artery.
   o. Clamp and divide transverse colon at rectosigmoid junction.
   p. Ensure adequate vascularization and tension-free bowel ends.
4. *Restoration and closure*:
   a. Restore bowel continuity with 3/0 PDS interrupted seromuscular sutures.
   b. Alternatively, perform a stapled anastomosis using circular stapler and 2/0 Prolene purse-string suture.
   c. Perform leak test with sigmoidoscope and air insufflation.
   d. Wash peritoneal cavity and close in layers.
5. *Postoperative care and complications:*
   a. Monitor for complications such as bleeding, infection, and anastomotic leaks.
   b. Provide supportive care including pain management and early ambulation.
   c. Ensure appropriate follow-up to monitor recovery and manage any postoperative issues.

TENSION-FREE MESH HERNIOPLASTY

In tension-free hernioplasty, posterior wall of inguinal canal is strengthened by a prolene mesh 10 × 15 cm in size. As the mesh is placed in between external oblique aponeurosis (EOA) and floor of the inguinal canal, contractions of the EOA on increasing intra-abdominal pressure such as coughing and straining applies center pressure over the mesh, thus using intra-abdominal pressure to protect repair. This operation basically comprises herniotomy and strengthening of posterior wall of inguinal canal by mesh (hernioplasty).

Anesthesia

Tension-free mesh repair can be performed under local, epidural, or spinal anesthesia. Local anesthesia is preferred for reducible inguinal hernias. For local anesthesia, 1% lignocaine is employed in the dose of 3–4 mL/kg body weight as the maximum dose. For local anesthesia, infiltration of the local anesthetic is done in subdermal, intradermal, deep subcutaneous, and subaponeurotic plane. Few milliliter of local anesthetic is also injected around pubic tubercle, near the neck of the hernial sac and inside the hernial sac in cases of indirect hernia. Spinal or epidural anesthesia is employed in cases of large hernias, sliding hernias, irreducible or strangulated hernias, or in uncooperative patients.

Position of the Patient

Patient lies supine on the operating table.

- A 5–7.5 cm long oblique incision is employed over medial two-thirds of inguinal ligament starting at the level of pubic tubercle, approximately 2–3.0 cm above it.
- After dividing skin, the subcutaneous fat, Camper's, and Scarpa's fascia are divided in the line of the incision. Superficial external pudendal and superficial inferior epigastric venous tributaries need ligation if encountered.
- EOA and superficial inguinal ring are exposed and divided in the line of the skin incision to open the inguinal canal. Cut margins of EOA are held in mosquito artery forceps.
- Upper flap is separated from underlying internal oblique muscle for a distance of at least one inch so that enough space is created to place a mesh over internal oblique. Iliohypogastric nerve comes into view at this stage, which should be safeguarded.
- Lower flap of external oblique is reflected downward till one sees the in turned portion of the inguinal ligament.
- Cord is lifted from the floor of the inguinal canal at the pubic tubercle, and the cremasteric fascia and muscle are divided along the whole length of the cord to expose the underlying sac.
- Cremasteric artery and vein usually need ligation or cauterization near deep ring.
- Indirect sac is anterolateral to the vas deferens and spermatic vessels and is separated from them till the neck of the sac. Indirect sac can be ligated at the neck and remaining portion excised or pushed back into the peritoneal cavity.
- Direct hernial sacs which are postero-medial to the cord are simply pushed back into the peritoneal cavity.
- If the sac is large, it is inverted with absorbable sutures.
- Strengthening of the posterior wall of the inguinal canal is performed by polypropylene mesh measuring 10 by 15 cm.

- Medial border of the mesh is rounded to correspond to the shape of medial corner of the inguinal canal and is overlapped at least by 1 × 1.5 cm over rectus sheath and sutured to it by prolene 2-0 sutures.
- Lower border of the mesh is sutured to the in turned portion of the inguinal ligament by continuous 2-0 prolene sutures till the level of the deep ring.
- A slit is made at the lateral end of the mesh creating two tails, upper wide (two-thirds) and lower narrower (one-third). Two tails of the mesh are overlapped, and the lower margins of both are stitched to the inguinal ligament. Crossing of the two tails creates an internal ring.
- Upper margin of the mesh is fixed to underlying internal oblique by means of interrupted sutures.
- Mesh should be lax, tented up or slightly wrinkled rather than lying flat to avoid tension on mesh when the patient stands and the fascia transversalis is pushed forward. Medially the mesh should lay 1.5–2 cm medial to the pubic tubercle, upper margin of the mesh should be 3–4 cm above Hesselbach triangle and 3–4 cm lateral to the deep ring.
- EOA is stitched by continuous prolene 1-0 sutures.
- Skin and subcutaneous tissue are closed and sterile surgical dressing applied.

HERNIORRHAPHY

In the era of modern surgical practice, tissue repair might be indicated in the following situations:

- In cases of strangulated inguinal hernia where bowel resection is carried out, mesh hernioplasty is contraindicated because of high chances of mesh infection.
- If the patient has a known allergy to mesh material.
- If the patient refuses to have foreign material implantation in his or her body.
- There are reports that in young males in their productive age with bilateral groin hernia, mesh repair on both sides may produce oligospermia or subfertility because of entrapment of vas in the mesh. Synthetic mesh, e.g., prolene mesh commonly used in hernia repair can cause an intense inflammatory response, leading to obstruction or narrowing of the vas. Prolene mesh in the young male, especially if bilateral hernia repair is needed, should be used with caution. Other alternatives such as tissue repair might be a better option.

Following tissue repairs are most popular:

- Bassini's repair
- Marcy repair
- Iliopubic tract repair
- McVay repair
- Shouldice repair
- Desarda's repair (tension-free mesh-free tissue repair).

Anesthesia

Majority of open groin hernia repairs can be performed under local anesthesia unless the hernia is very big, or it is a sliding hernia or reaching up to the scrotum. Commonly used agents for local anesthesia are 0.5–1% lignocaine with epinephrine or 0.25% bupivacaine with epinephrine or a combination of both. Sodium bicarbonate can be added in the solution to alter the pH, which is though to decrease the pain of injection.

10 mL of this preformed solution is injected just medial to the anterior superior iliac spine in a fan-shaped manner to block ilioinguinal and iliohypogastric nerves. Another 60 mL is injected as a field block along the line

of proposed incision in intradermal, subcutaneous, and subaponeurotic planes. After opening the inguinal canal, 5–10 mL is injected around the neck of hernia sac, and a few milliliter is instilled inside the hernial sac. 5–10 milliliter solution is also injected around the pubic tubercle to block genital branch of genitofemoral nerve.

Common Steps

1. Classically an oblique or horizontal skin incision is placed 2 cm above and parallel to the inguinal ligament over its medial two-thirds.
2. The incision is deepened through the Camper's and Scarpa's fascia till EOA is exposed.
3. EOA is incised in the line of incision through superficial inguinal ring.
4. After opening the inguinal canal, upper flap of the EOA is separated from underlying internal oblique and rectus muscle by blunt dissection. Iliohypogastric nerve is identified and safeguarded. Inferior flap is reflected down till the shelving edge of the inguinal ligament is seen.
5. Margins of the superior and inferior flaps of external oblique are held in artery forceps. Cord structures are lifted up away from the floor of the inguinal canal by blunt dissection near the pubic tubercle. After lifting the cord structures, they are held in an umbilical tape or in a penrose drain.
6. Cremasteric muscle is divided along the whole length of the cord to expose the underlying structures. The hernial sac is isolated from remaining cord structures till the neck of sac.
7. Once the sac has been isolated from cord structures, it is opened at the fundus to make sure that all contents have been reduced. Sac can either be reduced in the preperitoneal space without excision, or sac can be ligated at neck by transfixation and remaining part of the sac excised. If the hernia sac is complete and reaching up to the scrotum, there is no need to isolate it completely, rather it can be divided midway, and distal part of the sac can be left in situ along with cord structures after laying it open on its anterior wall.
8. Laying open of the distal remaining sac prevents the future hydrocele formation.

BASSINI'S REPAIR

Edwards Bassini advocated high ligation of the sac with reconstruction of posterior wall of the inguinal canal. Bassini emphasized the incision in the EOA superior to skin incision so that suture line of the repair does not lie in line with the line of closure of the external oblique.

- After handling the hernial sac fascia transversalis is opened from the internal ring to pubic tubercle.
- Upper flap of the fascia transversalis is dissected upward away from the pre-peritoneum, thus creating a flap comprising fascia transversalis, transversus abdominis, and internal oblique muscle.
- The first stitch in the Bassini's repair consists of flap of triple-layer superiorly and the periosteum of the pubic tubercle inferiorly.
- Repair is then continued laterally, and triple-layer flap is approximated to the reflected in turned portion of the inguinal ligament by means of interrupted sutures. Sutures are continued till the medial edge of the deep ring. Six to eight stitches are used to approximate the triple layer to the in turned portion of the inguinal ligament.
- Original Bassini's repair has been modified in North America where fascia transversalis is not incised. Only internal

oblique and transversus abdominis muscles are approximated to the inguinal ligament.

DESARDA REPAIR (TENSION-FREE MESH-FREE TISSUE REPAIR)

- This repair was first described by Dr Mohan Desarda from Pune, India.
- Skin and fascia are incised through a regular oblique inguinal incision to expose the EOA.
- The thin, filmy fascial layer covering it is kept undisturbed as far as possible and an assessment made about the strength of it and its thinned-out portion.
- The external oblique is cut in line with the upper crux of the superficial ring, which leaves the thinned out portion in the lateral leaf so a good strip can be taken from the medial leaf.
- Inguinal canal is opened. The cremasteric muscle is incised for the herniotomy, and the spermatic cord together with the cremasteric muscle is separated from the inguinal floor **(Fig. 6)**.
- The sac is excised in indirect hernias and inverted in direct hernias.
- Medial leaf of the external oblique aponeurosis is sutured to the inguinal ligament from pubic tubercle to abdominal ring using 1 or 0 monofilament polydioxanone absorbable continuous sutures **(Fig. 7)**.
- The first two sutures are taken above in the anterior rectus sheath where it joins the external oblique aponeurosis and below through the lacunar ligament or the medial most part of the inguinal ligament.
- The last suture is taken so as to narrow the abdominal ring sufficiently without constricting the spermatic cord. Each suture is passed first through the inguinal ligament and then the external oblique.
- A splitting incision is made in this sutured medial leaf, partially separating a strip with a width of 1–2 cm only.
- This splitting incision is extended medially up to the pubic symphysis and laterally 1–2 cm beyond the abdominal ring. The medial insertion and lateral continuation of this strip are kept intact. If some separation of fibers is seen in this sutured medial leaf, then splitting incision is planned through such site or separated fibers are sutured together with

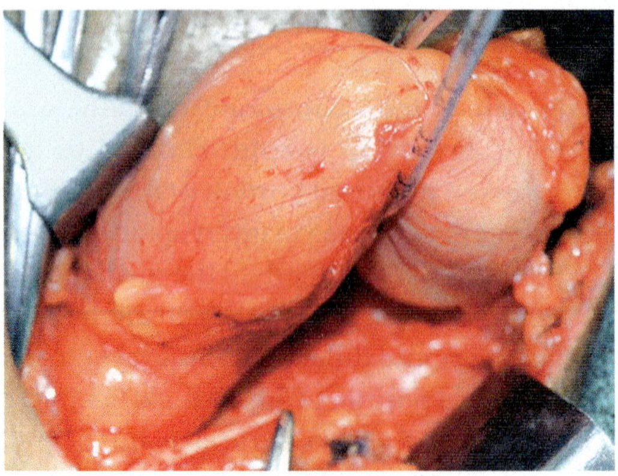

Fig. 6: Cord lifted.

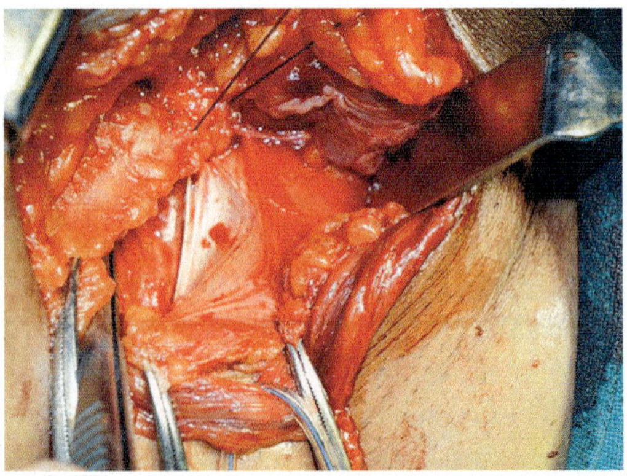

Fig. 7: Stitching upper leaf of external oblique aponeurosis to in turn portion of inguinal ligament.

few tiny sutures of 3 "0" monofilament polydioxanone.

- A strip of the external oblique is now available, the lower border of which is already sutured to the inguinal ligament **(Fig. 8)**. The upper free border of the strip is now sutured to the internal oblique or conjoined muscle lying close to it using 1 or 0 monofilament polydioxanone absorbable continuous sutures throughout its length **(Fig. 9)**.
- The aponeurotic portion of the internal oblique muscle is used for suturing to this strip wherever and whenever possible. This will result in the strip of the external oblique being placed behind the cord to form a new posterior wall of the inguinal canal.

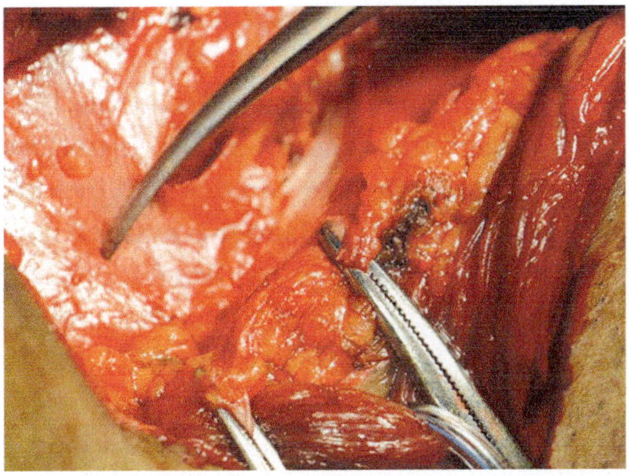

Fig. 8: Isolation of strip of upper leaf of external oblique aponeurosis.

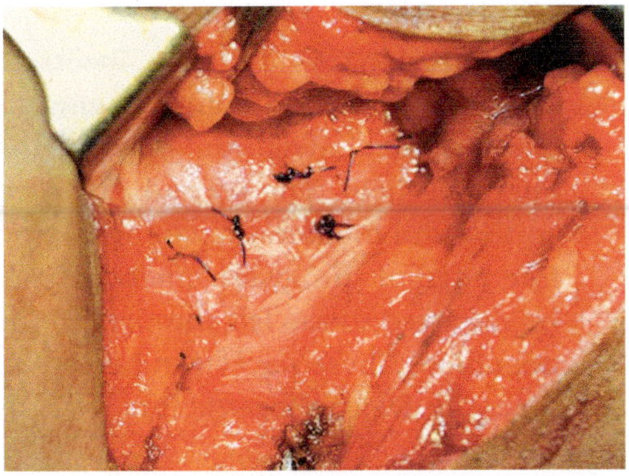

Fig. 9: Upper border of isolation strip stitched to underlying conjoint muscle.

- Spermatic cord is placed in the inguinal canal, and the lateral leaf of the external oblique is sutured to the newly formed medial leaf of the external oblique in front of the cord, as usual, again using 1 or 0 monofilament polydioxanone absorbable continuous sutures.
- The first stitch is taken between the lateral corner of this splitting incision and lateral leaf of the external oblique and carried medially toward the pubic symphysis, leaving behind a sufficient superficial ring for exit of the cord
- Closure of the superficial fascia and the skin is done as usual with subcuticular 3 "0" monofilament polydioxanone absorbable sutures or interrupted nonabsorbable sutures.

CHOLECYSTECTOMY

Introduction

Laparoscopic cholecystectomy has become a gold standard for symptomatic gallstone disease, and open cholecystectomy is being performed less often these days only in cases where safe laparoscopic cholecystectomy is not feasible.

Indications of Open Cholecystectomy

Indications for open cholecystectomy in the present era of laparoscopic surgery are following:

- Conversion from laparoscopic to open in following situations:
  - Elective conversion to open if there is anatomical obscuration in cholecystohepatic triangle with risk of injury to adjacent structures

- Forced conversion if there is an injury to common bile duct or duodenum or if there is bleeding which cannot be controlled by laparoscopic means
- Patient unwilling for laparoscopic surgery
- Patient with chronic obstructive airway disease
- Patient suffering from severe cardiac disease with low ejection fraction
- Gall stones associated with portal hypertension
- Gall stones associated with cirrhosis
- Refractory coagulopathy in which laparoscopic surgery should be avoided
- Empyema of gall bladder
- Emphysematous cholecystitis.
- Perforation of gall bladder or pericholecystic abscess
- Cholecystoenteric fistula
- Gallstone ileus
- Cholangitis
- Multiple past upper abdominal surgeries

▪ Third trimester of pregnancy
▪ Patient unfit for general anesthesia or laparoscopy
▪ Cholecystectomy is undertaken "prophylactically" in patients having a catheter inserted into the hepatic artery for hepatic perfusion chemotherapy.
▪ Carcinoma gall bladder
▪ Diffuse peritonitis with hemodynamic compromise.

Steps

1. The subcostal incision is placed 4 cm below and parallel to the right costal margin and usually extends from close to the midline to the tip of ninth costal cartilage.
2. Once the skin and subcutaneous tissue have been incised, the anterior rectus sheath and muscle are divided with a diathermy in the line of the skin incision with coagulation of any vessels which are encountered.
3. A Mayo or Roberts's forceps can be passed behind the muscle so that it is placed on a slight of vessels and their formal coagulation or ligation before they retract into the muscle.
4. The peritoneum is next opened with a knife between forceps. The incision can then be lengthened with scissors or diathermy.
5. The peritoneal cavity is explored systematically paying particular attention to the esophageal hiatus, stomach, duodenum, liver, gall bladder, small bowel, and colon.
6. The right hand is passed over the liver to break the vacuum and to introduce air so that the liver can descend into the wound. The gall bladder is grasped with two pairs of sponge-holding forceps, one pair being applied to the fundus, and the other to Hartmann's pouch.
7. The gallbladder is retracted downward and laterally. Any adherent structure with gallbladder which is generally omentum or colon or duodenum is carefully separated using dissecting scissors.
8. Two moist packs are then inserted. The first packs the colon downward and prevents bowel from entering the operative field. The second is placed so that the duodenum, stomach, and free edge of the lesser omentum can be retracted to the left throughout the operation. These packs can be kept in place by Deaver's retractors held by assistants.
9. The anterior layer of peritoneum overlying the hepatoduodenal ligament

is then incised near the region of neck of gallbladder using dissecting scissors.

10. Dissection is carried out in cholecysto-hepatic triangle using right angle dissection forceps or a pled get held in a pair of Mayo or Robert's forceps. The anatomy of the biliary tree is assessed carefully, noting the diameter of the cystic duct and common hepatic/ common bile duct.
11. The right-angle dissection forceps are used to sweep adventitial tissues carefully away from the cystic duct and to display the triangle bounded by the cystic duct, common hepatic duct, and inferior edge of the liver. This maneuver usually brings the cystic artery into view.
12. The cystic duct is securely tied with polyglactin or silk suture. Two sutures are applied on common bile duct side and one on the gallbladder side.
13. The cystic artery is also doubly ligated, and both structures are then divided.
14. The gall bladder is kept under tension by gentle traction from the surgeon's left hand, and the fold of peritoneum attaching the gall bladder to the liver is divided using a combination of sharp dissection and electrocoagulation.
15. On occasion, it may be safer to remove the gallbladder using a "fundus first" approach, particularly when inflammation or adhesion formation makes it difficult to display the common bile duct, cystic duct, and cystic artery.
16. Regardless of whether the gallbladder is removed fundus first or by the more conventional method, a small swab is placed in the gallbladder bed to control oozing.
17. Any small bleeding vessels are coagulated, and if bleeding is troublesome and persists, a gauze swab or small pack is left in the gallbladder bed for 3–5 minutes.
18. If this does not produce adequate hemostasis, under running of the bleeding points with a fine absorbable suture may be needed.
19. Once hemostasis is achieved, the right upper quadrant is lavaged with warm saline, which is then removed.
20. A drain is not inserted routinely, although many surgeons use a small suction drain (e.g., Redivac), if there are lingering anxieties about hemostasis.
21. The incision is closed using a mass suture technique, and the skin edges are approximated with metal clips.

LAPAROSCOPIC CHOLECYSTECTOMY

- Patient is placed supine, and parts are cleaned and draped.
- Pneumoperitoneum is created using open or closed technique,
- 10-mm port is most often inserted at the subumbilical site where the laparoscope (0 or 30°) is introduced **(Fig. 10)**.

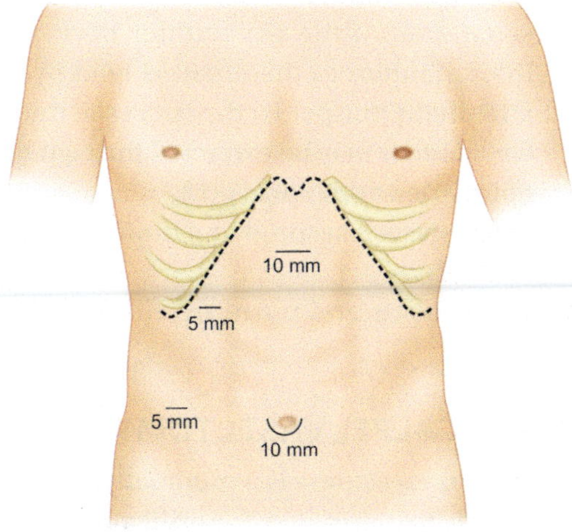

Fig. 10: Placement of ports for laparoscopic cholecystectomy.

- A systematic inspection of the contents of the four quadrants and pelvis is done.
- Operating port of 10–12 mm port through epigastrium to the right of falciform ligament is inserted directed toward gallbladder.
- One 5-mm port is inserted in midclavicular line to hold the neck of the gallbladder.
- Another 5-mm port is inserted in anterior axillary line 4 cm below the costal margin.
- Fundus of the gallbladder is held by a grasper with a ratchet or spring locking device and is pushed in a cephalad direction and laterally toward right shoulder exposing the Calot's triangle.
- Dissection of the cystic pedicle can be performed within the exposed Calot's triangle.
- Dissection of cystic duct is performed followed by dissection of cystic artery near the neck of gallbladder.
- Clips are applied at right angles to the long axis of the duct and to ensure that the lateral wall of the common bile duct is not included in the clip.
- The gallbladder is removed from the liver bed in a plane of dissection in the loose fibrous layer. Detachment starts by separation of the gallbladder neck and infundibulum as the organ is held by an atraumatic grasper by the cut cystic duct.
- Gallbladder may be extracted through the epigastric or umbilical port.
- Hemostasis is secured and drain placed if needed.
- Instruments and ports are closed under vision.

NO SCALPEL VASECTOMY

No scalpel vasectomy is a minimally invasive approach to permanent sterilization. It is usually performed in the supine position under local anesthesia.

- Vas is isolated using the three-finger technique. The middle finger and thumb fix the vas, and the index finger is used to stretch the skin overlying the vas.
- It is brought to the midline at the junction of upper one-third and lower two-thirds of the anterior scrotal raphe.
- A 1-cm wheal is raised on the overlying skin with 2% lignocaine solution.
- Needle is advanced toward the superficial inguinal ring in the perivasal plane, and 2 mL of anesthetic solution is deposited.
- The second side vas is similarly brought to the midline and anesthetized.
- The vas is fixed perpendicular to the line of the vas with a ringed clamp or extracutaneous vas fixation forceps.
- The vas dissecting forceps is inserted into the lumen of the vas.
- The forceps is gently opened, and all the overlying layers separated until vas are exposed.
- The vas is grasped between the blades of the dissection forceps, and the wrist is supinated. The vas is thus delivered out of the wound. The ringed clamp is released simultaneously.
- The vascular structures and fascia surrounding the vas are stripped using the vas dissection forceps.
- The ends of the vas are ligated and a 1-cm segment removed. The ligature on the abdominal end is kept long.
- The cut ends are deposited back, and the abdominal end is brought up again by pulling the tie attached to it.
- The re-emerging end is enclosed in fascia around which another tie is taken for fascial interpositioning.
- The other side is similarly operated through the same wound.
- An antiseptic dressing is applied on the midline wound.

TRENDELENBURG'S OPERATION

The Trendelenburg's operation is performed for saphenofemoral valve incompetence, leading to varicose veins. It is done in the supine position under spinal or general anesthesia.

Position of Patient

- Patient lies supine with the table tilted head down to an angle of 15°.
- A curved or hockey stick incision is made with the outer half lying in the gutter of the groin and inner half curving toward the thigh. Alternatively a 7–8 cm long oblique incision centered over anatomical marking of saphenous i.e., 3.75 cm below and lateral to pubic tubercle is made parallel to the fold of the groin.
- Incision is carried deeper till the superficial fascia is seen, which is then incised. Gauze is used to separate the fat and exposes the saphenofemoral junction. Saphena magna is dissected gently using a Mayo's tissue cutting scissors.
- Femoral vein is exposed 1 cm above and below the saphenofemoral junction.
- The all tributaries joining the termination of saphenous vein are defined and ligated.
- The end of the long saphenous vein is flush ligated at saphenofemoral junction with silk, and a second ligature is transfixed to avoid hemorrhage.
- Femoral vein is inspected above and below the junction and long saphenous divided.
- Incision is closed in layers.

KEY POINTS

- Basic surgical operations are the operations which surgical light learn first.
- To learn these operations the surgical trainee should understand the basics of these operations throughly.
- After understanding basics trainee should assist senior surgeon.
- After assisting they should these operations under guidance and then perform independently.
- Complications of these operations should be under stood including management.

CHAPTER 23

General Surgical Instruments

Mrunal Bharat Kshirsagar, Sudhir Kumar Jain

"Know your instruments well to get the best out of them"

INTRODUCTION

Instruments used in general surgery play a pivotal role in ensuring precision, efficacy, and safety during surgical procedures. These instruments are meticulously designed and engineered to facilitate a wide range of surgical tasks, from simple procedures to complex operations requiring intricate maneuvers.

The evolution of surgical instruments parallels advancements in medical knowledge, technology, and surgical techniques throughout history. From the early developments of basic cutting and dissecting tools to the sophisticated instruments of modern surgery, each device serves a specific purpose in the hands of skilled surgeons.

Today, the arsenal of instruments used in general surgery includes scalpels, forceps, retractors, scissors, clamps, and specialized devices for hemostasis, suturing, and tissue manipulation. These instruments are crafted from durable materials such as stainless steel and titanium alloys, ensuring durability, sterility, and precision in the operating room.

Understanding the function, handling, and maintenance of these instruments is essential for surgical teams to achieve optimal outcomes and minimize complications. As surgical techniques continue to evolve, so too do the instruments used, reflecting ongoing innovations aimed at enhancing patient care and surgical outcomes.

This introduction sets the stage for exploring the diverse array of instruments that form the backbone of general surgery, highlighting their critical role in the pursuit of surgical excellence and patient well-being.

Instruments are made of stainless steel.

COMMON STAINLESS STEEL GRADES IN SURGICAL INSTRUMENTS

Table 1 shows stainless steel grades in surgical instruments.

Benefits of Stainless Steel

Benefits are as follows:

- Corrosion resistance (against alkaline solutions, chlorine, acids, and water)
- High temperature resistance
- Easy to clean, making it ideal for medical environments
- Cost-effective
- 100% recyclable.

Summary of Alloys

- *Stainless steel and inox:*
    - *Usage:* General-purpose surgical instruments

TABLE 1: Stainless steel grades in surgical instruments.

Grade	*Composition*	*Characteristics*	*Common uses*
304	18% chromium and 8% nickel (also known as 18-8)	Corrosion-resistant, and not heat hardenable	General-purpose surgical instruments
316	16% chromium, 10% nickel, and 2% molybdenum	Enhanced resistance to saltwater corrosion	Surgical instruments for harsh environments
410	11.5% chromium	Good corrosion resistance, can be heat hardened	Cutting tools and surgical instruments
409	10.5% chromium	Similar to 410 but with slightly lower corrosion resistance	Less demanding surgical applications

  - *Pros:* Good corrosion resistance, cost-effective, and durable
  - *Cons:* Less resistant to extreme conditions compared to some other alloys
- *Dumoxel®:*
  - *Usage:* Instruments exposed to acidic environments
  - *Pros:* Excellent corrosion resistance, highly flexible, and 95% antimagnetic
  - *Cons:* More likely to bend than break
- *Dumostar®:*
  - *Usage:* Laboratory tools
  - *Pros:* Superior elasticity and corrosion resistance, 100% antimagnetic
  - *Cons:* Higher cost compared to other alloys
- *Titanium:*
  - *Usage:* Premium surgical instruments, especially for magnetic resonance imaging (MRI) applications.
  - *Pros:* Lightweight, very strong, 100% corrosion-resistant, and temperature stable.
  - *Cons:* Softer compared to other alloys
- *Antimagnetic:*
  - *Usage:* General-purpose surgical and laboratory tools
  - *Pros:* Good corrosion resistance, 80% antimagnetic
  - *Cons:* Not as hard as inox, less resistant to extreme conditions
- *Tungsten carbide:*
  - *Usage:* High-wear applications
  - *Pros:* Extremely durable and longer lifespan than stainless steel
  - *Cons:* Typically more expensive
- *Black titanium coated:*
  - *Usage:* Precision and microsurgical tools
  - *Pros:* Hard coating, excellent corrosion resistance, and antireflective
  - *Cons:* Higher initial cost, but cost-effective in the long run due to durability.

Choosing the Right Alloy

- *For general use:* Stainless steel and inox or antimagnetic
- *For corrosive environments:* Dumoxel® or titanium
- *For extreme durability:* Tungsten carbide or Dumostar®
- *For precision work*: Black titanium coated.

Selecting the appropriate alloy depends on the specific needs of your applications, including the environmental conditions, required durability, and budget constraints.

STAIN GUIDE FOR STAINLESS STEEL

Even though stainless steel is highly resistant to corrosion, it can still experience staining

TABLE 2: Stain guide for stainless steel.

Stain color	*Cause*	*Identification*
Brown/orange	High pH	Stain may appear due to exposure to alkaline substances
Dark brown	Low pH	Stain may be caused by acidic substances
Bluish/black	Reverse plating due to mixed metals during cleaning	Stain from reactions between different metal residues and cleaning agents
Multicolor	Excessive heat	Stains may result from overheating during use or cleaning
Light/dark spots	Water droplets drying on the surface	Stains may occur if water is left to evaporate without wiping
Black	Contact with ammonia	Stain caused by exposure to ammonia or ammonia-based cleaners
Gray	Excessive use of rust remover solution	Stain due to overuse or improper application of rust removers
Rust	Dried-on blood or biodebris	Rust-like stains from organic Matter that has dried and adhered to the surface

or rusting if not properly maintained. Here is a guide to understanding and identifying different types of stains on stainless steel **(Table 2)**.

How to Determine the Cause

- *Pencil eraser test:*
    - *Stain removal:* Use a pencil eraser to gently rub the stained area.
    - *No pitting:* If the discoloration is removed and there is no pitting, the stain was likely a surface issue, not corrosion.
    - *Pitting present:* If there is pitting or etching under the discoloration, it indicates corrosion, which is a more serious issue.

Recommendations for Cleaning and Maintenance

- *Routine cleaning:* Use mild detergent and water to clean stainless steel. Avoid abrasive materials that can scratch the surface.
- *Avoid extreme conditions:* Prevent prolonged exposure to high or low pH environments.
- *Immediate cleaning:* Clean off any biodebris or blood promptly to prevent rusting.
- *Proper use of chemicals:* If using rust removers or cleaners, follow the manufacturer's guidelines to avoid overuse or improper application.

By understanding the types of stains and their causes, you can take appropriate measures to maintain the appearance and performance of your stainless steel instruments.

STERILIZATION METHODS FOR SURGICAL INSTRUMENTS

Here is a table summarizing the procedures for autoclaving and cold sterilization, including key considerations and cautions **(Table 3)**.

Summary

- *Autoclaving:* Preferred for complete sterilization. Ensure proper lubrication,

TABLE 3: Sterilization methods for surgical instruments.

Sterilization method	***Step***	***Details***	***Cautions***
Autoclaving	1. Lubrication	Apply surgical instrument lubricant (WPI #500126) to instruments with metal-to-metal action (scissors, hemostats, needle holders, etc.)	• Do not use WD-40, oil, or other industrial lubricants • Do not lock instruments during autoclaving
	2. Preparation	• Place a towel on the bottom of the sterilization tray to absorb excess moisture • Arrange instruments in the tray to ensure proper steam circulation	Ensure proper arrangement to avoid overloading
	3. Loading the autoclave	Load the autoclave chamber, ensuring it is not overloaded to allow adequate steam penetration	Avoid overloading to ensure effective sterilization
	4. Running the autoclave	Follow the manufacturer's instructions for operation • Open the door slightly (about 3/4 inch) at the end of the cycle before the drying cycle • Run the drying cycle as recommended	Opening the door fully before the drying cycle can cause condensation and water stains
Cold sterilization	1. Immersion time	Immersion in cold sterilization solutions for 10 hours for complete sterilization or 10 minutes for disinfection	• Prolonged immersion may damage instruments • Do not use solutions with benzyl ammonium chloride for tungsten carbide inserts
	2. Chemical solutions	Use appropriate cold sterilization solutions that do not damage the instruments	Avoid solutions containing benzyl ammonium chloride for instruments with tungsten carbide inserts

loading, and drying procedures to maintain instrument quality.

- *Cold sterilization:* Suitable for disinfection; however, prolonged chemical exposure can be damaging. Avoid using harmful solutions for certain instruments.

Proper adherence to these sterilization methods will help ensure the safety and longevity of surgical instruments.

INSTRUMENTS

Scissors (Fig. 1)

Standard Scissor Tips

Standard scissors are available in a variety of lengths and patterns with straight, curved, or angled blades. Heavy duty patterns are for blunt dissection. Fine, thin blades are used for delicate cutting **(Fig. 2)**.

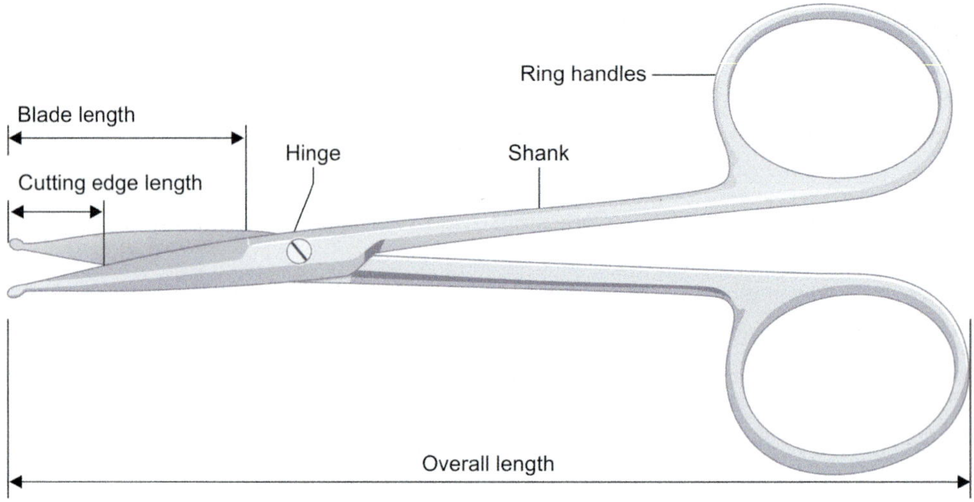

Fig. 1: Scissors.

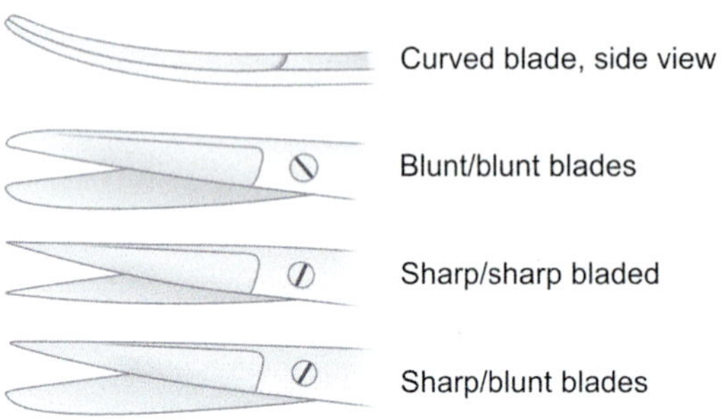

Fig. 2: Types of scissor tips.

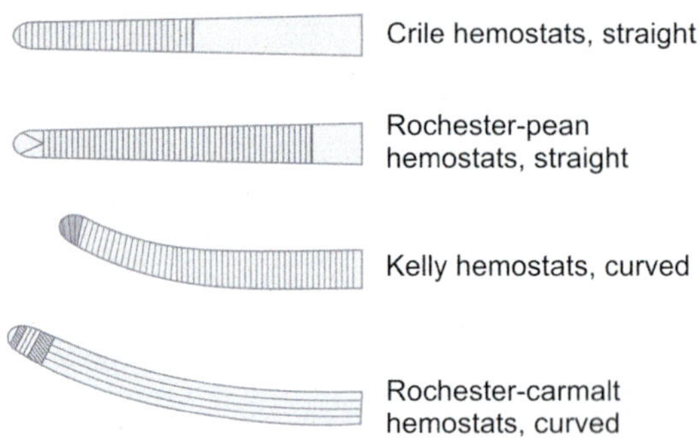

Fig. 4: Hemostat tips.

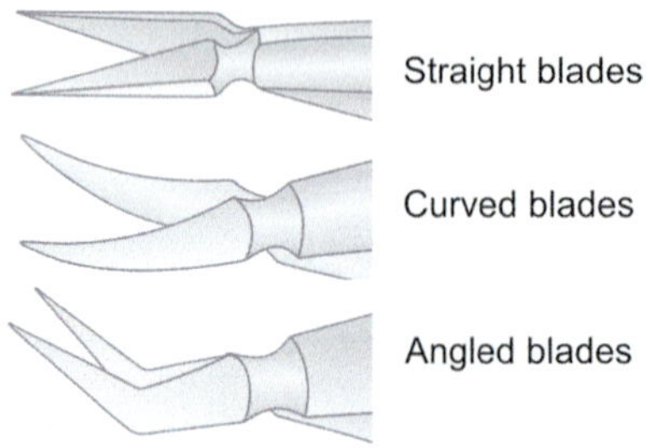

Fig. 3: Micro scissor tips.

Micro Scissor Tips

Micro scissors are often called vannas or spring scissors. They are excellent for left hand users **(Fig. 3)**.

Hemostat Tips (Fig. 4)

Surgical instruments have undergone rapid changes with advances in technology. These advances include discovery of newer and better materials, minimal ways of access, and development of gadgets to handle and dissect tissues. This has led to expansion of the surgical armamentarium, which a surgical student or trainee is expected to be familiar with. This chapter aims to introduce the conventional general surgical instruments along with their modern and laparoscopic counterparts.

Surgical instruments are made of stainless steel alloys with different grades (most common is 304) and properties. These alloys are inert, resilient, and allow construction of sharp edges. However, during surgery, they can get heated up or can conduct electricity and also can reflect the glare of OT lighting system upon the operating surgeon if not used with proper etiquette. Other problems with stainless steel alloys include poor galling resistance, loss of the sharpness of edges, and wear/tear on repeated use. Although stainless steel is relatively resistant to rusting, its durability is increased by a process called passivation, which is an engineering or physical chemistry, which makes the material passive to the effects of environmental factors such as air or water. During passivation, a light layer of metal oxide is coated over the equipment.

Stainless steel equipment is durable if cared for properly. They tend to lose sharpness with passage of time, but their exterior can be maintained if cleaned regularly. Most hospitals have a specific protocol for the care of their equipment. This protocol usually involves the following steps:

- Thorough cleaning with tap water to remove gross contamination
- Gross inspection care for left over soiling, misalignment, loose screws or joints, rough-ness, dullness, gross physical damage, staining, or corrosion.
- Soap-/detergent-based cleaning of grease and body fluids
- Deionized water is used for last round of cleaning
- Ultrasonic cleaning by cavitations if available for adherent tissue fat.

Following the cleaning process, instruments can be sterilized by one of the following methods:

- By autoclave
- Ortho-phthalaldehyde (OPA)
- Glutaraldehyde
- Ethylene oxide
- Formalin.

STORAGE OF INSTRUMENTS

Instruments in bulk are kept in ramps and trays such as the DIN tray or OP wash cart for multiple sets. Small or single instruments are kept in cassettes or peel pouches for sterilization. Mesh trays can be used for cleaning and sterilizing small detachable and reusable parts. It is advised that all jaws be opened before cleaning. Towels are used to separate instruments, with the larger ones kept below the smaller instruments. Tips of all instruments must be aligned in the same direction to avoid damage.

The operating room personnel are usually proficient at defining set of instruments for a particular procedure. Most operating rooms have a set of instruments predefined for upcoming cases, e.g., there would be a laparotomy set, or a laparoscopic cholecystectomy set and a gastrectomy set. These sets will have multiples of all the commonly required instruments for that particular procedure. This is one of the most convenient ways of organizing instruments and also makes possible customization from a common pool of instruments after the elective surgery list has been posted.

SECTION I: SURGICAL INSTRUMENTS

General surgical handheld instruments can be conveniently classified into:

- *Forceps:*
    - *Tissue holding forceps:* For surgical dissection
    - *Hemostatic forceps:* For control of bleeding vessels
- *Thumb forceps:* For holding and dissection

- Needle holders
- Retractors
- *Sharps:* Needles, trocars, and blades
- *Scissors:*
    - *Tissue cutting:* Employed for dividing tissue
    - *Material/suture cutting:* Employed for cutting sutures, dressing, plaster cast, etc.
- *Others:* Probes, blade handles, etc.

Tissue Holding Forceps

Tissue holding forceps most frequently used surgical instruments which can be used:

- For traction
- For retraction
- Holding tissues
- Occasionally for dissection.

They consist of ring handles, shafts converging at a box or screw joint which acts as a fulcrum and the working ends which have tips designed for specific functions. Common examples of tissue holding forceps are Kocher's forceps, Laheys forceps, Mixters forceps, Towel clip, Rochester Pean clamp, etc.

Hemostatic Forceps (Fig. 5)

Hemostatic forceps are used:

- For achieving control over bleeding vessels
- Sometimes to hold tough tissue.

The advantage with hemostatic forceps is the high shaft to working end ratio, which magnifies the force applied at the rings to about 3–5 times and is utilized in achieving a good and sometime destructive force. Hemostatic forceps that are commonly used include the mosquito forceps, Robert's artery forceps, Kelly's forceps, Bulldog clamp, Satinsky forceps, etc.

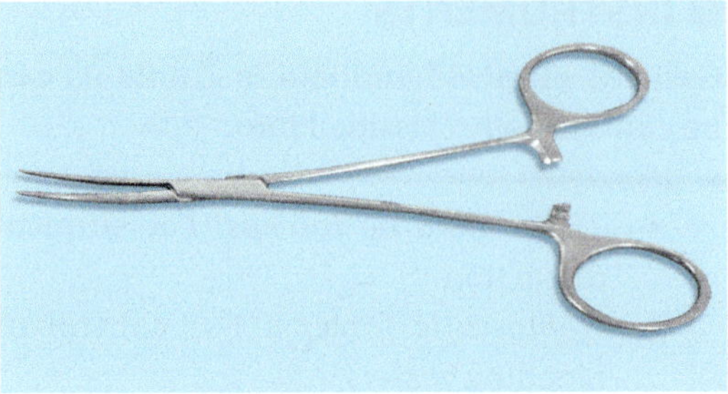

Fig. 5: Mosquito artery forceps.

Thumb Forceps

The thumb forceps aid in dissection and tying sutures by holding the tissue or suture and retraction using the left hand while the right hand does the dissection or suturing actively. The thumb forceps consists of four parts: the tip, shafts, handle, and a spring joint at the end. Thumb forceps have their tips designed specifically according to their use. They can be simple, serrated, toothed, and pointed for fine dissection. Russian tissue forceps have a cup and surrounding spike/serrations at the working end, designed specifically to dissect the biopsy specimen. Thumb forceps are available in a variety of sizes, making tissues at all possible depths accessible. Commonly used thumb forceps are the Adson's pickups, toothed dissecting forceps, DeBakey's forceps, St. Martin forceps, Colibri forceps, etc.

Needle Holders (Fig. 6)

Needle holders are designed with a very high mechanical advantage. The working tip is placed very close to the box joint, and the ringed handles quite far such that a force 8–10 times of that applied at the handles is transmitted to the needle holding tip. This, along with the multiple striations and a small pit, holds the suture needle firmly. Mayo-Hegar is the most commonly used type of needle holder.

Other needle holders that are also used include the Hegar-Baumgartner needle holder, Crile-Wood needle holder, Halsey

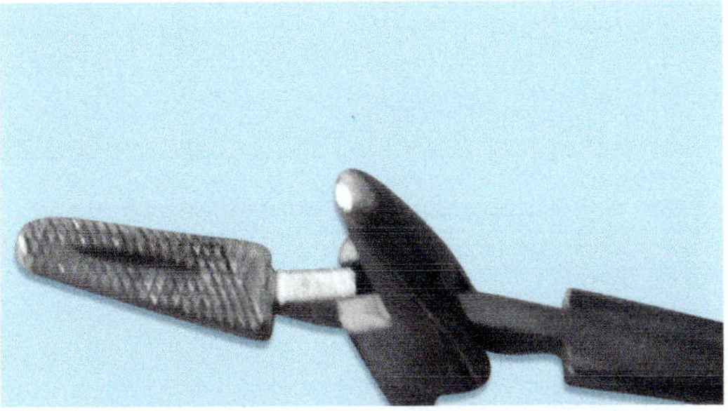

Fig. 6: Tip of needle holder with crisscross serrations and a small pit in the center.

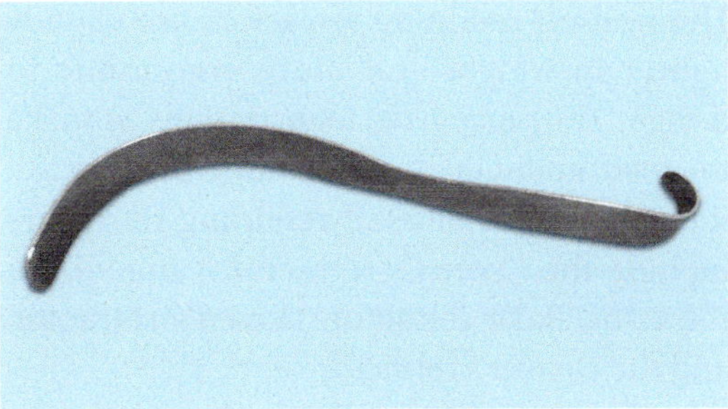

Fig. 7: Deaver'sretractor.

needle holder, Webster needle holder, and the Olsen-Hegar needle holder, which is a combined scissors and needle holding forceps. Apart from the regular ringed needle holders with a lock, spring action needle holders such as the Kalt needle holder, Paton needle holder, Castroviejo needle holder, and the McPherson needle holder are also used, more commonly in the microsurgery or other surgical subspecialties.

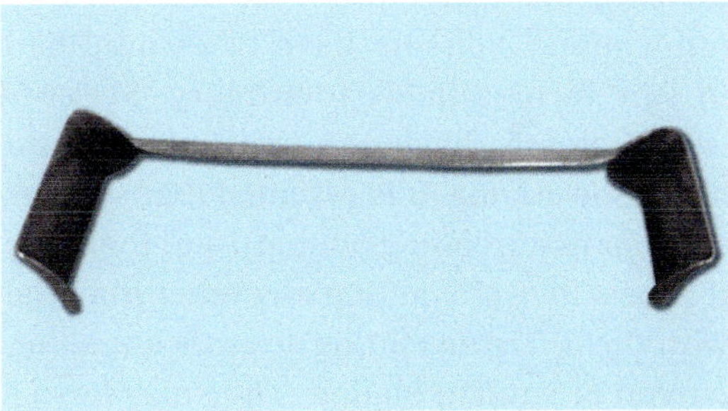

Fig. 8: Morris retractor.

Retractors (Figs. 7 to 10)

Compared to the era where fingers and hands were used for retraction, modern day retractors provide a more ergonomic environment letting the assistant work more actively in helping the operating surgeon. Retractors have been classically divided into self-retaining and nonself-retaining retractors. They can also be divided on whether they have blades on one side or both sides. While the self-retaining retractors avoid the need of an assistant, nonself-retaining ones also help immensely by reducing surgical fatigue and providing a better field of view compared to the hand. Commonly employed self-retaining retractors include the Jolls thyroid retractor, Balfour self-retaining retractor, Goldstein retractor, Agricola retractor, Barraquer retractor, Davis retractor, McKinney retractor, etc.

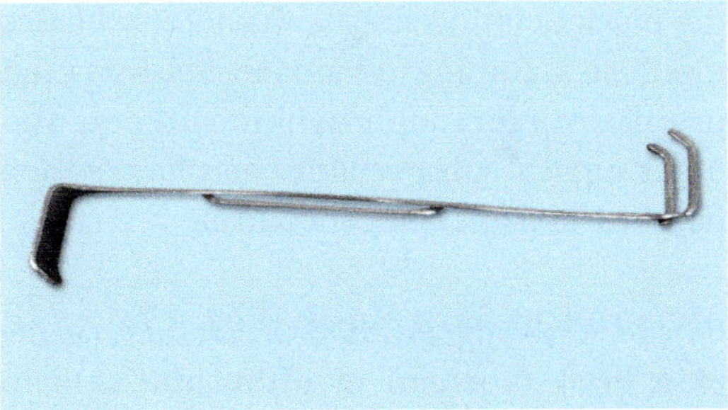

Fig. 9: Czerny's retractor.

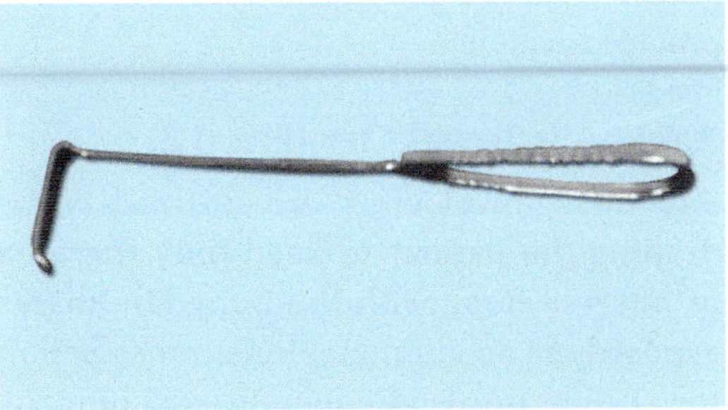

Fig. 10: Langenbeck's retractor.

The nonself-retaining retractors are usually lighter in weight and more ergonomic in design. They may have fenestrations to make the instrument lightweight and grips to make it easy to hold. Nonself-retaining retractors include the Czerny's retractor, Langenbeck retractor, Rake retractor, Doyen's retractor, and the Deaver's retractor.

Scissors

A wide variety of scissors are available to the surgeons with a constant influx of new innovations. Scissors have been modified to suit various fields to surgery. Scissors can be grossly divided as tissue cutting and nontissue cutting. It is essential that scissors used for tissue cutting be sharp and therefore it is best to avoid cutting any other material with them. Tissue cutting scissors are either curved or straight bladed. They may have a screw or a box joint. Nontissue cutting scissors such as the gauze cutting, suture cutting, or the plaster cutting scissors have their blades modified according to function. Scissors used in microsurgery, ophthalmic surgery, and other surgical subspecialties may have spring handles for a finer pincer control.

McGannon Skin Hook (Fig. 11)

Skin hook is useful in lifting the skin in surgeries of the subcutaneous tissue such as in modified radical mastectomy (MRM). It is usually held at right angles to the surface to provide traction.

Backhaus Towel Clip (Fig. 12)

Backhaus towel clips are utilized while draping the patient to keep only the area of interest along with the bony landmarks exposed. As an alternate, Jones cross-action towel clips are also frequently used in many centers.

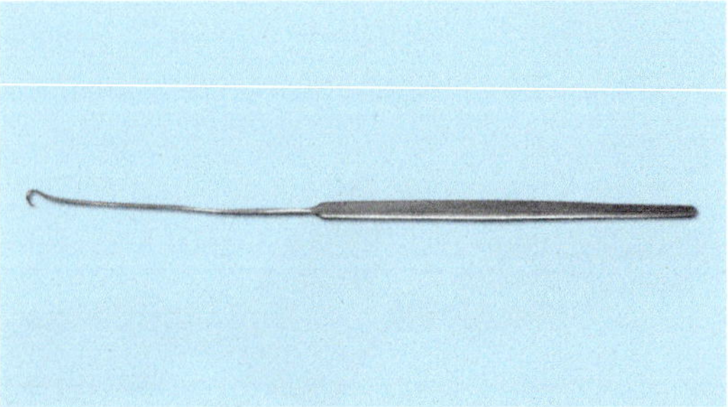

Fig. 11: McGannon skin hook.

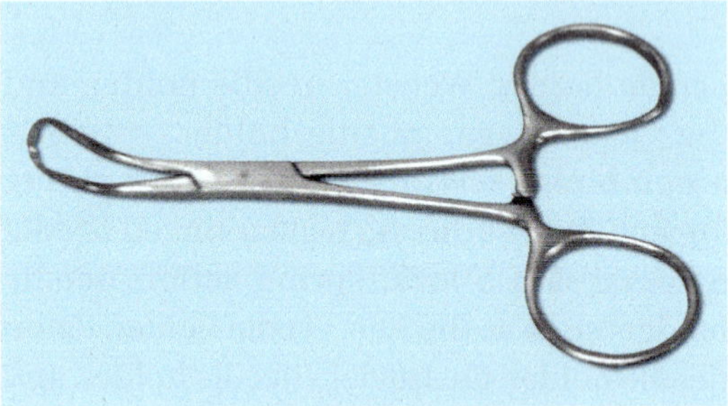

Fig. 12: Backhaus towel clip.

Towel clips have the following uses:

- Used to hold the drapes together at the points of intersection
- Can be used to lift umbilical pillar during the creation of pneumoperitoneum by open method
- Used to fix the cables and tubes during laparoscopic procedures.

Lahey's Right Angled Forceps (Fig. 13)

Lahey's right angled forceps are used during surgical dissection and hemostasis as described in the earlier sections of this book. They are frequently used for passing sutures in deeper regions as tip can be easily kept under vision avoiding injury to the deeper structures, which may not be well visualized. They are also used sometimes to hold a peanut swab.

Longer variants of the Lahey's right angled forceps (20 cm) are commonly called Heiss right angled forceps. Lahey's right angled

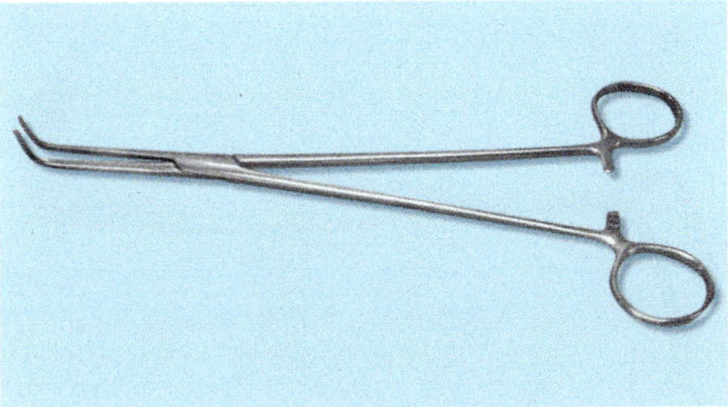

Fig. 13: Lahey's right angled forceps.

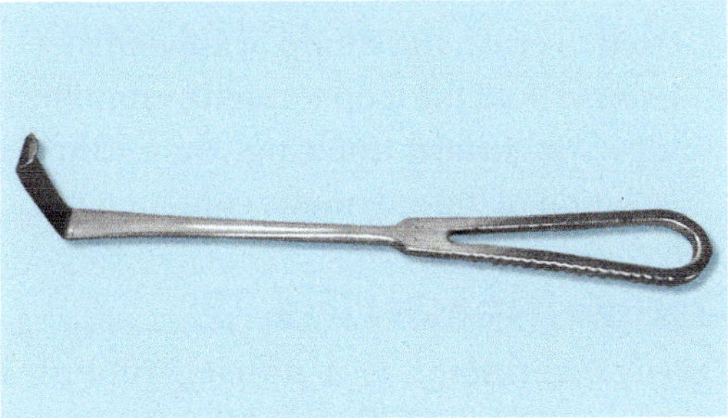

Fig. 14: Langenbeck retractor.

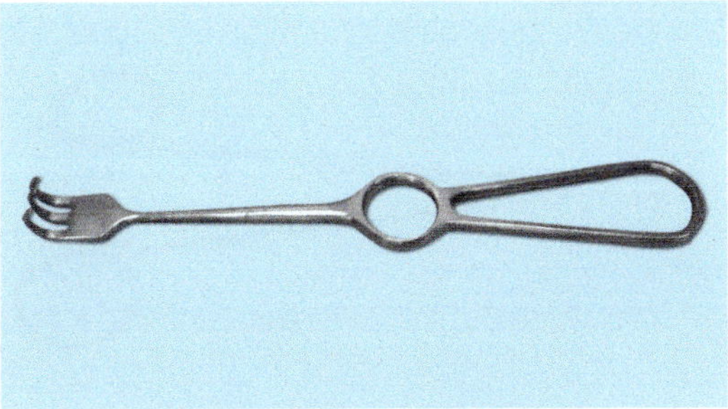

Fig. 15: Volkmann's retractor.

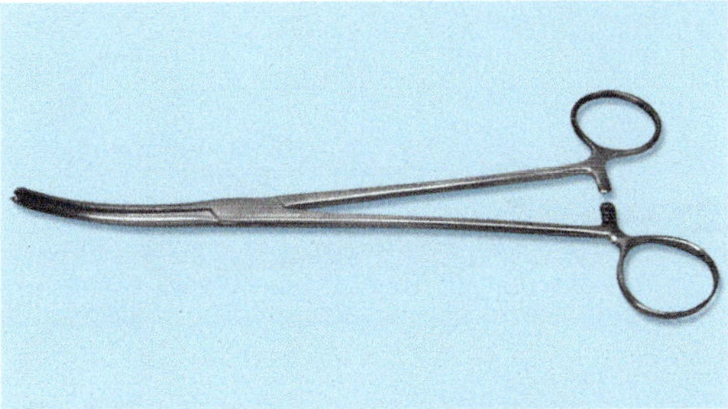

Fig. 16: Roberts artery forceps.

forceps can be commonly confused with the curved angle forceps. These forceps called the Mixters forceps are curved but not to a right angle.

Langenbeck Retractor (Fig. 14)

The Langenbeck retractor is one of the most commonly used retractors in minor and superficial surgeries. This retractor has its blades at right angles to the instrument. It can be used to retract the soft tissue during surgery such as hernia repair or appendectomy. The handle has a gap in between to make the instrument light weight. It resembles the "L" letter. A variant of the Langenbeck retractor is the *Richardson retractor*, which has similar blades at both the ends.

Volkmann's/Cat Paw/Rake Retractor (Fig. 15)

Volkmann's cat paw retractor is also used in superficial surgeries involving the skin and subcutaneous tissue. Some of its common application is to retract soft tissue during venesection or excision biopsy. The Volkmann's retractor has multiple small hooks at its end which retracts the superficial flap. One of its variant with a single hook is called Vicky's retractor. When the rake retractor is combined with a Langenbeck blade at the other end, it is commonly referred to as the *Senn retractor.*

Roberts Artery Forceps (Fig. 16)

Roberts artery forceps is a pair of long artery forceps useful for dissection and assisting in hemostasis in deeper regions of the abdomen. Some of its common uses are:

- Insertion of abdominal drains or inter-costal drainage tubes
- It can be used to pass free ties, especially in the pelvic surgery.

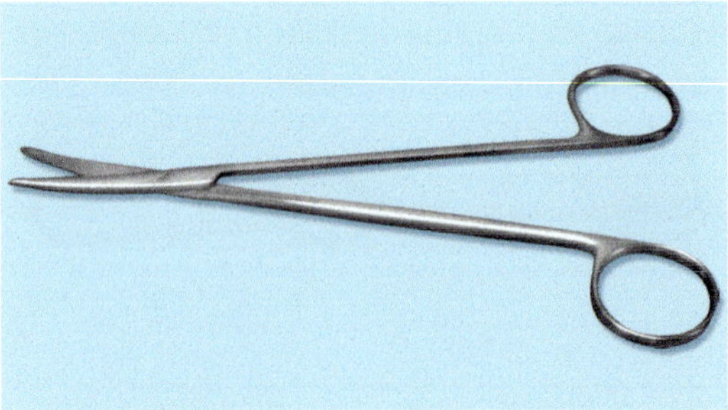

Fig. 17: Metzenbaum dissection scissors.

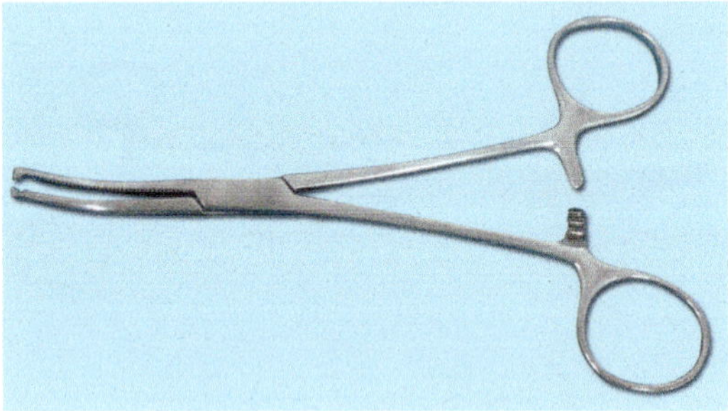

Fig. 18: Kocher's forceps.

Metzenbaum Dissection Scissors/ Tissue Cutting Scissors (Fig. 17)

Named after the American surgeon Myron Firth Metzenbaum, these scissors are used for cutting delicate soft tissue. They are different form the heavy Mayo scissors in being lighter, slender, and having a longer handle. Metzenbaum scissors may be coated with tungsten carbide cutting edges that provide a finer cut and are recognized by their gold-plated ring handles.

Kocher's Forceps (Fig. 18)

Named after Emil Kocher, a German born Swiss surgeon, Kocher's forceps are a type of toothed forceps with a long flat area to crush tissue in between. It is commonly:

- Used to hold tough fascia such as the rectus sheath during laparotomy.
- Used for artificial rupture of membrane.
- Used to crush the stump of appendix.
- Used to hold the loop formed by umbilical tape or infant feeding tube during isolation of the spermatic cord, ureter.

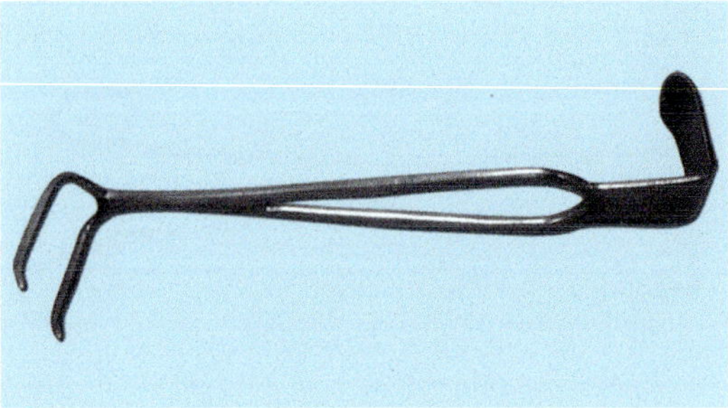

Fig. 19: Czerny's retractor.

Czerny's Retractor (Fig. 19)

Czerny's retractor is a nonself-retaining retractor with a biflanged hook at one end and a blade at the other end, both perpendicular to the instrument. The center is fenestrated to make the instrument light weight. It has a biflanged hook at one end and can be used to retract the wound in the tail end of the wound while sutures can be placed in the space between the two hooks. Czerny's retractor is used to retract the margins of the incision during laparotomy, cholecystectomy, etc. It is mainly used for superficial retraction. Its shape resembles the English alphabet "Z".

Desjardin's Gallstone Forceps (Fig. 20)

Desjardin's forceps have a screw joint with the tip designed to firmly hold the stone. They do not have serrations but have a central fenestration which helps in the lodgment of the stone. Desjardin's forceps are used to extract gallstones from the common bile duct of gallbladder.

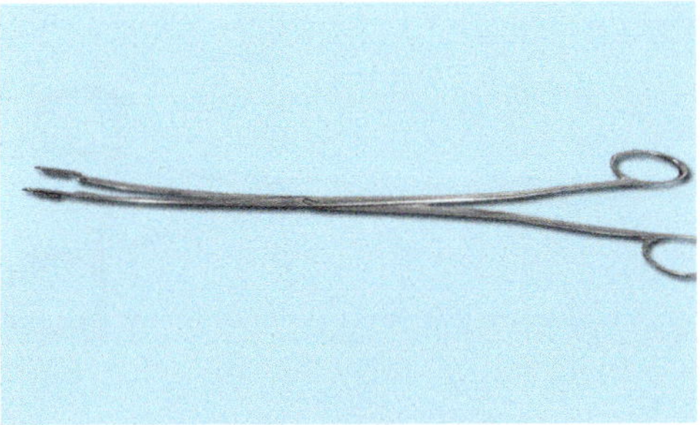

Fig. 20: Desjardin's forceps.

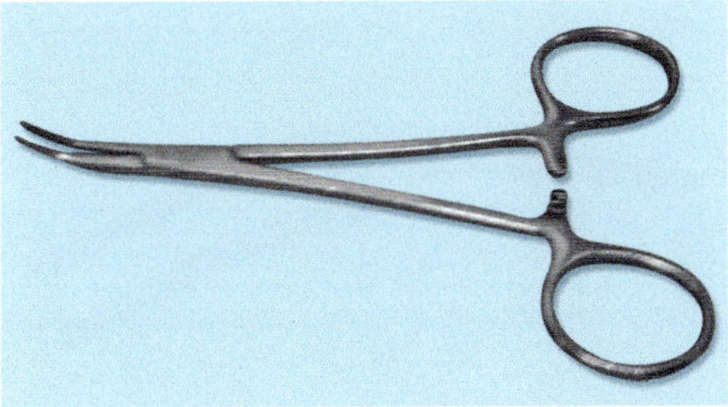

Fig. 21: Spencer Wells hemostatic forceps.

Randall's Stone Holding Forceps

Randall's stone holding forceps are very similar to the Desjardin's forceps in construction with the only differences being the serrations on the tips and the curved working ends. The Randall's forceps are available with working ends in various angles ranging from 60° to 270°. These angles facilitate the approach and removal of stones from calyces which are placed at varied angles in relation to the pelvis. Serrations provide a better grip for these harder renal calculi.

Spencer-Wells Hemostatic Forceps (Fig. 21)

These forceps are very commonly used as a hemostat or a pedicle clamp and are perhaps the most versatile forceps available to the general surgeon. They can be employed for tissue holding, hemostasis, dissection, and even holding a suture needle in the case of dire emergencies of when applying fine sutures. Spencer-Wells forceps can also be used to drain an abscess cavity in the same fashion as a Hilton's abscess forceps but with greater care to avoid damage to the deeper structures. Due to their versatility, they are available in various sizes ranging from very small (Mosquito/Halsted) to large (Kelly's).

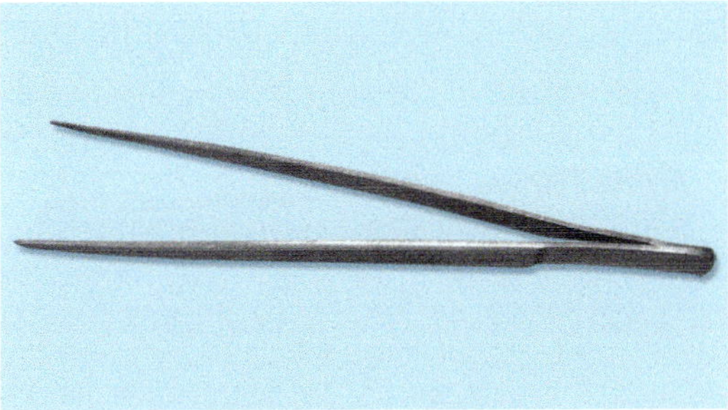

Fig. 22: Adson's forceps.

Tissue Dissection Forceps/ Pickups/ Adson's Forceps (Fig. 22)

Tissue dissection forceps is used to hold delicate tissue for traction and counter traction during dissection. The Adson's forceps has some transverse serrations in the tips to provide a better hold but is nontoothed. The toothed variants are also available and used to hold tough structures such as the sheaths and thick fascia.

Bulldog's Vascular Clamp (Fig. 23)

The Bulldog's vascular clamp is a spring-loaded cross-over clamp for vessels, to stop blood flow distal and proximal to the site of ongoing vascular repair. It is the most versatile clamp used in vascular surgery and has longitudinal striations along its tips such as the DeBakey's forceps and other vascular instruments. The working ends have been modified to suit all kinds of vessels and

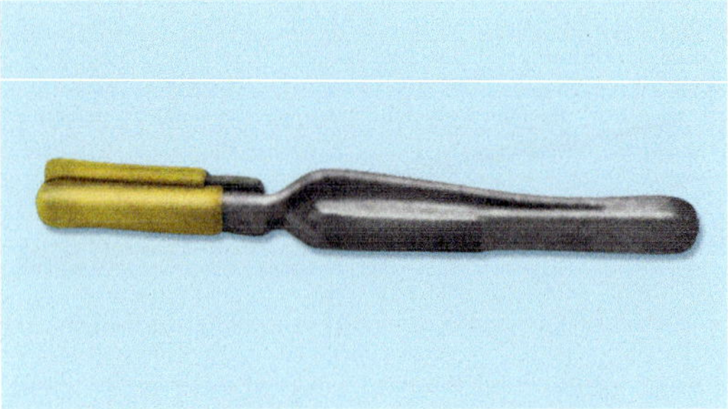

Fig. 23: Bulldog's vascular clamp.

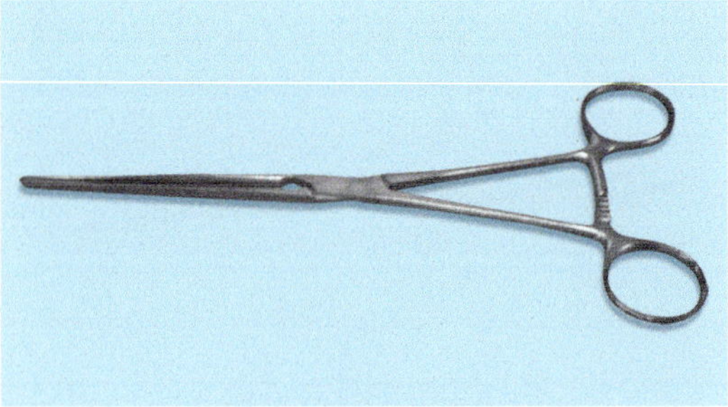

Fig. 24: Doyen's intestinal clamp.

maybe long, curved, or straight. In **Fig. 23**, the ends here are covered with rubber shots to prevent damage. This is how the instrument is usually stored to protect the fine striations at its tip.

Doyen's Intestinal Forceps/ Noncrushing Intestinal Clamps (Fig. 24)

Doyen's intestinal forceps or clamps are used to temporarily occlude lumen of the bowel. These clamps are designed to only occlude the lumen of the bowel without causing any physical damage to the wall of the gut. Compared to the crushing intestinal clamps which are more heavy duty and apposed very tightly, space is appreciable between the two blades of the Doyen's clamp until the instrument is locked. The blades are light weight and fit snugly into each other. They have longitudinal striations which cause minimal pressure necrosis and damage.

Payr's Crushing Intestinal/ Pyloric Clamp (Fig. 25)

Payr's crushing clamps use a double level mechanism to occlude and crush the bowel lumen while performing resection of gut. The instrument closes in two stages, the first wherein the bowel lumen is occluded, and the second lock where in the wall is crushed between the blades. To resect a part of the gut, two crushing clamps are applied to the ends of the diseased gut and two noncrushing clamps applied 5 cm from the crushing clamp on both the ends on the healthy part of the gut. The gut is transected between the crushing and noncrushing clamp, and the healthy gut is anastomosed to each other or brought out as a stoma. Another variant of the crushing intestinal clamp used in gastric resection is known as the *Rochester-Pean clamp*.

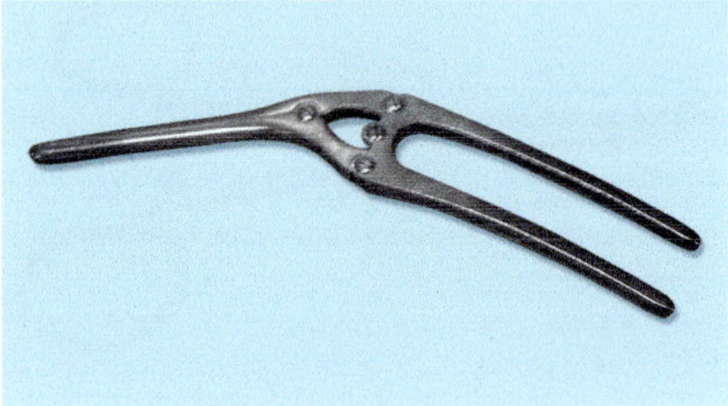

Fig. 25: Payr's crushing intestinal clamp.

Allis Forceps (Fig. 26)

Allis forceps is a hemostatic forceps used to hold fibrous structures such as the rectus sheath during laparotomy. It can also be used as a hemostat. The Allis forceps has splayed out tips with fine serrations which grip the tissue.

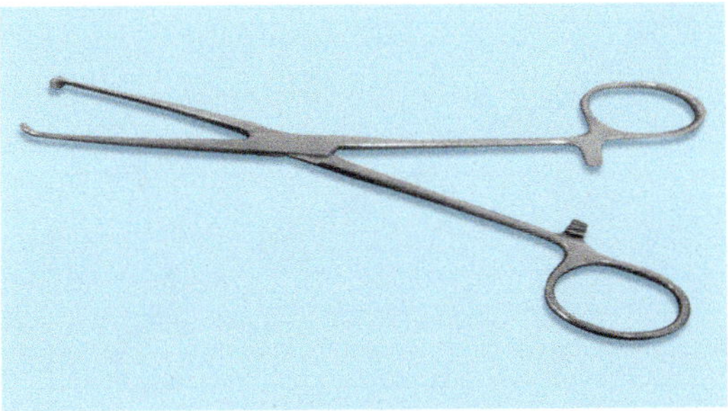

Fig. 26: Allis forceps.

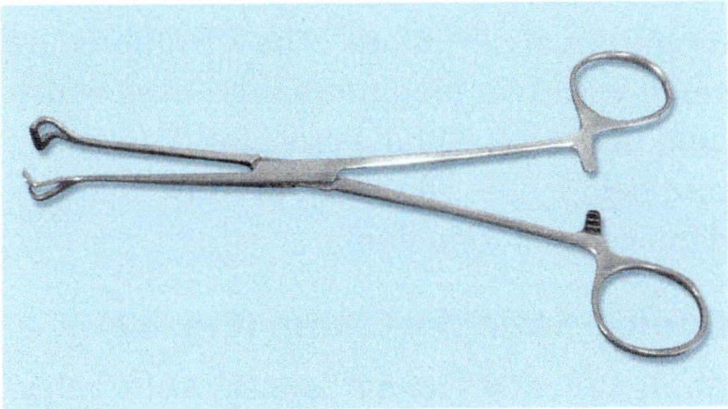

Fig. 27: Babcock's forceps.

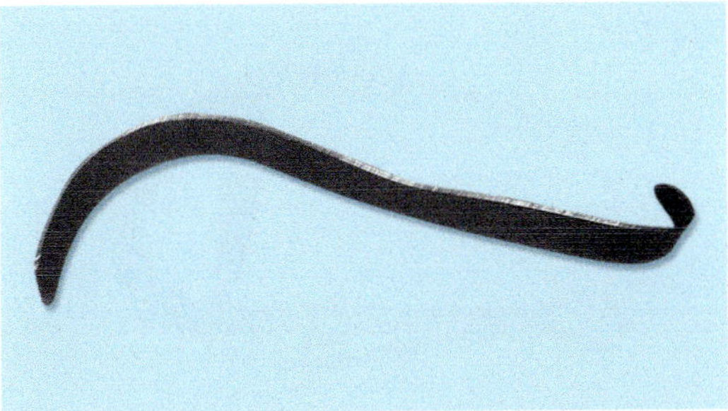

Fig. 28: Deaver's retractor.

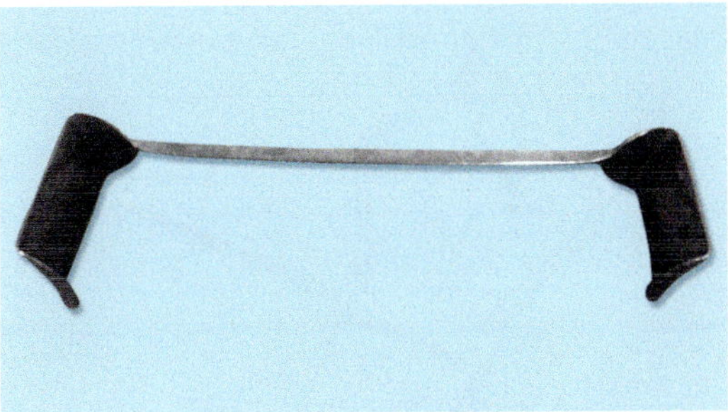

Fig. 29: Morris retractor.

Babcock's Forceps (Fig. 27)

Babcock's forceps is designed to handle tubular structures, such as the appendix, the ureter, and the fallopian tubes. The working end should have the tubular structures with minimal tension such that the intraluminal effects are minimal.

Ben Parker Handle and Blades

The Ben Parker handle consists of a stainless steel handle with a mount on which a surgical blade is placed. Commonly used sizes are handle number 3 and 4. Blades of series 11–15 are mounted on the handle number 3, while blade number 20–30 which are larger blades are mounted on handle number 4. The mounted BP handle is grasped such as a pen and always transferred in a kidney dish.

Deaver's Retractor (Fig. 28)

Deaver's retractor is a single blade curved retractor used to retract deep abdominal or chest incisions and viscera such as the liver during cholecystectomy. It is available in various sizes and used widely in upper abdominal surgeries. A wet mop may be used as an interface when applying it to solid viscera such as the liver or the spleen.

Morris Retractor (Fig. 29)

The Morris retractor is used to retract wound edges during deep abdominal procedures. It has a blade at both ends, which can snugly fit over the wound edge. Morris retractor is widely employed in laparotomy, pelvic surgeries, and gynecological surgeries.

Jolls Thyroid Retractor (Fig. 30)

Jolls thyroid retractor is a screw adjustable retractor bearing two spring action clips on its ends. Its width can be actively adjusted by a central roll over screw mechanism. The spring action clips have a release button at their lateral margins to demount the

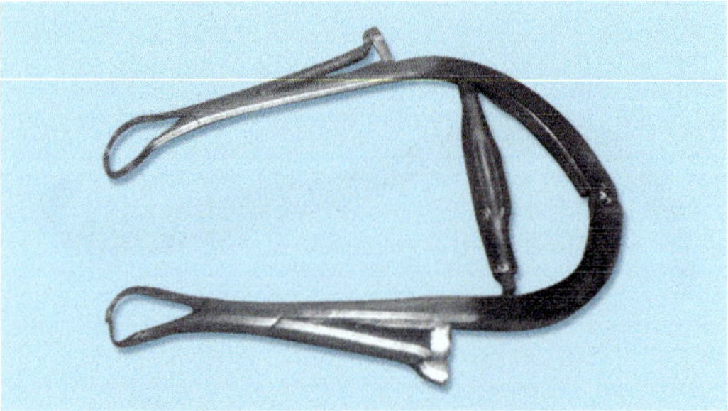

Fig. 30: Jolls thyroid retractor.

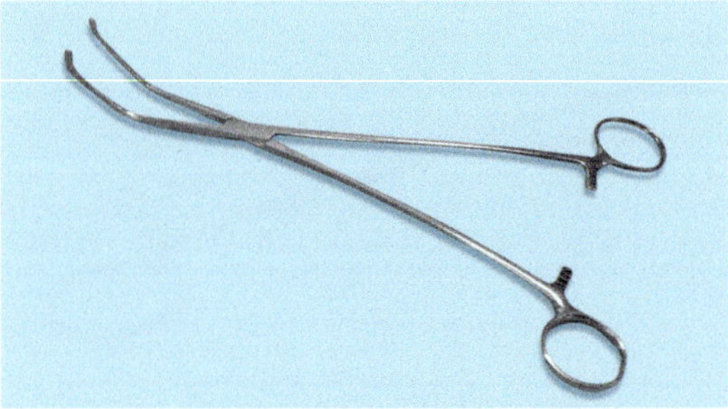

Fig. 32: Satinsky clamp.

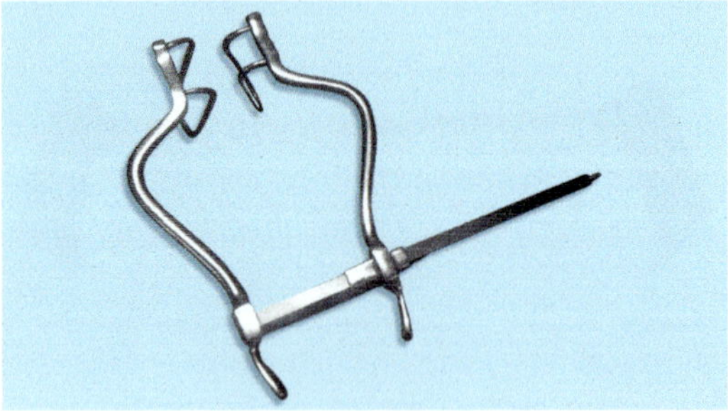

Fig. 31: Balfour self-retaining abdominal wall retractor.

apparatus. This retractor is widely used in thyroid surgeries and other neck surgeries. Other commonly employed retractors for thyroid and neck surgery are the green goiter retractor and the *Weitlaner retractor.*

Balfour Self-retaining Abdominal Wall Retractor (Fig. 31)

Balfour abdominal retractor consists of two blades over a pair of channels with a lock, of which one is fixed and the other one can be slided over the channel and retained in its position. This instrument is used in laparotomies and lower abdominal surgeries. It eliminates the use of active traction by the assistant.

DeBakey's Vascular Forceps

DeBakey's forceps belong to the DeBakey's series of instruments with characteristic longitudinal serrations. The serrations are small with two longitudinal grooves which hold the vessel without crushing. Vessels are best held by the adventitia to cause minimal damage to endothelium.

Cooley-Satinsky Clamp (Fig. 32)

Named after Dr Victor P Satinsky, the Cooley-Satinsky clamp is used to clamp the vessel and repair or perform vascular end-to-side or side-to-side anastomosis. The section to be repaired is placed in the concavity of the clamp, and the distal and proximal flow is occluded by locking the clamp. The working ends have longitudinal serrations to gently occlude the lumen.

Rampley's Sponge Holding Forceps (Fig. 33)

Rampley's sponge holding forceps has ringed tips with transverse serrations that provide a good grip for holding objects. It is commonly used for:

- Swabbing the operative field for disinfection
- Holding the sponge and swabbing the vagina
- Applying medication to deep seated areas
- Pressure over the small areas which are oozing
- Grasping the gall bladder during open cholecystectomy.

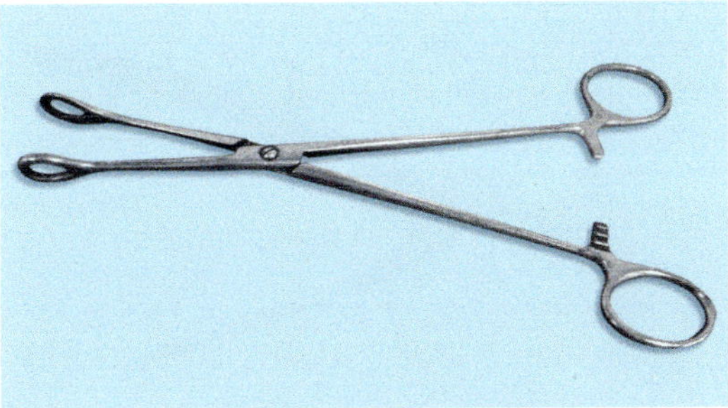

Fig. 33: Sponge holding forceps.

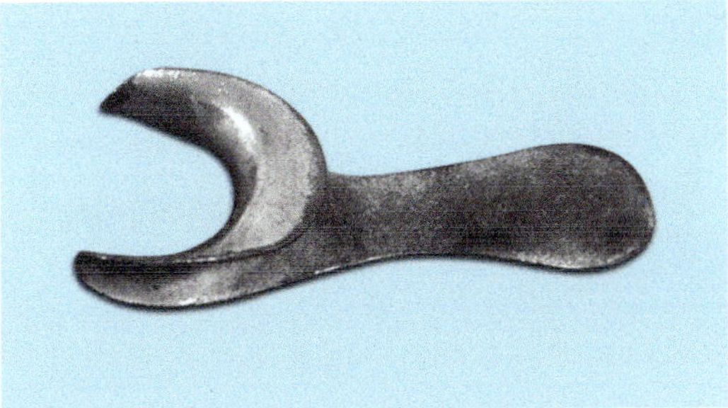

Fig. 34: Cheek retractor.

Lister/Bandage Scissors

Lister's or bandage cutting scissors have a broad blade on one side and a normal second blade. One of its variant used to cut plaster or thick dressings has a blunt tip in front of one of its blades, which is broader than the second blade. These scissors are heavier, and the blunt tip prevents from accidental injury to the body when the blade is introduced between the skin and the dressing.

Cheek Retractor (Fig. 34)

Cheek retractors are available in a variety of designs, being self-retracting as well as nonself-retracting. These retractors are useful in surgeries on the cheek, oral cavity, tongue, and the maxilla. The blades of the cheek retract or fit in the vestibular area between the lips and the gums and the self-retaining mechanism, usually in the form of a spring keeps the oral cavity wide open. The classical single piece nonself-retaining cheek retractor is also applied in a similar fashion, and traction is applied laterally by the assistant.

Cystolithotomy Forceps (Fig. 35)

The cystolithotomy forceps are designed with a cup-shaped working end with multiple spikes in the concavity to firmly grip the stone during open cystolithotomy. One of the rings is open, and the other ring is complete.

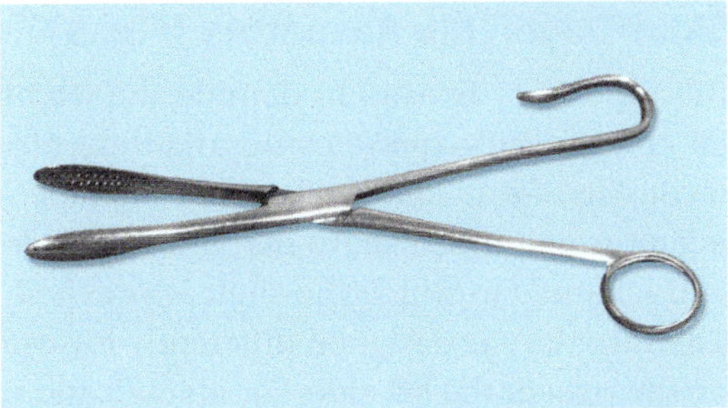

Fig. 35: Thomson Walker's cystolithotomy forceps.

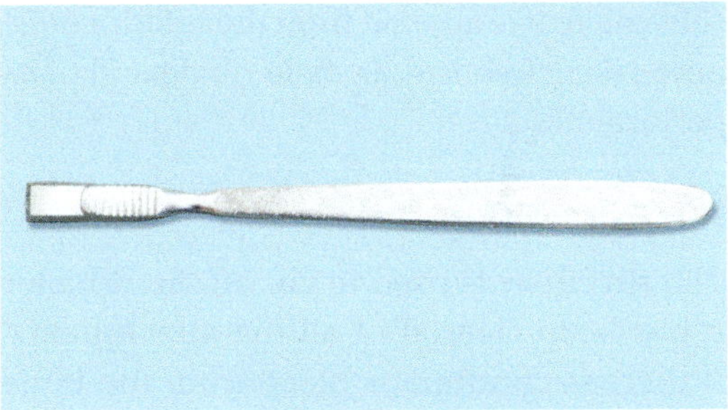

Fig. 36: Periosteal elevator.

Alexander Farabeuf's Periosteal Elevator (Fig. 36)

Farabeuf's periosteal elevator is used to elevate the periosteum from the underlying boon. It has a sharp edge which peels off the periosteum along with attached muscles and ligaments from the bone. The edged end is connected to a shaft with a grip. It is commonly used in renal surgeries where the ligaments and muscles are shaved off the ribs during the flank approach.

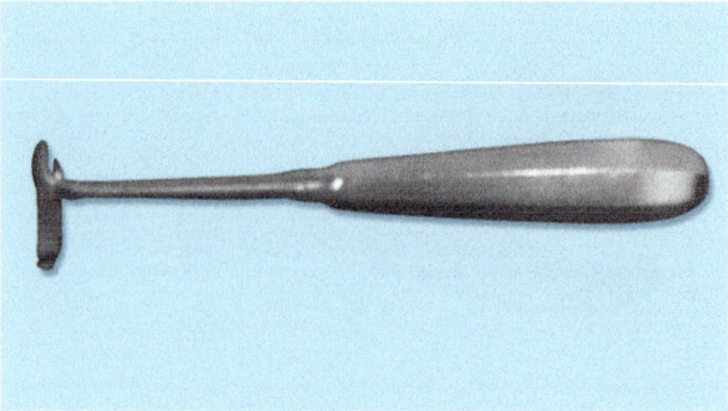

Fig. 37: Rib raspatory.

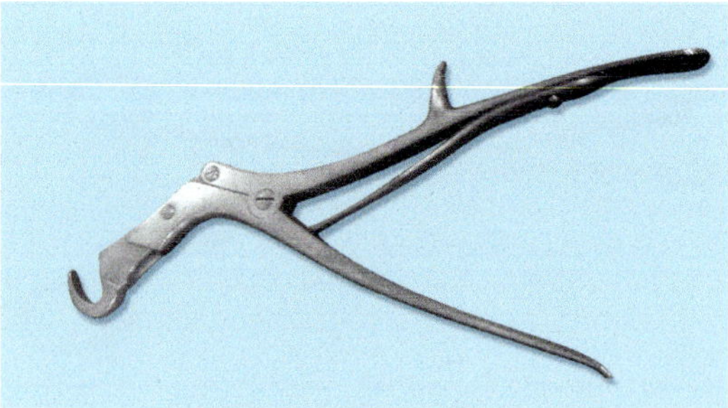

Fig. 38: Rib cutter.

Sklar Doyen Rib Raspatory (Fig. 37)

Rib repository is used to denude the rib of all the musculoaponeurotic attachments. It consists of a tubular shaft coiling and tapering at its end into a sharp marginated blade and a handle to which the shaft is attached. The raspatory is designed differently for use on the right or the left side. For identification, the raspatory is placed on the level surface, and the side to which the coil is open is the side where it is applied from the inferior edge onward encircling the whole rib devoid of its periosteum.

Rib Cutter (Fig. 38)

The rib cutter is used to cut off the rib after it has been cleared of all the attachments. If there is continuous bleed from the bone ends after cutting the rib, bone wax may be applied to the fresh end. Rib is cut during the flank approach if the exposure of the kidney is compromised otherwise.

Finochietto Chest Wall Retractor (Fig. 39)

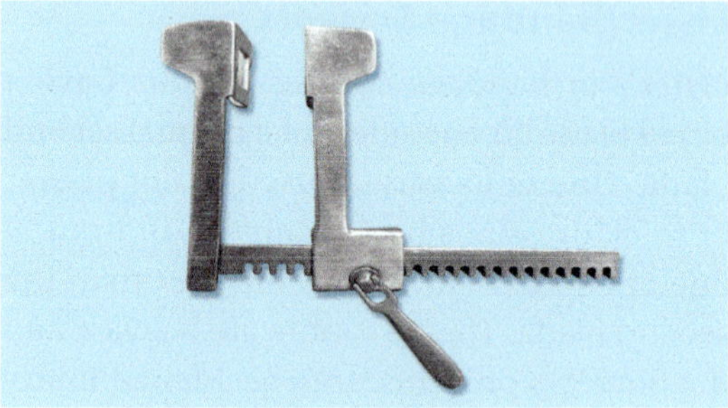

Fig. 39: Chest wall retractor.

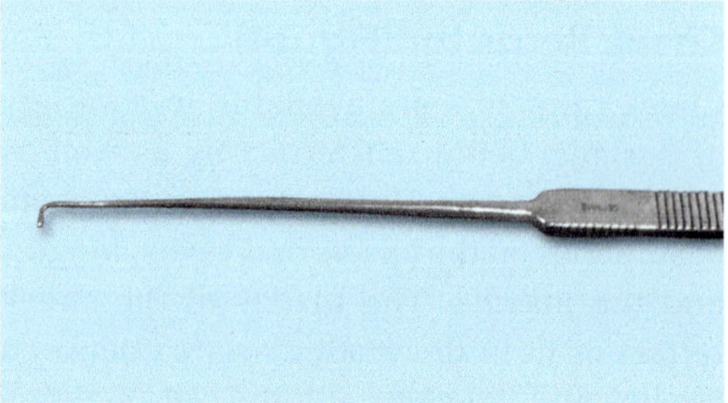

Fig. 40: Nerve hook.

Unlike the abdominal wall which is flexible, the thoracic wall is much less pliable and requires much stronger retraction. This is possible with the Finochietto chest wall retractor, which is a self-retaining retractor with two blades and a rack and pinion arrangement to retract them as required. Being a strong mechanical device, it is important to prevent damage to delicate viscera.

Nerve Hook (Fig. 40)

This is used to hook and raise nerve, e.g., lumbar sympathectomy and transposition of ulnar nerve. This helps in dissection of nerve.

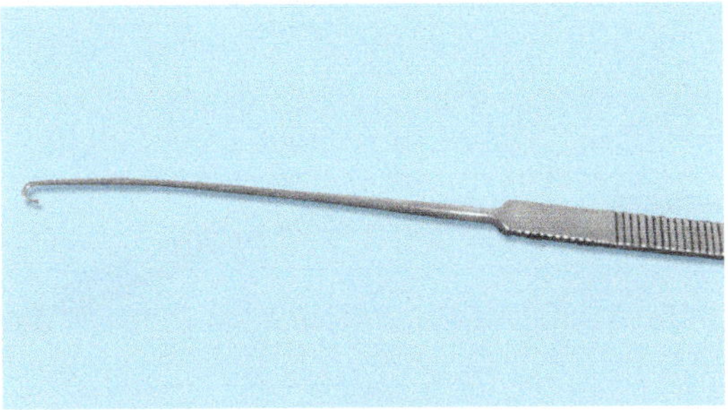

Fig. 41: Vein hook.

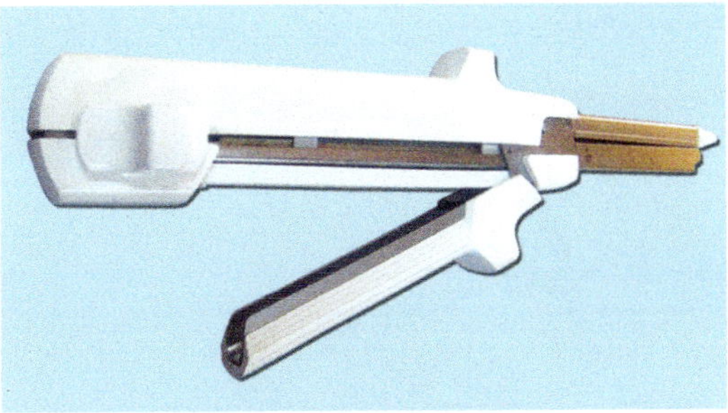

Fig. 42: Linear cutter.

Vein Hook (Fig. 41)

This instrument is useful in dissecting and lifting the veins during avulsion of veins.

SECTION II: STAPLERS

Staplers and their applications in surgery have already been discussed in the earlier sections of this book. In this section, the commonly used stapling devices have been arranged to induce familiarity with these new advancements in the field of surgery.

Disposable Linear Cutter (Fig. 42)

The disposable linear cutter has two halves and a cartridge. The two halves are engaged into each other and the cartridge is loaded between the two blades. The various cartridges have color codes which determine the depth to which the stapler can penetrate. The vascular structures can be anastomosed using the gray and white cartridges, while thicker structures such as the intestine require the blue or green cartridge. Once engaged over the tissue to be divided, the instrument is locked and fired by closing the bar on the right side of the instrument and cut by sliding the handle over the groove. While engaging the stapler on the tissue to be divided, the slider must always face the surgeon. The slider is dealt with the thenar aspect of the hand. Once the stapler is fired, some surgeons would advocate a waiting period of 30 seconds to achieve hemostasis before the tissue is cut. After the completion of the division, the tissue cavity must be inspected for any active bleeding, which can be dealt with active compression by a gauze or electrocautery. The linear cutter can be used for performing side-to-side anastomosis.

The linear cutter is also available in usable stainless steel variant **(Fig. 43)**.

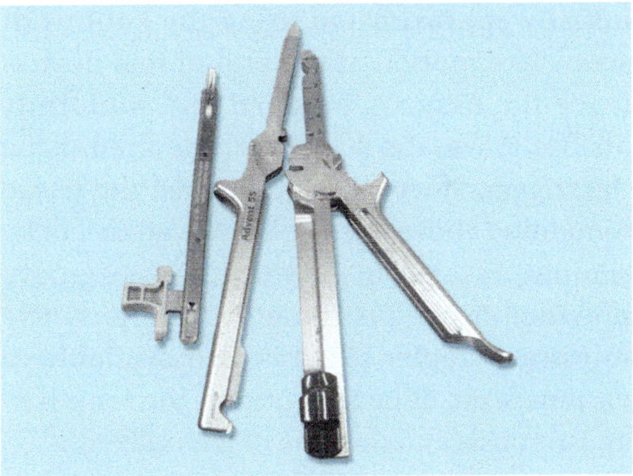

Fig. 43: Reusable stainless steel variant of the linear cutter.

Transverse Intestinal Stapler (Fig. 44)

Transverse stapler is also employed while fashioning a side-to-side anastomosis. The open ends of the anastomosed tissue (performed initially using the linear cutter) are engaged in the groove between the two parts of this stapling device. The ends are

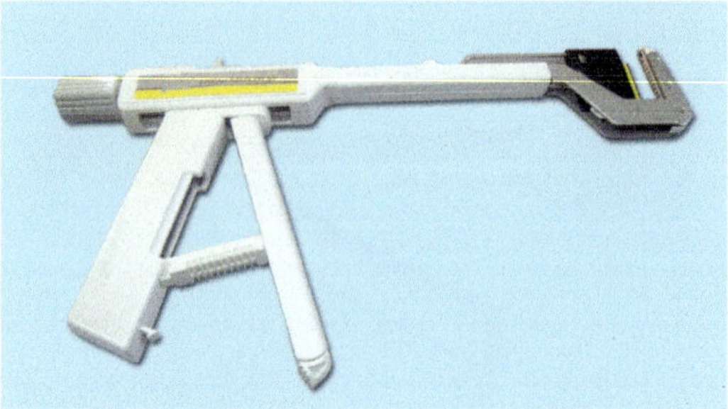

Fig. 44: Transverse interstitial stapler.

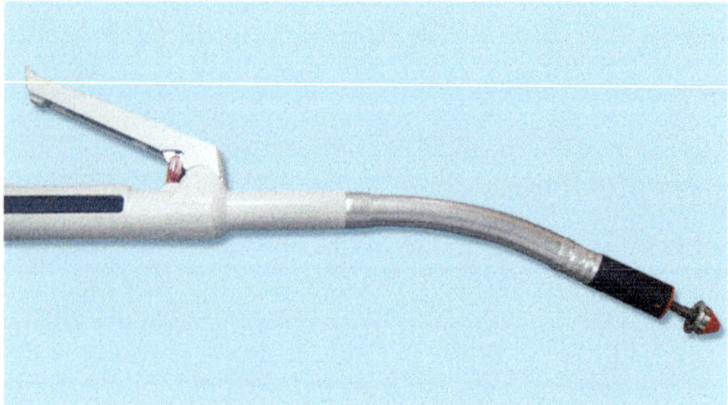

Fig. 45: Circular stapler.

initially approximated using the knob with screw like motion at the end of this device. Once the tissue is engaged and uniformly fits the grove, the stapler can be fired using the trigger. Since it is not a cutter, the tissue remaining above the staple line can be cut by running a scalpel in the stainless steel groove provided in the instrument. The transverse intestinal stapler (TIA) is also available in various sizes depending upon the length of anastomosis and the type of gut utilized.

Circular Stapler (Fig. 45)

The circular stapler is devised to perform the end-to-end anastomosis. It has two essential components: The anvil and the stapling device. The anvil is first engaged in the proximal part of gut and purse string sutures applied to secure it in the lumen. The distal part of the device is introduced through the distal gut or the anal canal the lumen of which is already occluded in the proximal aspect. The sharp end of the anvil pierces the occluded end of the distal gut and engages into the stapler. Once the device is engaged, the screw knob at the distal end of the device is turned to bring the two ends in the firing safe zone, which is indicated by a colored indicator incorporated in the handle of this device. When the indicator turns green, indicating that the anastomosis is safe to perform, the stapling device is fired by using the trigger. The anastomosis is performed also which cutting of the excess gut tissue in the form of a donut which is checked for adequacy and complete circumference once the device is disengaged. As with other types of stapling devices, the hemostasis and adequacy of anastomosis are essentially confirmed intraoperatively.

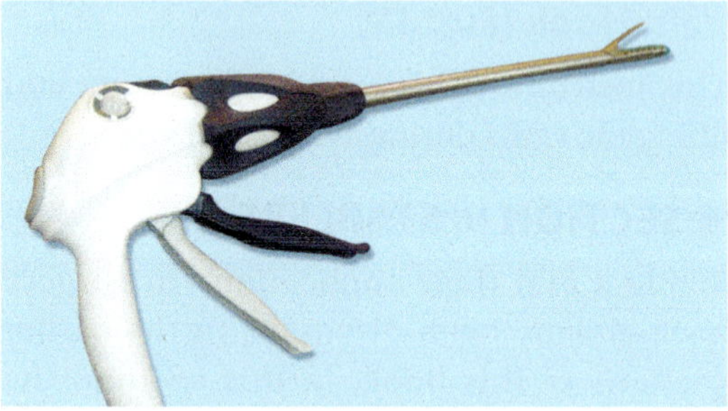

Fig. 46: Laparoscopic linear stapler.

Laparoscopic Linear Stapler (Fig. 46)

Introduced through a 12-mm port, this device functions in essentially the same way as the linear cutter. It has two triggers: One to engage the stapler and the other to cut the tissue. It is a disposable and costly device available in various sizes and cartridge lengths.

Laparoscopic Transverse Stapler (Fig. 47)

This is the laparoscopic variant of the TIA, which has the same construction as the laparoscopic linear stapler with two triggers

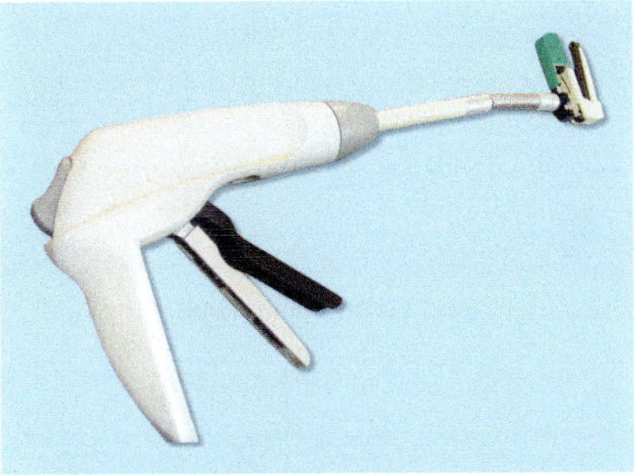

Fig. 47: Laparoscopic transverse stapler.

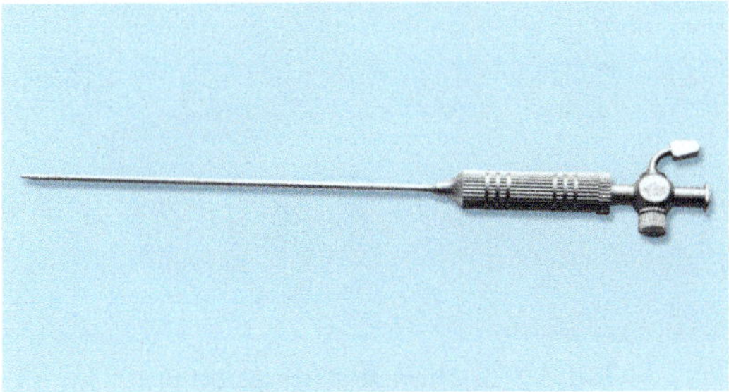

Fig. 48: Veress needle.

and an additional flexible head to engage the open ends for transverse stapling.

Basic Laparoscopic Instruments

Veress Needle (Fig. 48)

The Veress needle is a specially designed needle used for creating pneumoperitoneum by the closed method. This needle was devised by Janos Veress in 1932 and consists of a spring-loaded stylet in a 14-gauge needle, which is about 15 cm long. The blunt tip recedes back exposing the sharp outer sheath when it encounters resistance. On hitting soft tissue such as the viscera, it is the blunt needle that is encountered, thereby protecting these tissues from penetrating injury. The needle has high flow stop cock which can allow gas flow up to 2 L/min.

Laparoscope

The laparoscope consists of a Hopkins Rod Lens system with intervening vacuum encased in a stainless steel tube. Around this system is a series of fiberoptic cables that transmit light from the light source. The laparoscope can be a straight viewing one which is also called a 0° scope and identified by a green ring on the light cable port. Other widely used angles are the12° (black ring), 30° (red ring), and the 70° (yellow ring). The angle scopes are especially useful in single-port surgeries and are an effective solution to the rollover problems. The laparoscope is connected to the camera and a fiberoptic cable for transmitting images to the monitor and light to the abdominal cavity. The new generation laparoscopes feature a flexible tip and the charge-coupled device (CCD) camera at the tip of the scope rather than the end.

Trocars (Fig. 49)

Trocars provide a sheath for introduction of laparoscopic instruments and minimize tissue damage and complications in laparoscopic surgery. A variety of trocars are available to the minimal access surgeon and include the solid core pointed trocars, bladed trocars, and the new generation nonbladed and see through trocars. The shielded and nonshielded bladed trocars have largely been replaced by the bladeless trocars. These trocars are made up of plastic and can be safely inserted using a corkscrew movement. Apart from minimizing the risk of injury to bowel or vessels, these trocars obviate the need of fascial closure of port sites. Apart from closing the midline 12-mm port sites, all other sites can be left open. The see through ports allow the operator to see the abdominal wall layers as the port passes through them making them an excellent

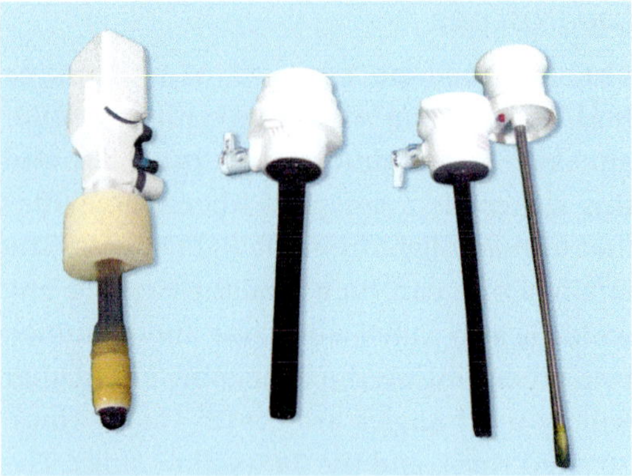

Fig. 49: Various types of laparoscopic trocars.

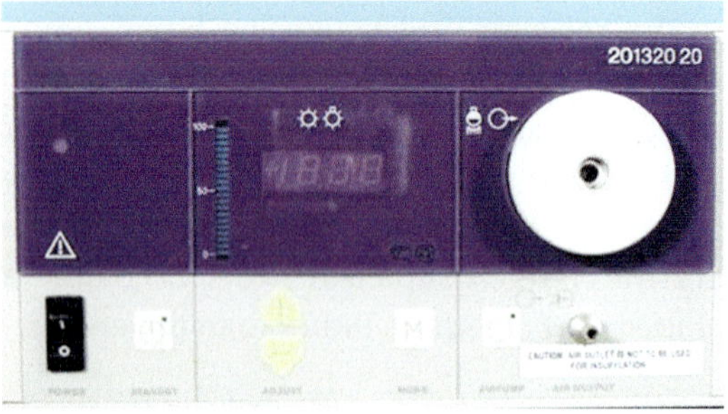

Fig. 50: Light source.

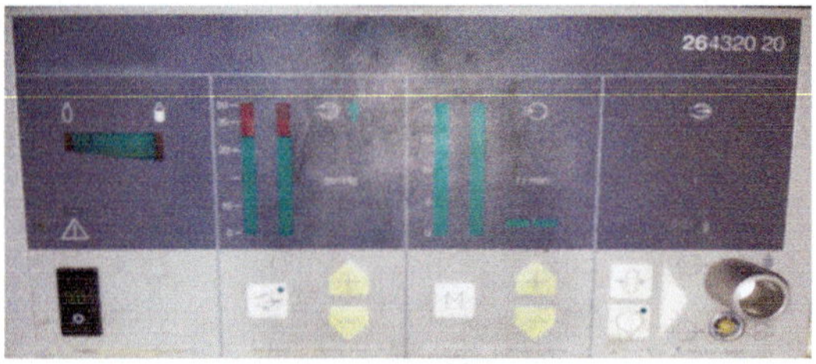

Fig. 51: Insufflation unit.

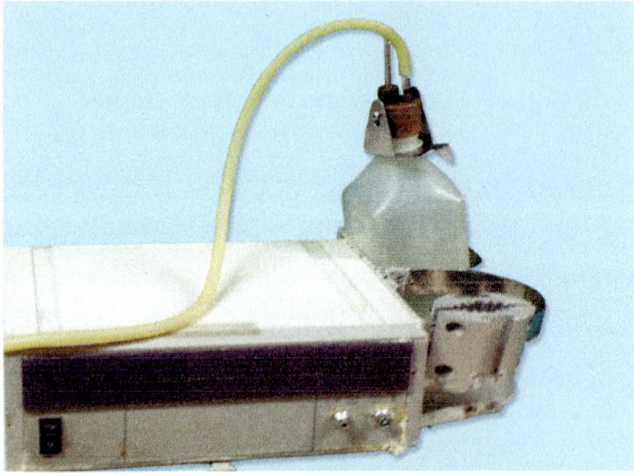

Fig. 52: Suction and irrigation unit.

option of establishing pneumoperitoneum by the open method. Once the trocar is inserted, it can be connected to the gas inflow.

Light Source (Fig. 50)

Light is generated by a high-power light bulb. This can be a white light source such as xenon or incandescent light from a halogen lamp. Light is made to pass through special filters, and its temperature is reduced as it exits the light source unit. By means of fiberoptic cables, the light reaches the laparoscope and illuminates the working space.

Insufflation Unit (Fig. 51)

The insufflation unit is responsible for inflation of gas in the peritoneal cavity, maintenance of intraperitoneal pressure at a desired value, and a feedback loop to constantly monitor the abdominal pressure. The insufflation unit is connected to a gas cylinder.

Suction and Irrigation Unit (Fig. 52)

The suction irrigation unit connects a suction irrigation cannula to a suction bottle and a sterile saline solution which can be used for suction and irrigation respectively at the touch of a button placed on the cannula. The irrigation fluid can be delivered at specified flow rates and suction done at low, medium, or high pressures.

Forceps Overview

The gamut of laparoscopic instruments today is essentially a modification of the contemporary open surgical instruments. The working ends remain the same buy the

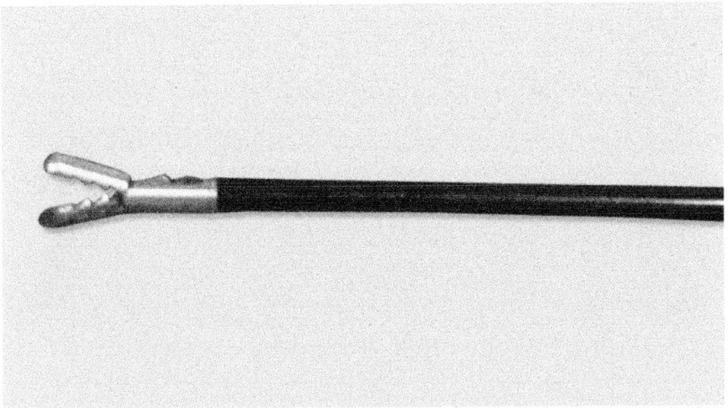

Fig. 53: Short rat tooth grasping forceps.

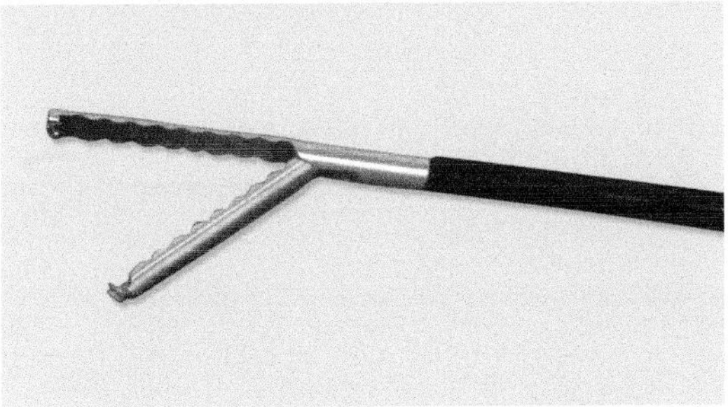

Fig. 54: Long rat tooth grasping forceps.

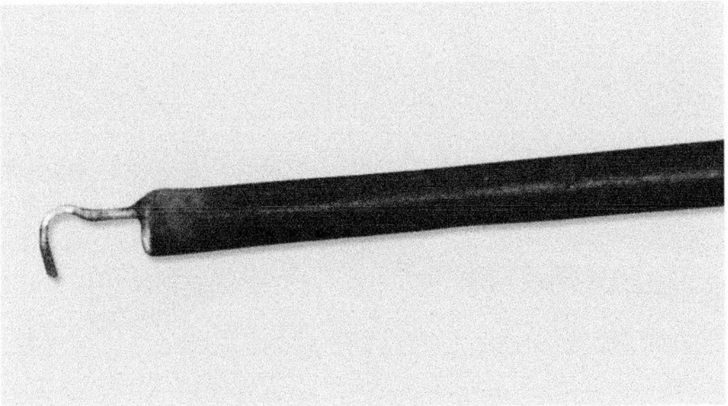

Fig. 55: Electrosurgical hook.

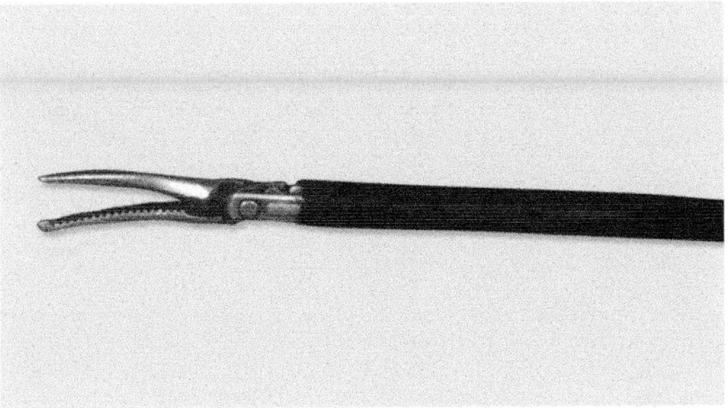

Fig. 56: Maryland's dissector.

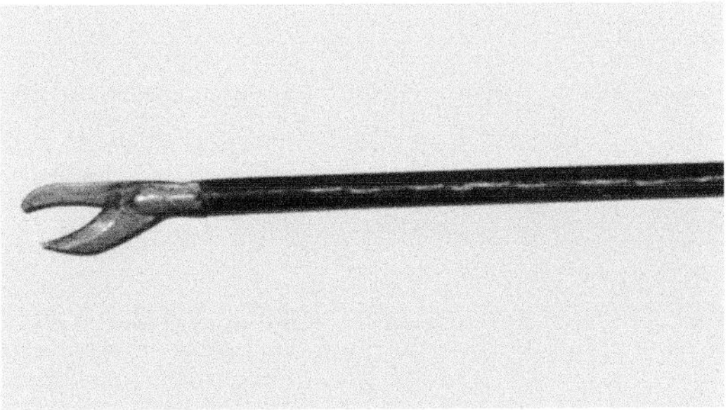

Fig. 57: Hook scissors.

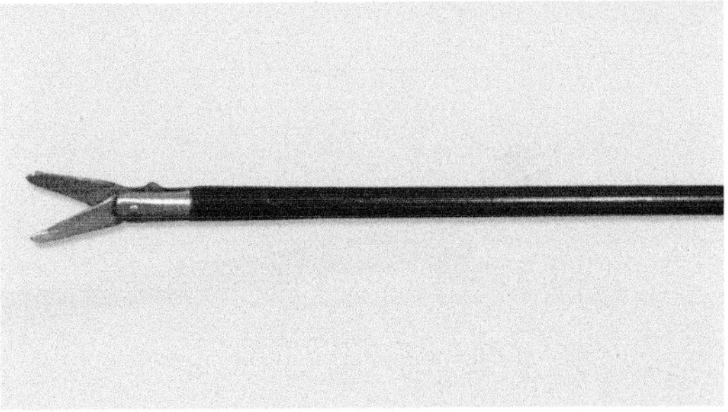

Fig. 58: Metzenbaum scissors.

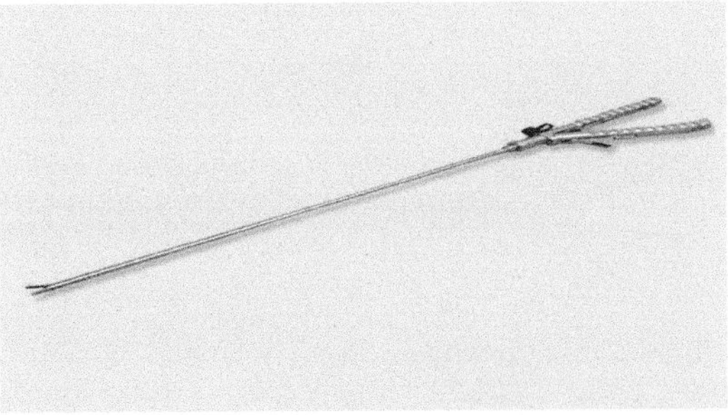

Fig. 59: Needle holder.

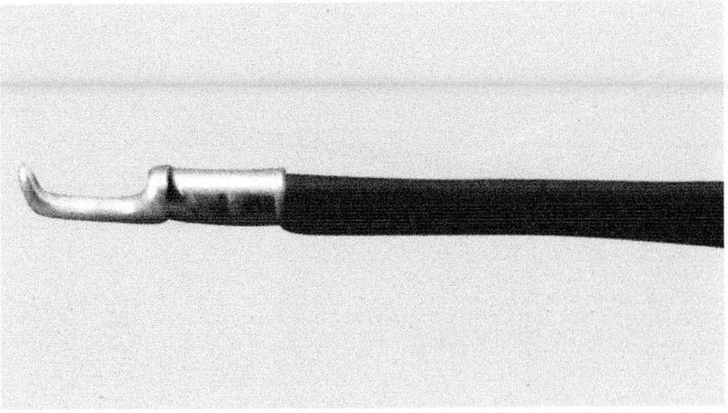

Fig. 60: Crile dissection forceps.

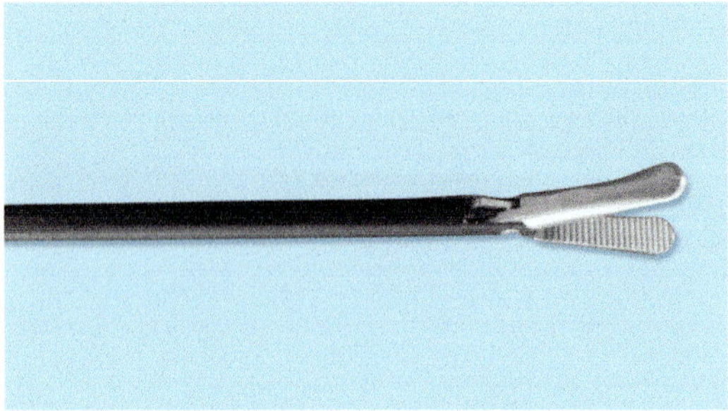

Fig. 61: Duckbill grasper.

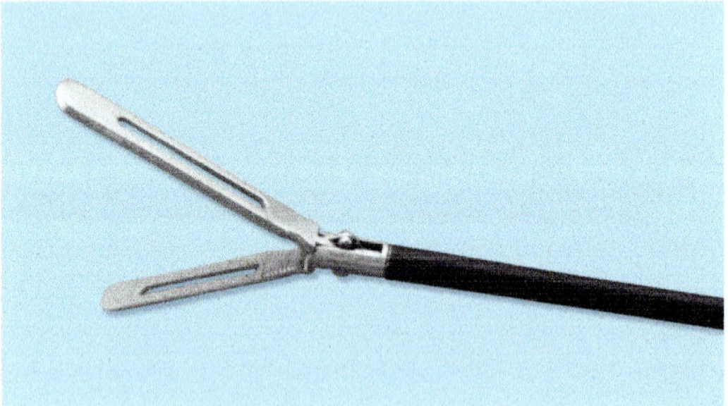

Fig. 62: Dorsey intestinal forceps.

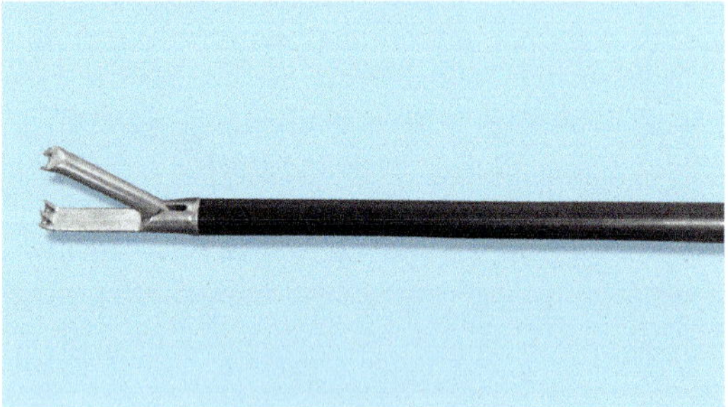

Fig. 63: Claw grasper.

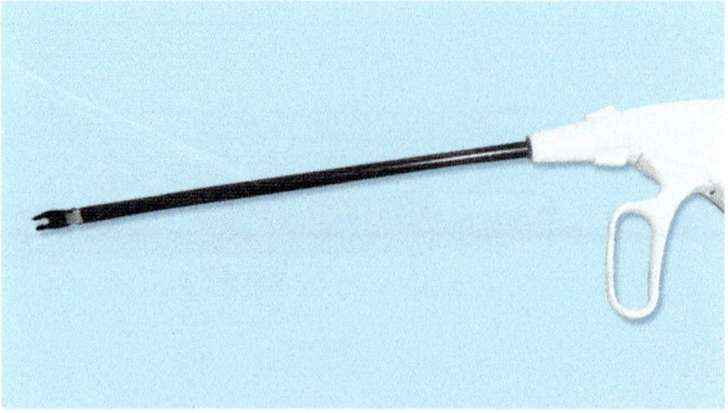

Fig. 64: Clip applicator (disposable).

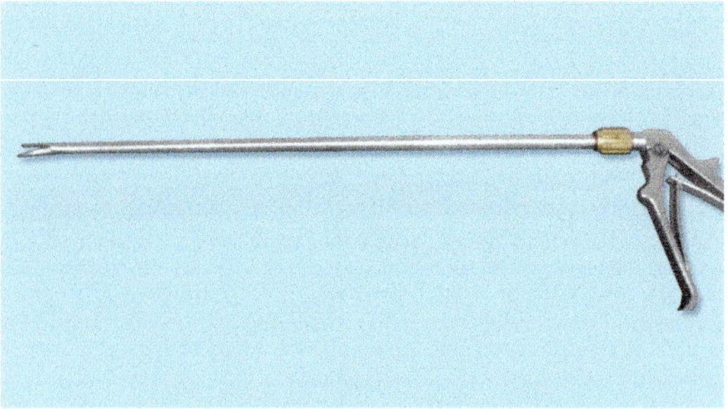

Fig. 65: Reusable clip applicator.

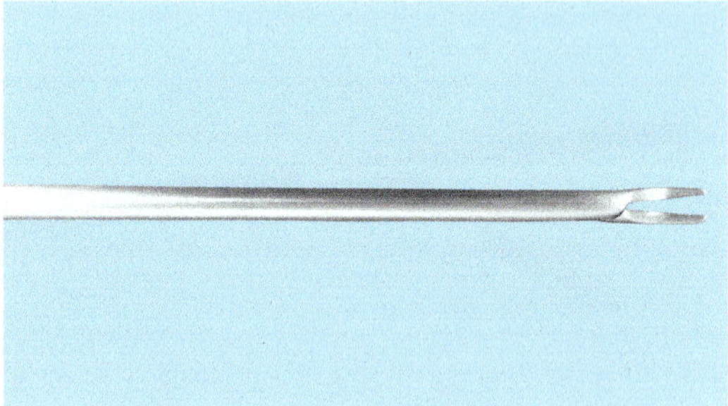

Fig. 66: Reusable clip applicator tip.

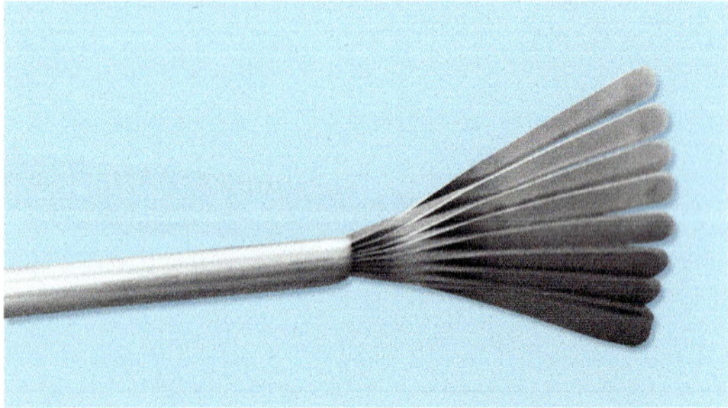

Fig. 67: Fan-shaped retractor.

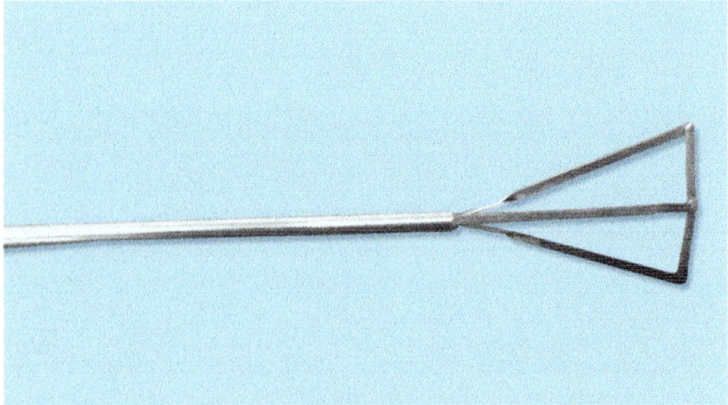

Fig. 68: Triflange retractor to retract liver, intestine, etc.

overall construction consists of a handle with a trigger, rotation knob, an outer insulated sheath, an inner metal sheath, and a jaw insert bearing the working end. The handle may be ratcheted or nonratcheted with a toggle switch to lock the jaws of needed. These instruments are 20–35 cm long with their fulcrum at the midpoint. Bariatric instruments may be up to 45 cm long.

The various laparoscopic instruments are depicted in **Figs. 53 to 68**.

KEY POINTS

Key points on sterilization methods:

- *Autoclaving lubrication:* Apply surgical instrument lubricant (e.g., WPI #500126) to metal-to-metal instruments like scissors and needle holders.
  **Caution:* Avoid using WD-40 or other industrial oils; do not lock instruments during autoclaving.
- *Autoclaving preparation:* Place a towel at the bottom of the sterilization tray to absorb moisture and arrange instruments for proper steam circulation.
  **Caution:* Avoid overloading the tray to ensure effective steam penetration.
- *Autoclave loading:* Load the autoclave chamber carefully, ensuring instruments are not packed too tightly to allow adequate steam flow.
  **Caution:* Overloading may prevent effective sterilization.
- *Autoclave operation:* Follow the manufacturer's guidelines for running the autoclave.
  **Caution:* Open the autoclave door slightly (about 3/4 inch) before the drying cycle to prevent condensation and water stains.
- *Cold sterilization immersion time:* For complete sterilization, immerse instruments for 10 hours; for disinfection, 10 minutes.
  **Caution:* Prolonged immersion can damage instruments.
- *Cold sterilization solutions:* Use appropriate chemical solutions for sterilization that do not harm the instruments.
  **Caution:* Avoid solutions containing benzyl ammonium chloride for tungsten carbide instruments.
- *Instrument handling:* Properly arrange instruments during autoclaving and cold sterilization to avoid damage and ensure full exposure to the sterilizing agents.
- *Avoiding damage:* Be mindful of the specific requirements for different sterilization methods to prevent instrument wear, such as avoiding harsh chemicals for delicate components like tungsten carbide inserts.

CHAPTER 24

Recent Developments in Energy Sources in Surgery

Raman Tanwar, Sudhir Kumar Jain

"Use of energy sources reduces surgical time and causes fewer complications"

INTRODUCTION

The field of surgery has seen a vast expansion with the amalgamation of technical advances with surgical principles. Energy in its various forms has been controlled and selectively applied in facilitating and minimizing surgical trauma. Aim of this chapter is to outline the principles of various devices which use energy sources. These forms of energy include:

- *Electric current is used in:*
  - Conventional monopolar and bipolar electrodes
  - Feedback equipped bipolar systems, e.g., Ligasure®
  - Radiofrequency ablation
- *Ultrasonic waves:* Ultrasonic dissector
- *Electromagnetic waves:* Used as microwaves, radiosurgery
- Cryoablation
- *Light energy:* Lasers, argon beam coagulation, photodynamic therapy, and infrared coagulation with the advances in minimally invasive surgery are commonly used, and the aim of this chapter is to outline the basic principles of these energy sources.

APPLICATION OF ELECTRIC CURRENT

With the advent of technological advances such as incorporated impedance monitoring and feedback regulation of current, it is possible to perform safer and reliable coagulation of tissue with minimal damage to surrounding tissue as the spread of current is minimal due to impedance monitoring. The commonly used devices employing these principles are ENSEAL®, PKS®/Thunderbeat®, and LIGASURE® **(Fig. 1)**. They are basically bipolar low-voltage high-current electrocautery devices, which are activated after grasping the tissue to send electrical current in a computer-controlled fashion followed rapidly by a cycle of sensing tissue impedance and temperature at the site of action. Such cycles of monitoring the process of coagulation and providing appropriate energy in the next cycle take place hundreds or thousands of times depending upon the device specification. These devices give audible signals to inform the operator of completion of the process of coagulation.

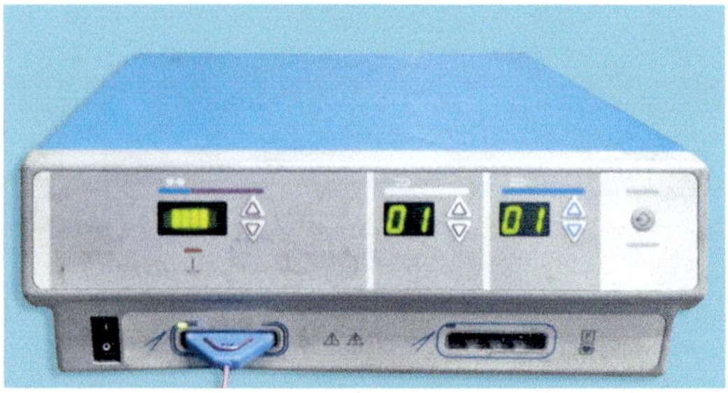

Fig. 1: Ligasure generator.

The use of offset electrodes prevents lateral spread of current and minimizes thermal damage to surrounding tissues.

Mechanism of Action

These bipolar impedance devices act by a combination of bipolar current and pressure. A uniform pressure is applied to the tissues held between the soft jaws of the applicator to coagulate them. The applicator is connected to the generator which senses the various tissue impedance variables and decides the amount of energy that needs to be delivered in the next cycle. The device can be handed or foot activated.

There is denaturation of proteins and coaptation of vessels which makes these devices excellent tools to seal vessels. They provide bloodless dissection and can effectively seal vessels of diameters as large as 7 mm. These devices are superior over the conventional electrocautery. The cost of these devices limits its widespread use and application. The use of these devices saves time as the surgeon does not have to tie vessels up to 7 mm.

RADIOFREQUENCY ABLATION

Radiofrequency ablation is a method for inducing tissue necrosis by using high-frequency alternating current ranging from 350 to 500 kHz. Alternating in this frequency generates ionic agitation and cellular friction producing temperatures in the order of 80–100°C, causing coagulative necrosis. The application can be controlled to generate areas of coagulation necrosis as large as 3–5 cm. Device work on the principle that temperatures generated above 50°C is sustained for more than 3 minutes leads to denaturation of intracellular proteins along with loss of the bilayered lipid membrane, leading to tissue death. This technology has been widely utilized for benign and malignant tumors and ablation of veins, nerves, and cardiac tissue. The principle for all these applications remains the same with the types of probes varying according to the site of application. Radiofrequency ablation bears the advantage of being combined with other modalities of treatment and being used more than once to treat a lesion. It can be used percutaneously, laparoscopically as well as for open surgical approach. Percutaneous management of liver and renal tumors under image guidance is being extensively used to realize the potential and limitations of radiofrequency ablation.

Radiofrequency ablation can be applied to the conscious patient with morbidity approaching that of a tissue biopsy. Radiofrequency ablation is limited in application by the problems of charring of tissue and limited area of damage, especially when applied close to a large vessel and therefore increased risk of residual disease. Addressing these issues, manufacturers have come out with various design modifications and employment of cooling tip to reduce the charring and burning of tissue from heat. Impedance feedback can be added to the probes to provide more adequate tissue destruction. When the impedance rises rapidly, the flow of current is cut off preventing further charring.

ULTRASONIC SHEARS (FIGS. 2 AND 3)

Ultrasonic shear is a safer multipurpose instrument, which can perform multiple tasks minimizing instrument change with minimal lateral damage. Ultrasonically activated scalpel is one of the essential instruments which are used in laparoscopic surgery. The ultrasonic scalpel is the descendant of the widely used Cavitron Kelman phacoemulsifier system used for

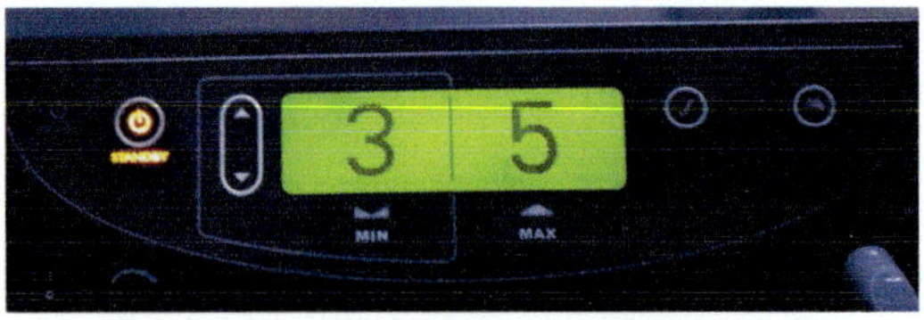

Fig. 2: Ultrasonic generator.

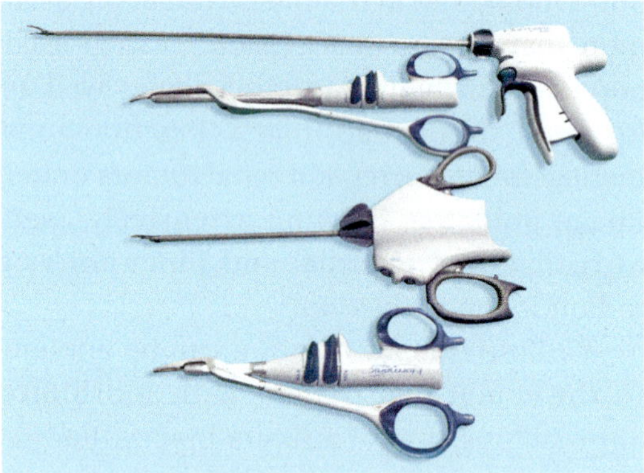

Fig. 3: Different probes of ultrasonically activated scalpel.

performing cataract surgeries. Ultrasonically activated scalpel is based on the mechanical propagation of sound or pressure waves from an active energy source to the tissues through an active blade element. Energy is supplied to either by piezoelectric or magnetic transducer which converts the electric energy or magnetic field to mechanical energy. This energy can be used for cutting and coagulation of tissue.

The ultrasonic scalpel which is available in the market as HARMONIC SCALPEL®, LOTUS®, SONOSURG®, SONICBEAT®, THUNDERBEAT® (combination of advanced bipolar and ultrasonic), etc. is composed of a generator, a hand piece, and an active blade. The generator device is a microprocessor which converts the AC current into a high-frequency operating current at 55,000 cycles/sec. Besides providing a constant high frequency, it also monitors the circuit constantly like the new generation of bipolar electric devices and breaks it whenever the delivered energy is below standards set for the generator by an inbuilt feedback system. This energy is transferred to the transducer through a high-conductivity cable. The transducer houses a number of piezoelectric ceramic plates bound under pressure between two metal plates. The metal plate is connected to a mount which is further attached to the blade extender and the blade. As the power is delivered to and fro, motion of the crystals is transmitted to the active blade which rests in close proximity to the passive blade. This way the entire system uniformly vibrates at 55 kHz with the blade displacing longitudinally by about 60–100 μm.

Mechanism of Action

The transfer of mechanical energy breaks the tertiary hydrogen bonds in the tissues and generates heat from internal cellular friction. Coaptation of vessels by tamponading occurs along with sealing by denatured protein coagulum. Vibrating protein further produces secondary heating which seals larger coapted vessels. Heat, pressure, and turbulence generate bubbles in tissues with high water content, leading to disruption. Another mechanism of cutting is by the movement of the blade to and fro, causing stretch of tissue beyond its elastic limit, leading to breakage of molecular bands. This effect is more prominent in areas of high protein density such as collagen-rich areas. The cavitation effect occurs ahead of the blade which facilitates dissection and makes it more precise. The whole apparatus is housed in sheaths of varying lengths and diameters. The ultrasonic scalpel can coagulate blood vessels in the range of 5 mm without difficulty. In the blunt mode, it can be used to coagulate vessels up to 6–7 mm in diameter. The laparoscopic variants of the ultrasonic scalpel have a vibrating blade with sharp and blunt edges, which rests along with a passive tissue pad between which the tissue is grasped and coagulated. This allows the unsupported tissue also to be coagulated with ease and without bleeding.

The propagation of sound waves though tissues which cause lower heat generation compared to electrocautery and laser devices prevents lateral damage to the surrounding structures. Charring and blackening of tissue occur at high thermal damage and are accompanied by carbonization and smoke generation. The ultrasonic scalpel does not reach such temperatures. Ultrasonically activated scalpel works by coaptation of vessel for sealing the two walls together and forming a protein coagulum within. Electrocautery on the other hand causes direct thermal damage. The luminal contents on application of conventional electrocautery act as a heat sink causing one side to coagulate more than the other with resultant increase in bleeding from one wall of the vessel. The random burning of tissues by lateral thermal damage causes more difficult differentiation of planes and forms a hard eschar and ischemia. The tissues thus heal poorly with more adhesion formation. There is concomitant sealing of vessels and lymphatics on using the ultrasonic scalpel through loose tissues such as fat which leads to better sealing of lymphatics and hemostasis. There is also no risk of muscle or nerve stimulation by transmitted sound energy.

Besides its own advantages, the ultrasonically activated shears keep the surgeon at bay from the ill effects of free current such as stray electric current injuries, pad grounding problems, bowel electric injury, and burns. The visual field which is crucial particularly in laparoscopic surgeries is also disturbed less with the ultrasonic shears at work, since less temperature production causes little smoke and minimal obscuration of the surgical field with tissue fog. With the back of the passive blade, blunt dissection is also possible side by side with making planes. Ultrasonic devices have also found favor among patients with pacemakers. The theoretical advantages of the ultrasonic scalpel have been put to test by number of surgeons all across the globe with encouraging results.

MICROWAVES

Microwave energy produced through a generator (usually 0.9–2.45 GHz) produces heat by generation of friction by the movement of water molecules. This energy is applied to the tissue by the means of 14 G microwave antenna which is placed directly into the tumor. This antenna transmits electromagnetic waves that have been produced by the generator. These waves cause the agitation of water in and around the tissue causing coagulation and necrosis due to production of heat by friction, reaching temperatures above 55°C. Microwaves can be applied in a fashion similar to radiofrequency ablation using percutaneous, laparoscopic, or open approach. Liver, lung, renal, adrenal, and bone tumors have been treated with the use of microwave technology with encouraging results. Microwave generators have reduced in size considerably and have made this technology more portable. Microwave ablation carries the same advantages and disadvantages as radiofrequency ablation but lesser tissue charring.

CRYOABLATION

Cryoablation is a process of inducing tissue death by rapid cooling. It has become a standard modality of treatment for management of solid organ tumors and superficial lesion. Cryoablation works by intracellular crystallization of the tissue to which it is applied and also by damaging the vasculature by forming thrombi and inducing a state of ischemia. A second wave of reperfusion injury damages the left overs. This can be achieved by utilizing a 14–16G probe similar to the ones seen with microwave and radiofrequency ablation but with different internal structure. The third-generation system utilizes rapidly flowing gases such as carbon dioxide and argon at extremely low temperatures that cause rapid cooling of tissue to as low as -40°C. Probes can achieve temperatures close to -200°C although such temperatures are rarely used in vivo. After a rapid freezing cycle, the tissue is left to thaw actively or passively. Thawing is important for inducing damage by restoring blood supply and allowing reperfusion injury to set it. After a slow thaw phase, the whole cycle is repeated to increase effectiveness of cryoablation. Nearby important tissues are protected using a warming device intraluminally. With the use of multiline cryoablation wherein multiple small probes are used, every nook and corner of the tumor can be covered.

Advantages of cryoablation over other minimally invasive and percutaneous therapies are the ability to monitor the ice ball formed by ultrasound or direct visualization when applied in a laparoscopic or open surgical setting. Therefore a complete coverage of tumor can be ensured. It causes minimal pain and morbidity and used as an office procedure in various settings. The application of probes near large vessels can cause a heat sink effect and is therefore ineffective in such lesions which lie adjacent to vessels such as the renal hilum. Compared to open surgery, these minimally invasive methods have a higher chance of recurrence. However, the ability to utilize them again and again gives a little advantage in this situation.

Combinations of various energy sources are mostly used for hemostasis and dissection utilizing the better of every available device to deliver the best results. Some devices such as the THUNDERBEAT® incorporate both bipolar electric energy and ultrasonic energy in one applicator and either can be used to dissect without switching instruments. It is the experience and skill of the surgeon along with the awareness regarding these new devices which ultimately delivers. Application of the right source at the right place is what makes a difference.

KEY POINTS

- Complex surgical procedure like radical cystectomy and Whipple procedure becomes much easier by use of ligasure and ultrasonic machine.
- Ultrasonic scissor is an essential adjunct for minimally invasive surgery.
- Cryoablation is being commonly used for treatment of T1a renal cell carcinoma and liver metastasis.

CHAPTER 25

Robotic Surgery

Sudhir Kumar Jain, Mrunal Bharat Kshirsagar, Raman Tanwar

"Robotics is not about making machines to serve us. It's about creating machines that can be our partners—Cynthia Breazeal"

HISTORY OF ROBOTIC SURGERY

The key milestones in the history of robotic surgery, from the early experimental use of robots such as the Puma 560 to the development and commercialization of systems such as Da Vinci and Zeus, which have significantly impacted modern surgical practices is shown in **Table 1**.

Here is the enumeration of the Food and Drug Administration (FDA)-approved robotic systems for general surgical use:

- *ROBODOC:* Developed by Integrated Surgical Systems (Sacramento, CA), initially approved for machining the femur during hip replacement surgeries.

TABLE 1: History of robotic surgery.

1985	*Puma 560* robot used by Kwoh et al. for neurosurgical biopsies
1988	Davies et al. perform transurethral resection of the prostate using Puma 560
Early 1990s	Development of PROBOT for transurethral resection of the prostate
Early 1990s	Development of *ROBODOC* by Integrated Surgical Supplies Ltd., *first FDA-approved surgical robot*
Mid-to-late 1980s	NASA Ames Research Center begins work on telepresence surgery
Early 1990s	Scientists from NASA-Ames join SRI and develop dexterous telemanipulator for hand surgery
Early 1990s	Exploration of surgical robots' potential in overcoming limitations of laparoscopic surgery
1990s	US Army funds development of telepresence surgical system for battlefield casualty care
Early 1990s	Formation of commercial ventures from Army-funded projects, leading to civilian adoption of surgical robots
Late 1990s	Computer Motion develops AESOP, a robotic arm for endoscopic camera manipulation
Late 1990s	SRI's Green Telepresence Surgery system licensed and redesigned as the *Da Vinci surgical system by Intuitive Surgical*
Late 1990s	Computer Motion introduces *Zeus surgical system* for robotic surgery

(AESOP: automated endoscopic system for optimal positioning; FDA: The Food and Drug Administration; NASA: National Aeronautics and Space Administration)

TABLE 2: Difference between Da Vinci Surgical System and Zeus Surgical System.

Feature	***Da Vinci Surgical System***	***Zeus Surgical System***
Development origins	Evolved from telepresence machines developed for NASA and the US Army	Developed independently by Computer Motion Inc.
Components	Vision cart, master console, moveable cart with instrument, and camera arms	Similar setup with vision system, master console, and moveable arms
Camera system	Dual 3-chip cameras providing a 3-dimensional image with depth of field	Utilizes advanced camera technology for enhanced visualization
Control interface	Master console with image processing computer, view port for 3D visualization, foot pedals, and master control grips	Equipped with controls for precise manipulation of surgical instruments and camera
Instrument arms	Features two instrument arms and one camera arm, all cable-driven with 7 degrees of freedom	Provides multiple arms with comparable degrees of freedom and capabilities for surgical tasks
Operational philosophy	Instruments operated from console to mimic surgeon's hand movements with enhanced dexterity	Focuses on enhancing surgical precision and control through advanced robotic technology
Surgical applications	Widely used across various surgical specialties for minimally invasive procedures	Applied similarly across surgical fields, aiming to improve surgical outcomes and patient recovery
Manufacturer	Developed by Intuitive Surgical Inc., based in Mountain View, CA	Developed by Computer Motion Inc., Santa Barbara, CA (later acquired by Intuitive Surgical)

- *AESOP:* Automated endoscopic system for optimal positioning, developed by Computer Motion Inc. (Santa Barbara, CA), a voice-activated robotic arm for endoscopic camera manipulation.
- *Da Vinci Surgical System:* Developed by Intuitive Surgical Inc. (Mountain View, CA), a comprehensive master-slave surgical robotic system widely used across various surgical specialties.
- *Zeus Surgical System*: Developed by Computer Motion Inc. (Santa Barbara, CA), a master-slave surgical robotic system similar to Da Vinci, aimed at enhancing surgical precision and control.

These systems have significantly advanced the field of robotic surgery, each offering unique capabilities and features approved by the FDA for clinical use **(Table 2)**.

DA VINCI ROBOTIC SYSTEM

Da Vinci Robotic System is shown in **Fig. 1**.

SSI Mantra Robot—First Indian Robot

The first Indian robot SSI Mantra is shown in **Fig. 2**.

Zeus Robotic System

ZEUS robotic system is shown in **Figs. 3A to C**.

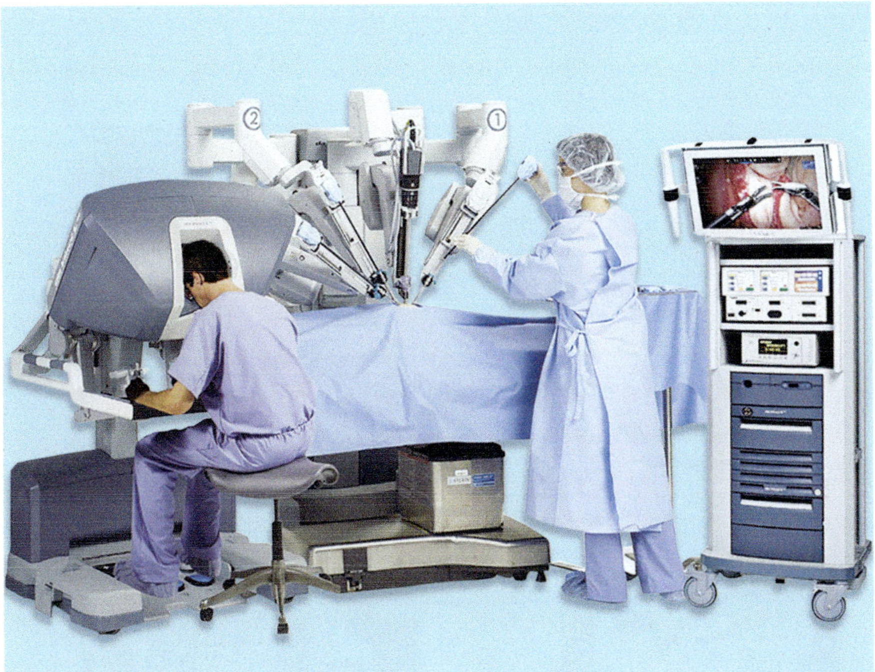

Fig. 1: Da Vinci robotic system.

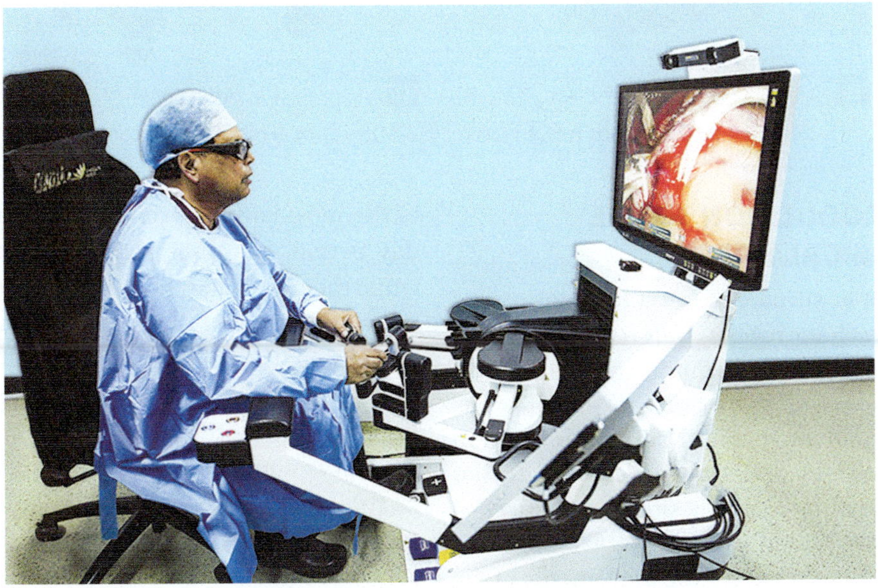

Fig. 2: First Indian robot—SSI Mantra robot.

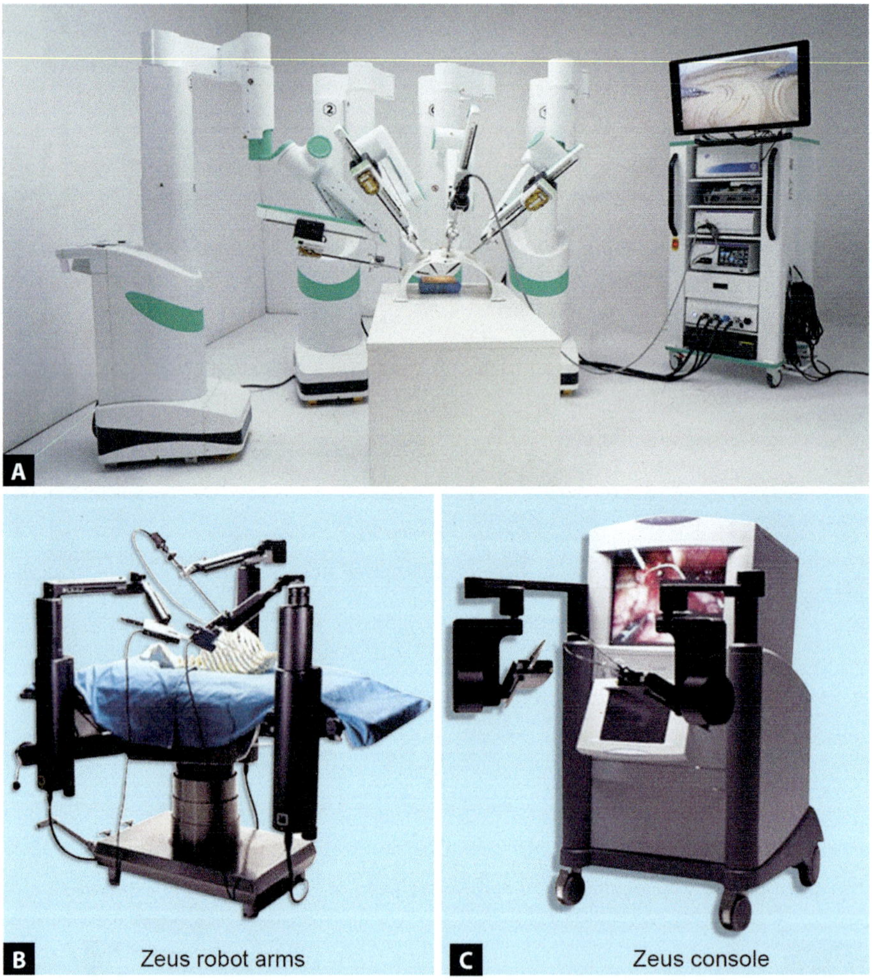

Figs. 3A to C: (A) Zeus robot system; (B): Zeus robot arms; (C) Zeus console.

INTRODUCTION TO THE SURGICAL ROBOT

Robotics in surgery is not a new entity and we have had robots before which were used to hold the camera and scope and also responded to voice. The scenario has become advanced with the introduction of the master and slave system such that the operating surgeon sits at the surgical console while the patient cart contains the arms that replicate the movements of the surgeon's hand as precisely as possible. One of the most common misconceptions to this day is that the robot performs the surgery while the fact is that the robot only replicates the movements of the surgeon's hands. We are far from the era where robots will gain the intelligence and be allowed to operate upon humans independently. The surgery where a robot is employed is thus only referred to as robotically assisted surgery. Robots may be of two types. Passive robot is essentially a retractor system where its role is to position the instrument and hold it there. Active robots allow guided movement which are controlled by the surgeon or replicated from the surgeon through a console.

Robotic surgery team consists of a group of health professionals of which the surgical robot can be viewed as a complex instrument with multiple attachments. The team is led by the robotic surgeon who performs the procedure through the master system or the surgical console. The assistant surgeon is responsible for the docking, introduction of the ports, surgical assistance through accessory ports in the form of application of clips, aspiration, specimen extraction, change of instrumentation undocking, and removal of the ports. Another important member of the core team is the scrub nurse who is responsible for the docking and draping of the surgical robot patient cart, instrument changes, and undocking.

The modern surgical robot provides some distinct advantages over conventional laparoscopic surgery **(Table 3)**:

- Better ergonomics with minimal surgeon fatigue
- 7 degrees of freedom and flexibility
- Possibility of telesurgery
- Trainee console for better training opportunities
- Enunciation of 90 degrees
- Finger-tip control and spontaneous movement control
- Decrease in tremor
- Motion scaling.

Disadvantages of the surgical robot to this day are the enormous cost, lack of long-term data, mechanical failures, and loss of tactile feedback. Visual resistance is the only means of haptic feedback **(Table 4)**.

The surgical robot consists of three essential segments namely the surgeon or master console, the patient cart, and the vision cart **(Table 5 and Fig. 4)**.

Master Console

Master console is where the surgeon sits and controls the movements of the arms.

TABLE 3: Advantages and disadvantages of robot-assisted surgery versus conventional surgery.

Human strengths	***Human limitations***	***Robot strengths***	***Robot limitations***
Strong hand-eye coordination	Limited dexterity outside natural scale	Good geometric accuracy	No judgement
Dexterous	Prone to tremor and fatigue	Stable and untiring	Unable to use qualitative information
Flexible and adaptable	Limited geometric accuracy	Scale motion	Absence of haptic sensation
Can integrate extensive and diverse information	Limited ability to use quantitative information	Can use diverse sensors in control	Expensive
Rudimentary haptic abilities	Limited sterility	May be sterilized	Technology in flux
Able to use qualitative information	Susceptible to radiation and infection	Resistant to radiation and infection	More studies needed
Good judgment			
Easy to instruct and debrief			

TABLE 4: Advantages and disadvantages of conventional laparoscopic surgery versus robot-assisted surgery.

	Conventional laparoscopic surgery	***Robot-assisted surgery***
Advantages	• Well-developed technology • Affordable and ubiquitous • Proven efficacy	• 3-D visualization • Improved dexterity • Seven degrees of freedom • Elimination of fulcrum effect • Elimination of physiologic tremors • Ability to scale motions • Micro-anastomoses possible • Tele-surgery • Ergonomic position
Disadvantages	• Loss of touch sensation • Loss of 3-D visualization • Compromised dexterity • Limited degrees of motion • The fulcrum effect • Amplification of physiologic tremors	• Absence of touch sensation • Very expensive • High start-up cost • May require extra staff to operate • New technology • Unproven benefit

TABLE 5: Types of special surgeries and procedures performed using robotics.

Surgical specialty	***Most common procedures performed using robotics***
General surgery	• *Cholecystectomy:* Removal of the gallbladder • *Hernia repair:* Repair of abdominal hernias • *Appendectomy:* Removal of the appendix
Gynecological surgery	• *Hysterectomy:* Removal of the uterus • *Ovarian cystectomy:* Removal of ovarian cysts • *Myomectomy:* Removal of uterine fibroids
Urological surgery	• *Prostatectomy:* Removal of the prostate gland for prostate cancer treatment • *Nephrectomy:* Removal of part or all of the kidney • *Pyeloplasty:* Reconstruction of the ureteropelvic junction for UPJ obstruction
Cardiac surgery	• *Coronary artery bypass grafting (CABG):* Revascularization of blocked coronary arteries • *Mitral valve repair/replacement:* Repair or replacement of the mitral valve • *Atrial fibrillation ablation:* Treatment of atrial fibrillation to restore normal heart rhythm
Orthopedic surgery	• *Total knee arthroplasty (TKA):* Knee replacement surgery • *Total hip arthroplasty (THA):* Hip replacement surgery • *Spinal surgery:* Various procedures including spinal fusion
Head and neck surgery	• *Transoral robotic surgery (TORS):* Surgery for head and neck cancers • *Thyroidectomy:* Removal of the thyroid gland • *Parathyroidectomy:* Removal of overactive parathyroid glands

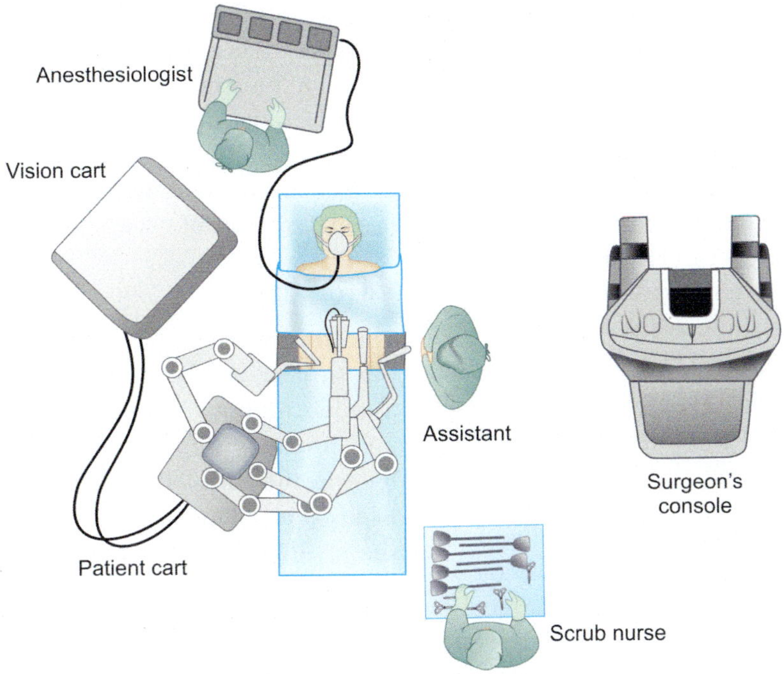

Fig. 4: Robotic surgery theater layout.

The latest versions provide a stereoscopic vision. Magnified 12× view with stereoscopic 3D vision is ensured by the endoscopic camera of the robotic system that houses two cameras in one. It also houses a microphone. Infrared sensors sense the head of the surgeon and as soon as the surgeon looks outside the movements of the instruments are frozen.

The armrest of the master console has two pods, one on each side. The da Vinci Si system has two buttons on the right pod, one for switching the system on, and the other for emergency shutdown. Once the emergency shutdown is pressed, the entire motion freezes to prevent any inadvertent harm to the patient. The left side pod has ergonomic controls, one to adjust the location of the foot pedal, other for the arm-rest height, third one for the movement of the master control shell and the tilt. This provides adjustment for ergonomic seating, thereby minimizing surgical fatigue. There are various foot pedals on the master console that are used for changing the active arms, camera control, and activation of cautery.

The surgical console is placed away from the sterile field in such a way that a clear view of the operative area is always available to the operating surgeon and whenever required he can communicate with the assistants and the anesthesiology team.

The surgical console has a driving handle at its back and can be used to reposition the console by pushing it using this handle. Once the position is confirmed, the wheels can be locked to ensure stability.

Patient Cart

The patient cart houses the arms of the robot which are controlled by the operating surgeon at the master console. There are four arms in the modern robot, one for the camera and three for the instruments. Any extra number of instruments can be introduced manually and controlled by the assistant using separate ports. Unlike the master console and the vision cart, the patient cart has to be kept in the sterile field and has to be draped. The patient cart is heavy and requires two personnel to position it. To facilitate this process, the patient cart has a driving motor which can be engaged by switching the main power button on the patient cart and then shifting the lever to D or drive mode. In order to move the cart, the throttle enable switch (TAB), located on the left-hand side of the driving bar has to be kept pressed and the throttle can be rotated to enable acceleration. Direction of the movement is changed by movement of the driving bar, which operates in a fashion similar to the handle of a bicycle. While one person drives the cart, the other person provides verbal directions to move the patient cart system. There is also a provision to move the patient cart manually by shifting the lever to the neutral (N) mode. Once the cart is parked in drive mode, the breaks are automatically engaged.

The instrument arms are numbered from one to three. The arms contain the port clutch and the arm clutch buttons. The port clutch button once pressed allows the proximal half of the arms to move grossly in any direction as long as it is kept pressed. The arm clutch button can be used to adjust the distal portion of the arm. It is activated by a single touch, and once the position is finalized, the clutch button can be pressed again to fix the arm in that position. Each arm is constructed of various pulleys and four motors drive the fine movements of the attached instruments.

The sweet spot indicator is a transverse mark on the proximal part of the camera arm. The sweet spot indicator must be checked for so that the clashing of instruments and the arms can be minimized. Once the marker is set in the range of the sweet spot indicator, the clashing is minimal. Ideally the arm should be placed such that the marker on the arms lies in the center of sweet spot indicator.

Vision Cart

The third part or the vision cart telecasts the surgery on the monitor. It consists of a video monitor which is touch enabled and provides opportunity for interaction by drawing various markers on the screen itself. The vision cart also houses space for the insufflator and electrosurgical cautery. The dual camera control unit (CCU) gets the feed from both the cameras located on the endoscope. It integrates them to create a 3-dimensional image and feeds into the monitor and the surgeon console stereoscopic head. The illuminator is also an integral part of the vision cart, and the cold light source illuminates the dark body cavities similar to as in laparoscopy.

The vision cart is placed close to the patient so as to allow the light, camera, and other cables to lie in easy access but essentially away from the sterile field. Once the location is decided, the cart is locked using the rear wheel locks on the vision cart. The cart must be visible from the master console at all times.

DRAPING THE SURGICAL ROBOT

Sterile drape sets are provided by the manufacturer. The set consists of a camera drape to drape the camera head and two instrument arm drapes. Before draping the arm is splayed and adjusted to the optimum height of the assistant who is draping the arm. The drapes are extracted, and the hand is

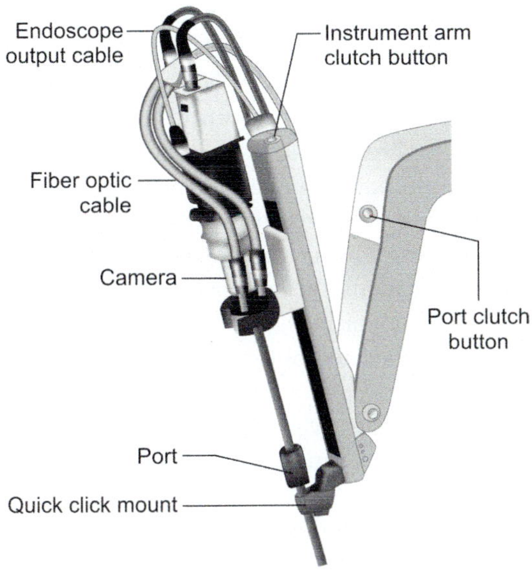

Fig. 5: The camera arm.

placed in the drape to catch hold of the sterile adapter. The drape is held as a sock, and the sterile adapter is placed over the camera arm socket and the drape subsequently spread to accommodate for the endoscope length. The rest of the drape is then opened and spread over the entire arm **(Fig. 5)**. The attached tapes are then applied to fix the drape at every part of the arm. The camera drape is different in that it contains the camera sterile adapter that is made to fit on the corresponding endoscope end. In the end, the endoscope and camera head are draped as far as possible to its CCU and rested on a sterile tray before it can be docked. The instrument arms are draped in a similar fashion except that there is an instrument adapter that needs to be fixed over the corresponding instrument plate on the arm. It is over this instrument adapter that the instrument slides over and locks itself.

DOCKING THE ROBOTIC INSTRUMENTS

Docking is the process of attaching the instrument into the arms and into the ports so that they are ready for action. It is necessary to insert the ports first as required by the surgeon before the draped patient cart is brought in. The ports should be placed 15–20 cm away from the area of interest, and there should be a gap of at least 8–10 centimeters between the various ports. Only the optional assistant port can be placed near to the robotic arm ports, but that distance too should be no <5 cm. The various types of available ports will be discussed in the instrumentation section, but irrespective of their length, the remote center technology allows the instruments to move around a fixed area, thus exerting minimal torque at the port site. Once the ports are in place, the arms are engaged using the clutch buttons to bring the arms close to the ports. The quick click mounts are used to hold these ports in place and move with the movement of the arms. Once all arms have been attached to the respective ports using the quick click mounts, the instruments can be engaged in the respective arms.

In order to load the instruments in the respective arms, the instruments must be in a semi open and neutral position. The instruments are introduced into the ports and slid into the instrument bracket which lies on the proximal aspect of the arm. Once the instrument is correctly engaged, the indicator light will be turned on indicating that the instrument is now ready for use. The guided instrument change is another feature which has been incorporated into the latest generation of surgical robot wherein the robot memorizes the location of the last instrument, and the new instrument which is loaded retains the place of the last instrument once the engagement has been completed. During the guided instrument change, a green light blinks on the respective arm, indicating that this function has been activated.

Docking the camera requires some special considerations. The endoscopic camera is fit into the special plastic adapter that is part of the surgical plastic drape, and the telescope is held with the quick click mount. The most important is that the axis of the port, the camera, and the arm should all lie in the same line, and the line should cross the area of interest. Similarly, the arms should also be at an angle of 45° from each other **(Fig. 6)**. Also, the angle at setup joint two must be about 90°.

BASIC ROBOTIC INSTRUMENTATION (FIG. 6)

Robotic instruments are based on the endowrist technology where four pulley systems help in providing 7 degrees of freedom to the instrument that closely simulate the movements of the human hand. The important and widely used instruments include hot shears, scissors, forceps, graspers, and certain specialized instruments. The most important instrument is the endoscopic camera. The 12-mm endoscope is available in 0° and 30°. An 8-mm endoscope is also available. The camera head which fits over the endoscope has two eyes. There are various controls on the camera head in the form of four buttons. The up and down arrow buttons control the focus, the light button controls the illumination settings, and the last button or the white balance button is common to all cameras.

Instruments available are used through a 5-mm or 8-mm port. 8-mm endowrist instruments are the ones mostly used. These instruments include **(Figs. 7 to 39)**:

- *Monopolar instruments:*
  - Hot shears
  - Cautery hook
  - Cautery spatula
- *Scissors:*
  - Round tip scissors
  - Curved scissors
  - Potts scissors

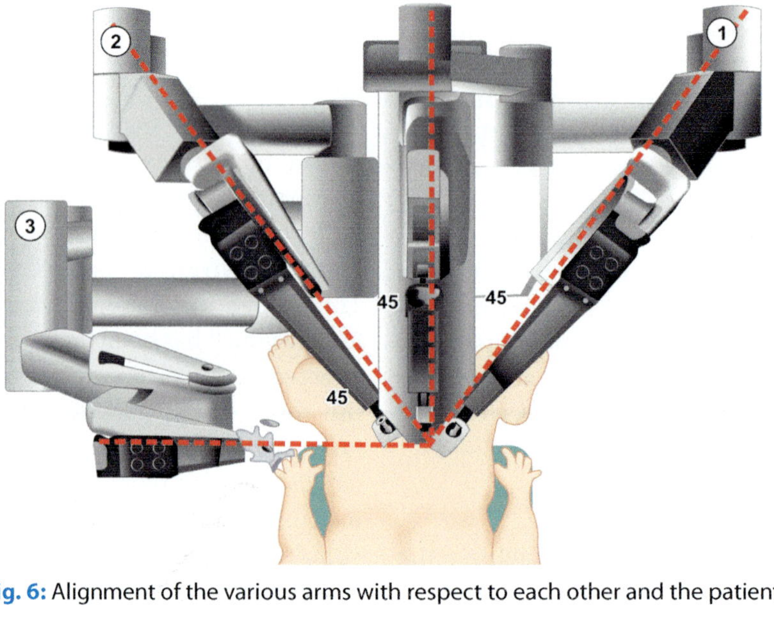

Fig. 6: Alignment of the various arms with respect to each other and the patient.

- *Forceps:*
  - DeBakey forceps
  - Long tip forceps
  - Resano forceps
  - Fine tissue forceps
  - Black diamond micro forceps
  - Tenaculum forceps
- *Graspers:*
  - Prograsp forceps
  - Cobra grasper
  - Cadiere forceps
  - Double fenestrated
  - Grasping retractor (graptor)
- *Needle drivers:*
  - Large
  - Large suture cut
  - Mega
  - Mega suture cut
- *Bipolar cautery instruments:*
  - Maryland bipolar
  - PK dissecting forceps
  - Fenestrated bipolar forceps
  - PreCise™ bipolar forceps
  - Micro bipolar forceps
  - Curved bipolar dissector
- *Other special instruments:*
  - Snap fit scalpel
  - Dual blade retractor
  - Valve hook
  - Pericardial dissector
  - Clip appliers
  - Harmonic shears
  - Vessel sealer
- 5-mm instruments include **(Figs. 40 to 47)**
  - Monopolar cautery
  - Harmonic ACE shears
  - Needle driver
  - Round tip scissors
  - Curved scissors
  - Maryland dissector
  - DeBakey forceps
  - Schertel grasper
  - Bowel grasper.

Ports of 11 cm and 16 cm are available. The 5 cm extra length is suggested for patients with high body mass index (BMI). These ports have a black band engraved in them. When the black band is placed at the level of fascia, then the remote center technology comes into play and any rotation of the arms, and the instrument happen with the black band as the focal point thereby avoiding any unnecessary stress and tension at the level of the fascia.

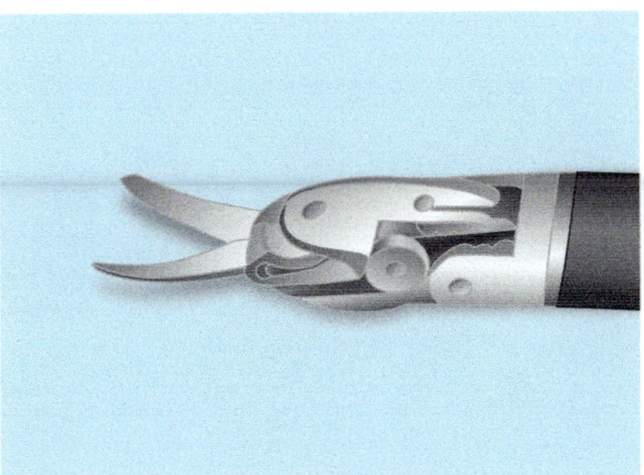

Fig. 7: An 8-mm monopolar curved Hot Shears™.

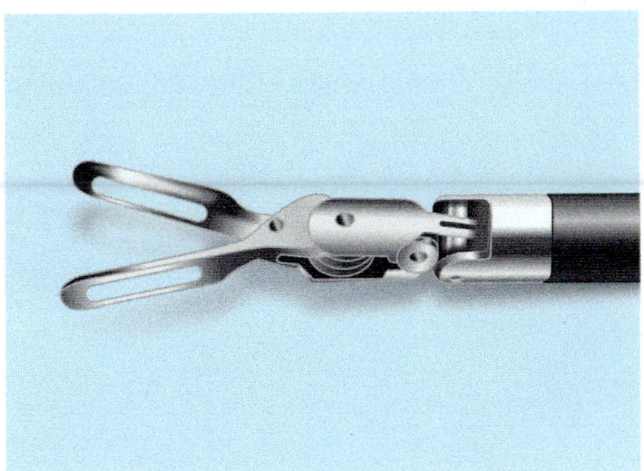

Fig. 8: An 8-mm ProGrasp™ forceps.

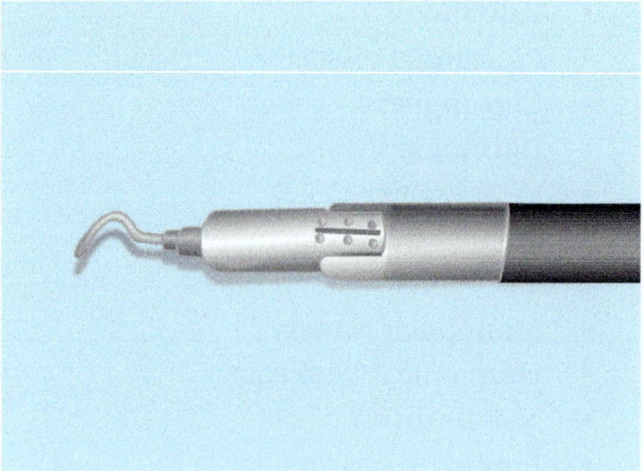

Fig. 9: An 8-mm cautery hook.

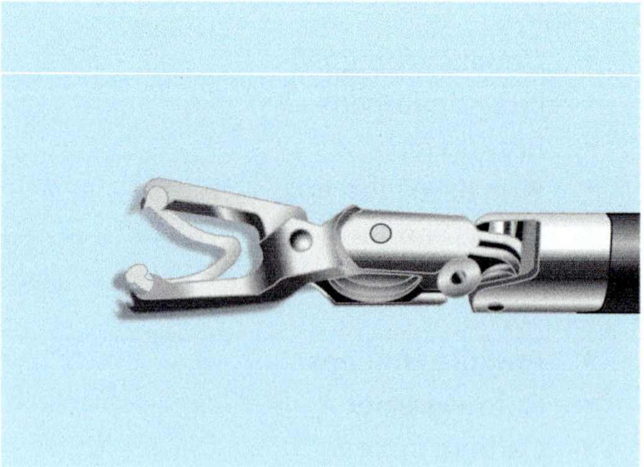

Fig. 12: An 8-mm medium clip applier.

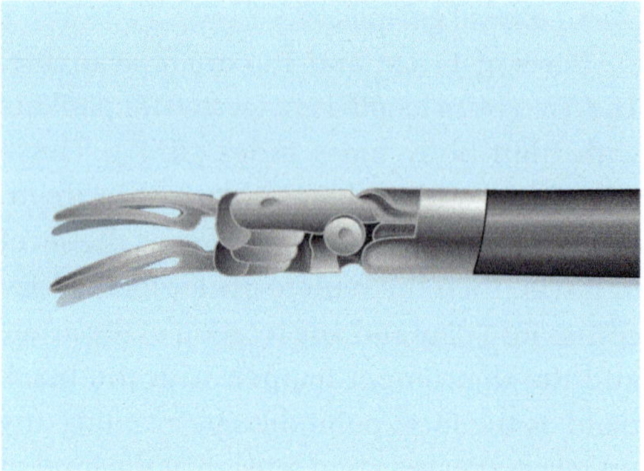

Fig. 10: An 8-mm Maryland bipolar forceps.

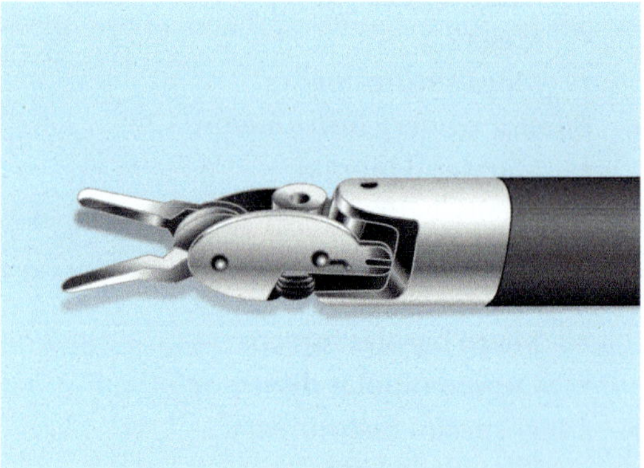

Fig. 13: An 8-mm large needle driver.

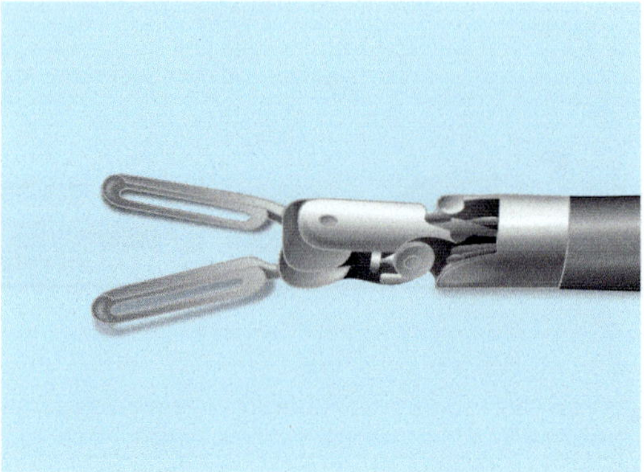

Fig. 11: An 8-mm fenestrated bipolar forceps.

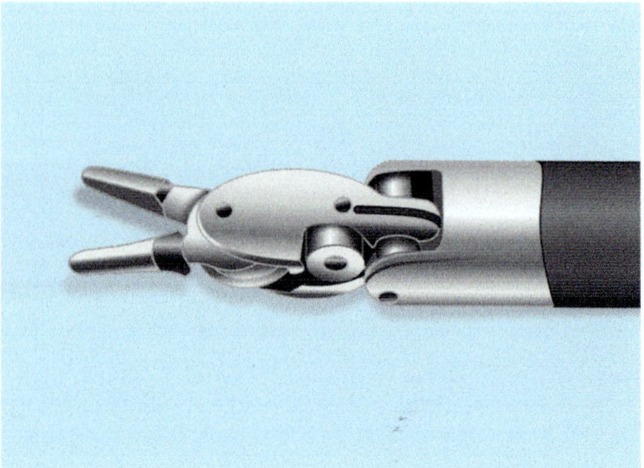

Fig. 14: An 8-mm large SutureCut™ needle driver.

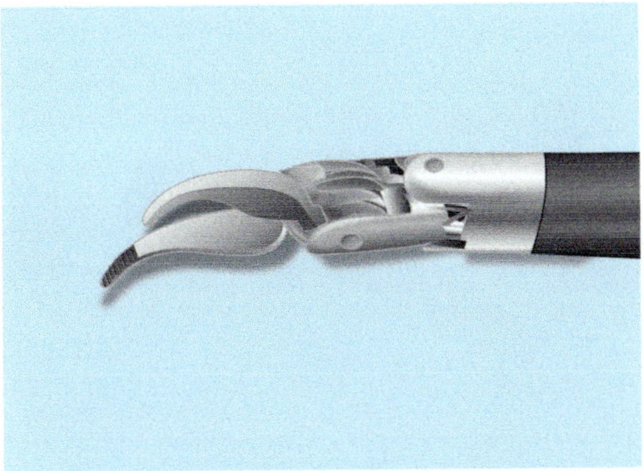

Fig. 15: An 8-mm curved bipolar dissector.

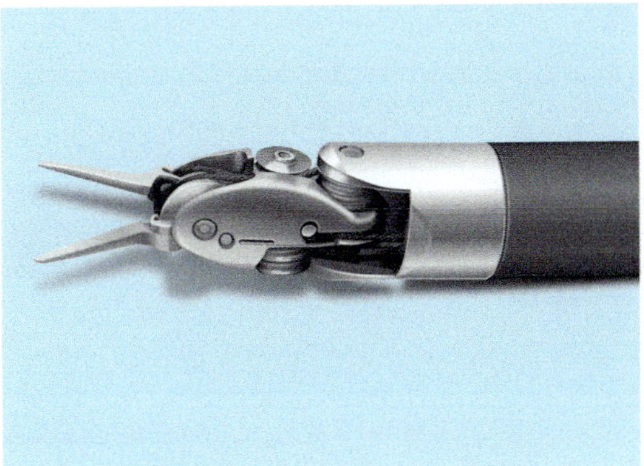

Fig. 16: An 8-mm fine tissue forceps.

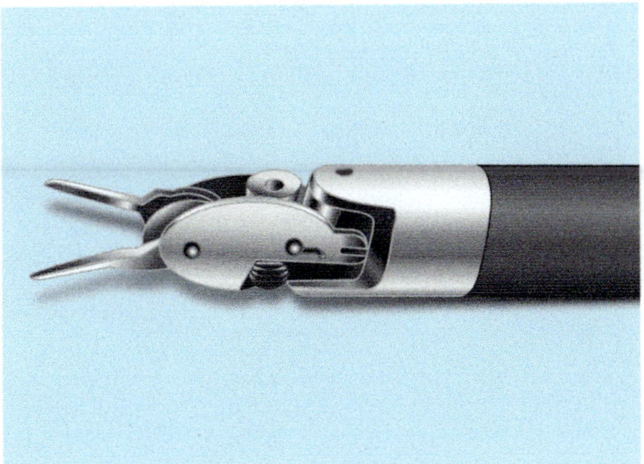

Fig. 17: An 8-mm micro forceps.

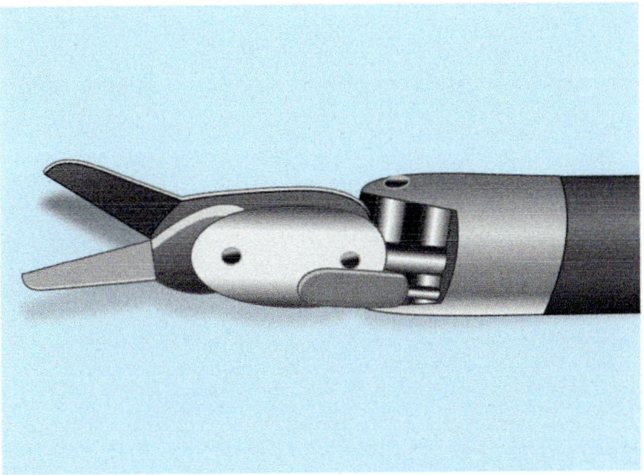

Fig. 18: An 8-mm round tip scissors.

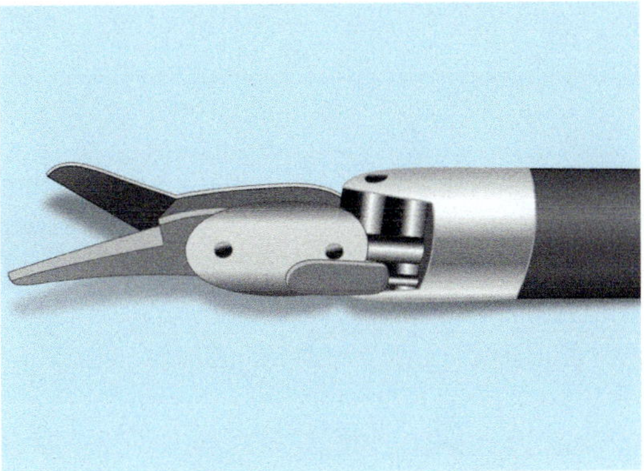

Fig. 19: An 8-mm curved scissors.

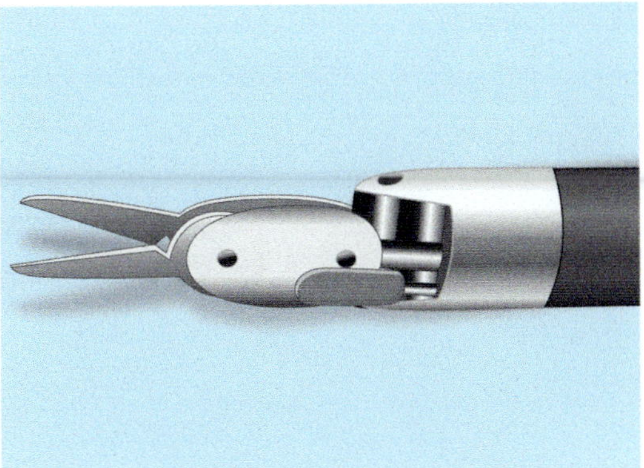

Fig. 20: An 8 mm Potts scissors.

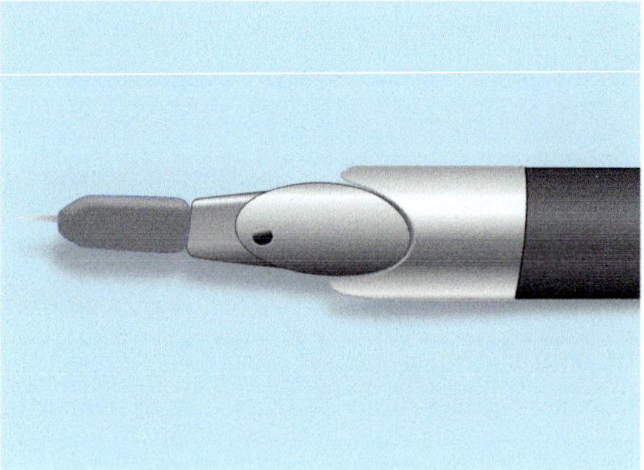

Fig. 21: An 8-mm scalpel instrument.

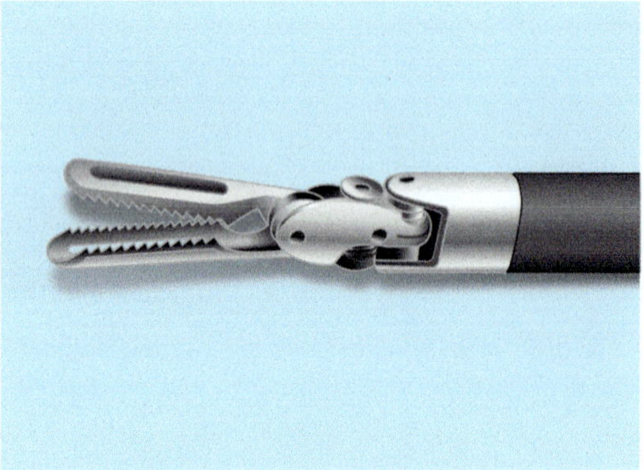

Fig. 22: An 8-mm Cadiere forceps.

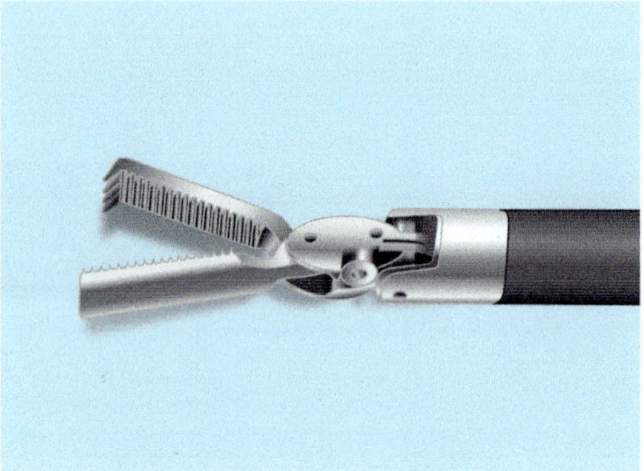

Fig. 23: An 8-mm cobra grasper.

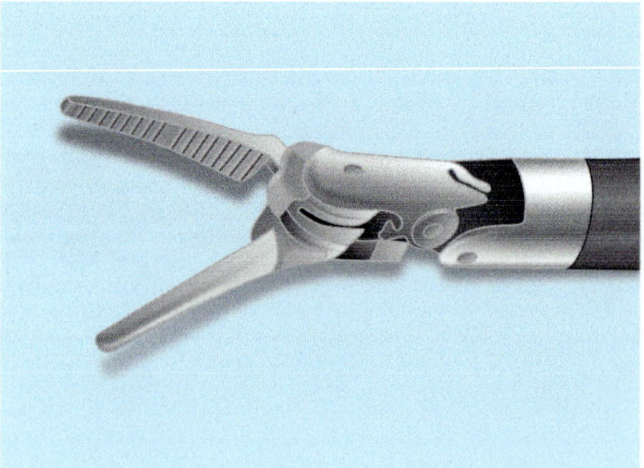

Fig. 24: An 8-mm PK dissecting forceps.

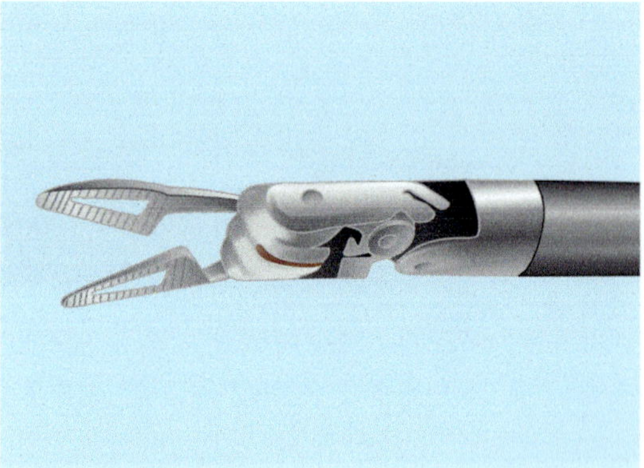

Fig. 25: An 8-mm PreCise™ bipolar forceps.

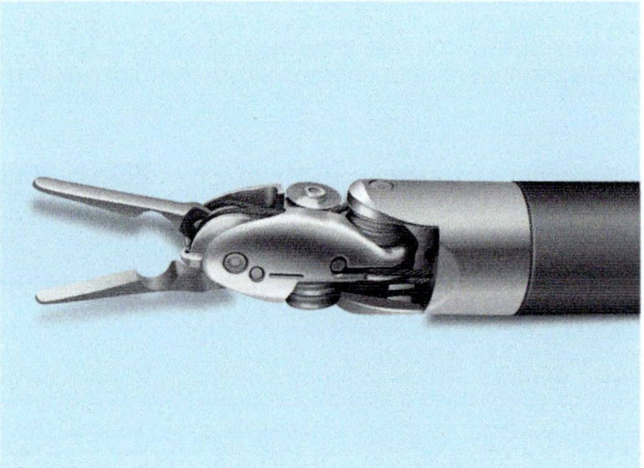

Fig. 26: An 8-mm DeBakey forceps.

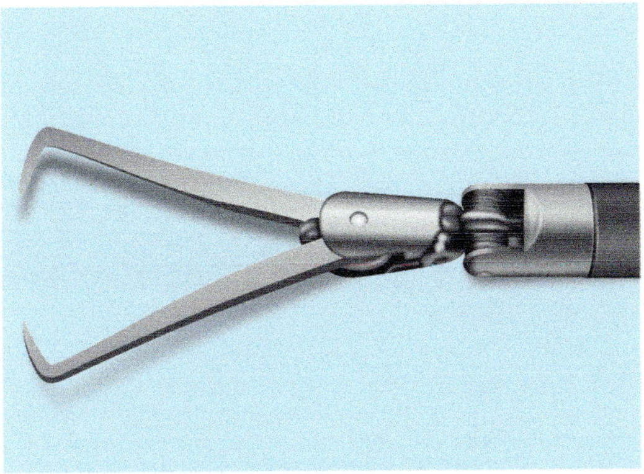

Fig. 27: An 8-mm tenaculum forceps.

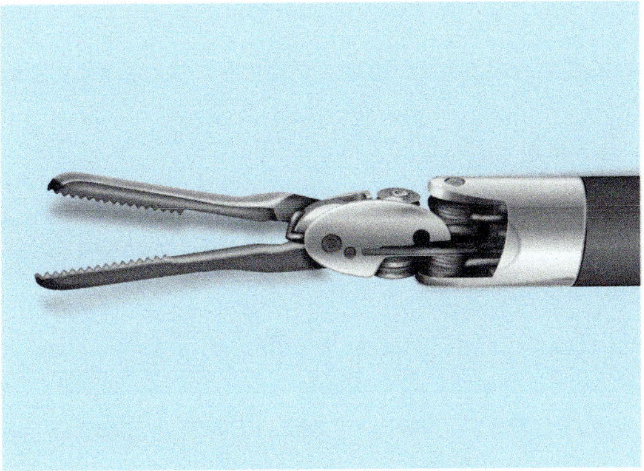

Fig. 28: An 8-mm long tip forceps.

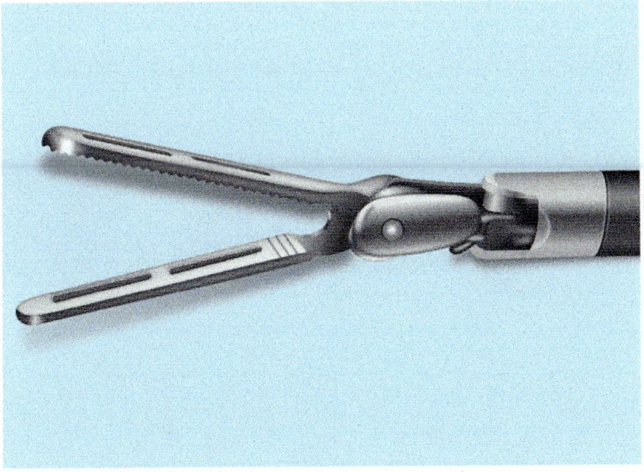

Fig. 29: An 8-mm double fenestrated grasper.

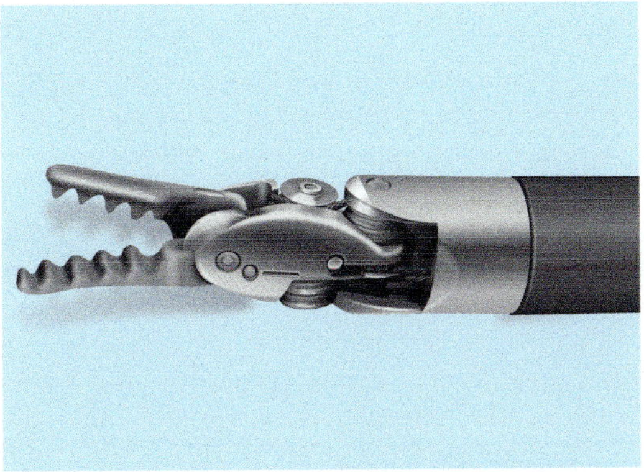

Fig. 30: An 8-mm Resano forceps.

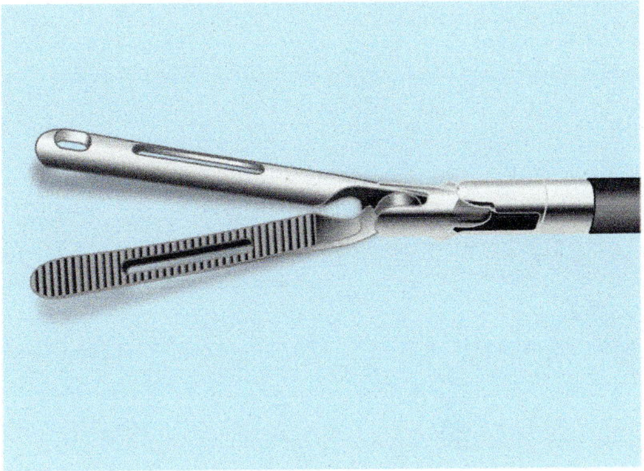

Fig. 31: An 8-mm grasping retractor.

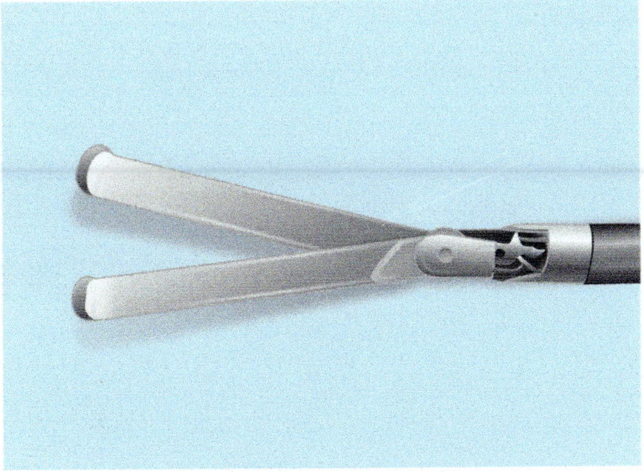

Fig. 32: An 8-mm atrial retractor.

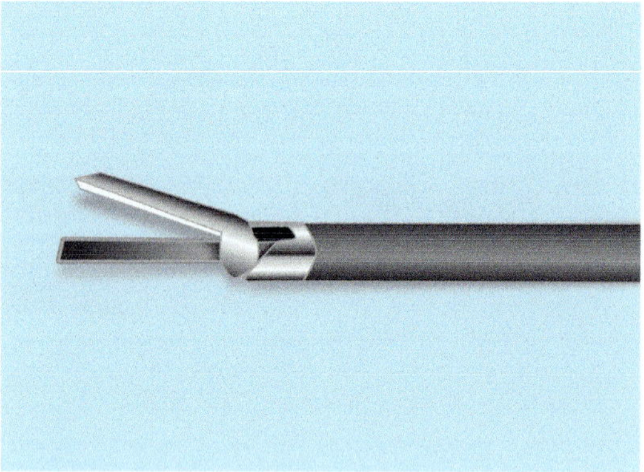

Fig. 33: An 8-mm Harmonic ACE® curved shears.

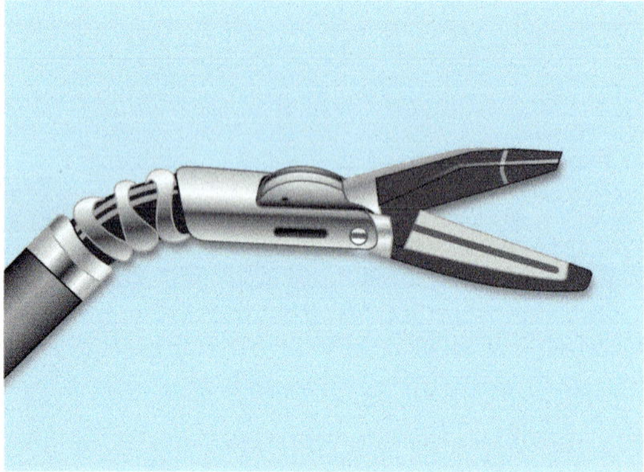

Fig. 34: An 8-mm vessel sealer.

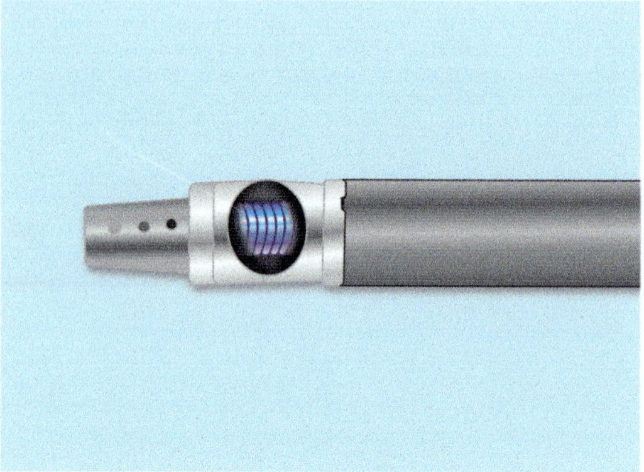

Fig. 35: An 8-mm suction/irrigator.

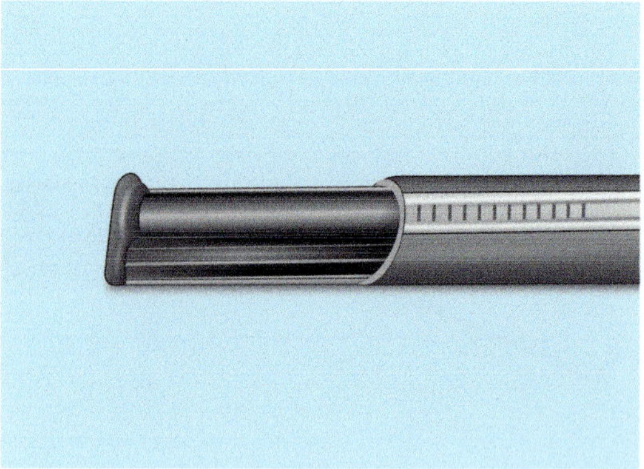

Fig. 36: An 8-mm EndoPass delivery instrument.

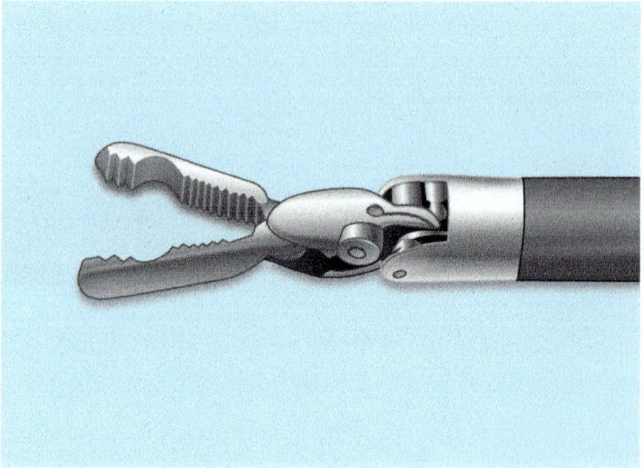

Fig. 37: An 8-mm cardiac probe grasper.

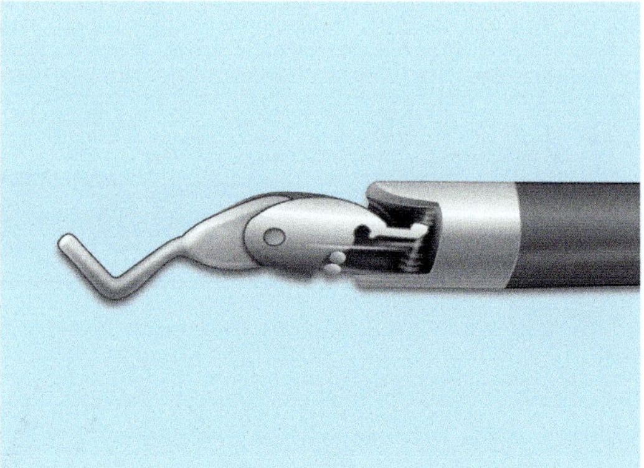

Fig. 38: An 8-mm valve hook.

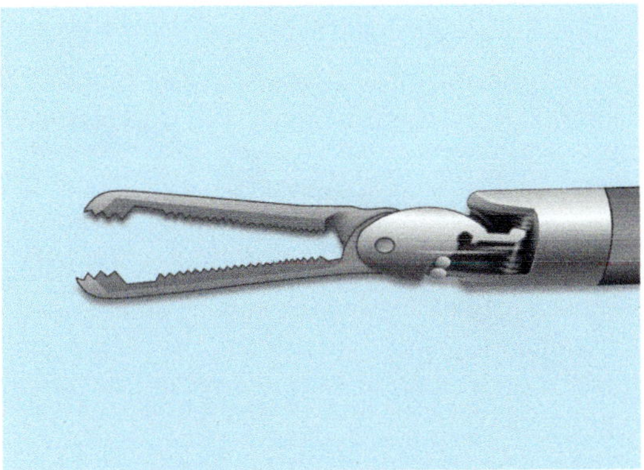

Fig. 39: An 8-mm pericardial dissector.

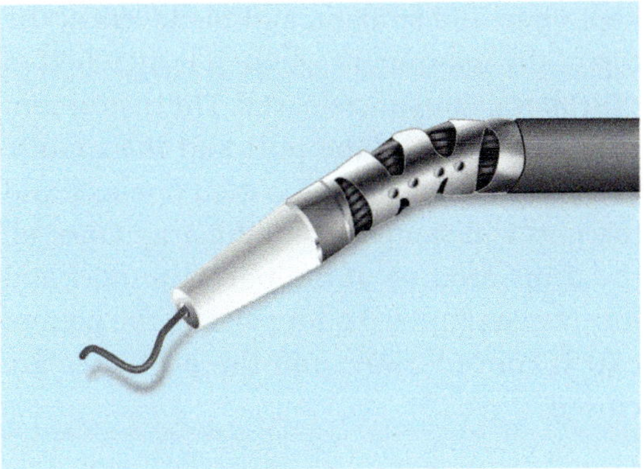

Fig. 40: A 5-mm monopolar cautery.

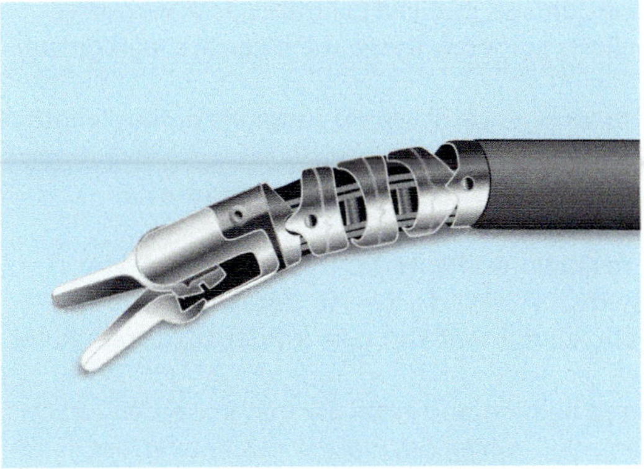

Fig. 41: A 5-mm needle driver.

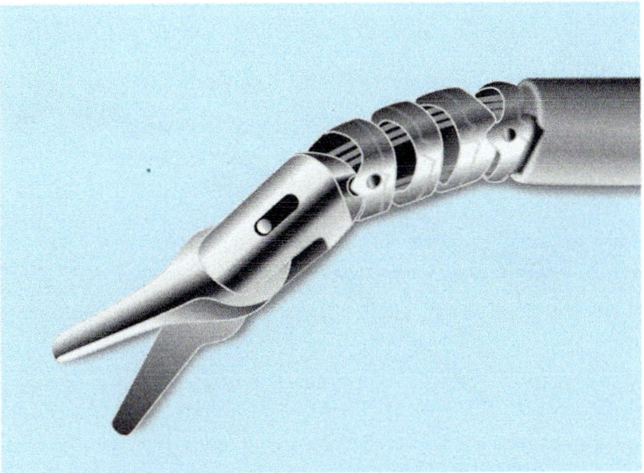

Fig. 42: A 5-mm round tip scissors.

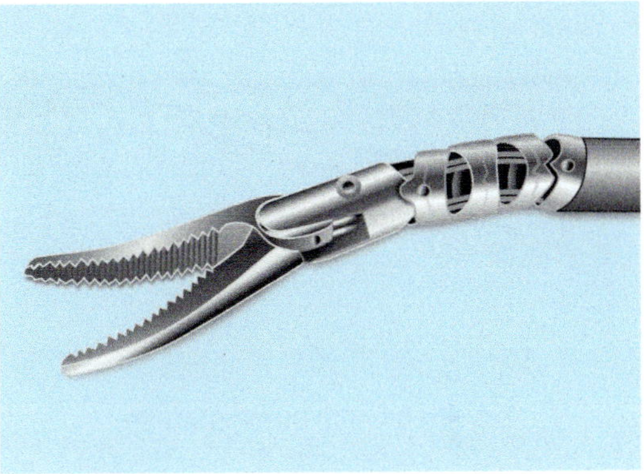

Fig. 43: A 5-mm Maryland dissector.

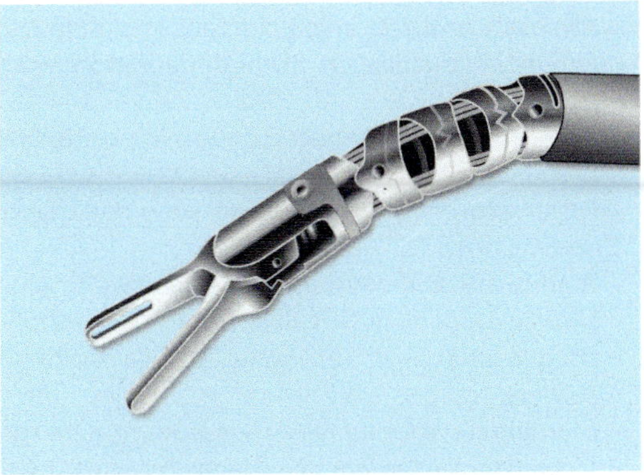

Fig. 44: A 5-mm DeBakey forceps.

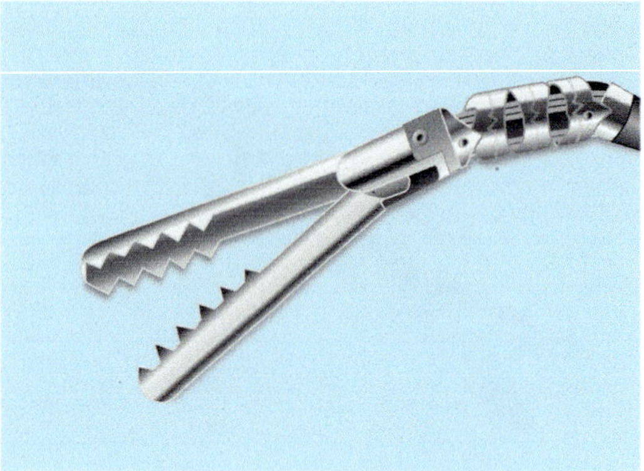

Fig. 45: A 5-mm Schertel grasper.

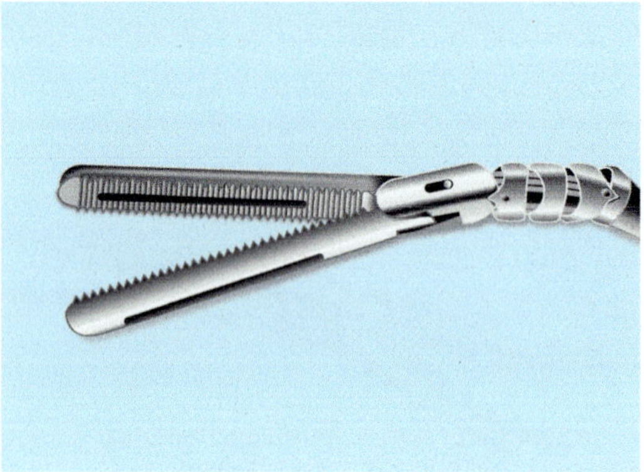

Fig. 46: A 5-mm bowel grasper.

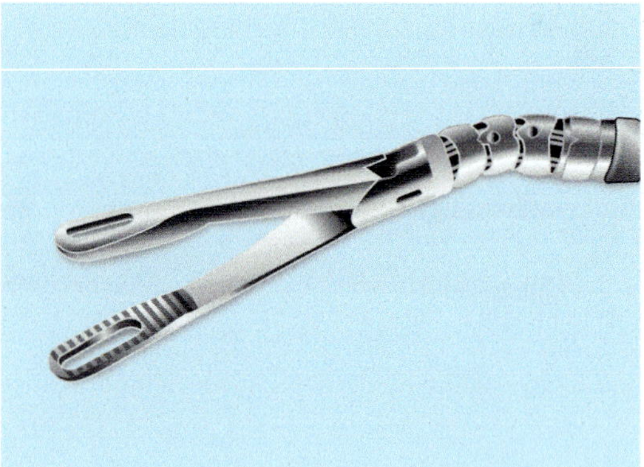

Fig. 47: A 5-mm thoracic grasper.

UNDOCKING

To undock the robot, the instrument is first kept open and straight, and the levers at the top of the instrument where it is attached to the robotic arms are released. The instrument is then slid out of the port and the robotic arm. Quick click mount is then opened, and the port is dislodged from the arm. Once all the arms are free of the port cannulas and have been removed under vision, the patient cart is moved away, and the port sites are closed.

KEY POINTS

Key Points on advantages and disadvantages of robotic surgery:

Advantages:

- *Precision and accuracy:* Robotic systems offer enhanced precision for complex and delicate procedures.
- *Minimally invasive:* Smaller incisions result in less tissue damage, reduced pain, and faster recovery.
- *Enhanced visualization:* 3D high-definition imaging allows surgeons to see the surgical site in greater detail.
- *Reduced surgeon fatigue:* Ergonomic positioning reduces physical strain on surgeons during lengthy procedures.
- *Faster recovery:* Shorter hospital stays and quicker recovery times due to less invasive surgery.

Disadvantages:

- *High cost:* Robotic systems are expensive to acquire, maintain, and operate.
- *Limited availability:* Not all hospitals have robotic systems, restricting access to certain patients.
- *Longer setup time:* Setting up and calibrating robotic equipment can take longer than traditional surgery.
- *Learning curve for surgeons:* Surgeons require specialized training, and initial use may impact efficiency.
- *Limited tactile feedback:* Surgeons have less tactile sensation, which can make it harder to assess tissue resistance.

CHAPTER 26

Basic Endoscopy

Raman Tanwar, Sudhir Kumar Jain, Mrunal Bharat Kshirsagar

"In the modern Era it is highly desirable to learn endoscopic techniques atleat diagnostic"

INTRODUCTION

The role of endoscopy in surgery is continuously evolving, and it has since its inception remained an essential surgical skill. Endoscopy at present is both diagnostic and therapeutic in many cases and miniaturization of the scopes and technological advances in terms of digitalization, addition of 3D vision and improved flexibility have allowed widespread use throughout the globe. Three important endoscopic procedures that we will acquaint the readers within this chapter are the upper gastrointestinal (GI) endoscopy, the lower GI endoscopy, and cystoscopy (with rigid scope) **(Fig. 1)**.

UPPER GASTROINTESTINAL ENDOSCOPY (FIGS. 2 AND 3)

Anatomy and Physiology of Digestive System

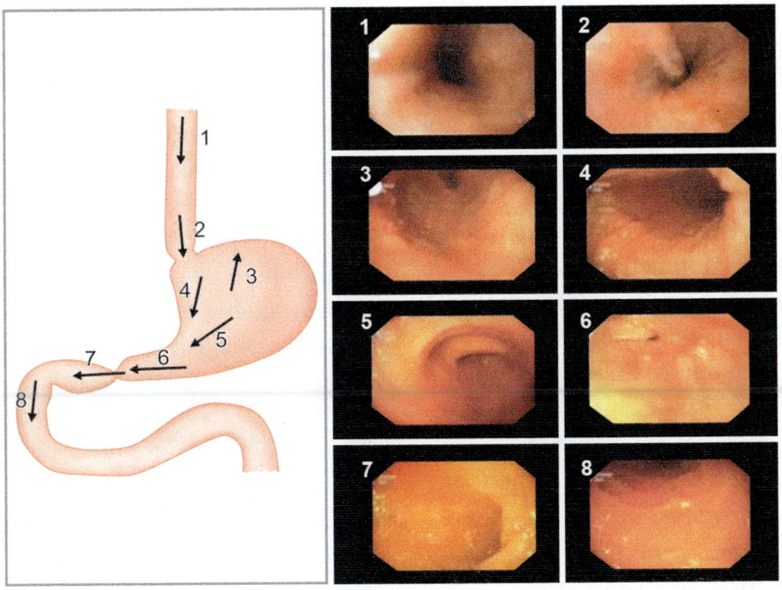

Fig. 1: Parts of digestive system.

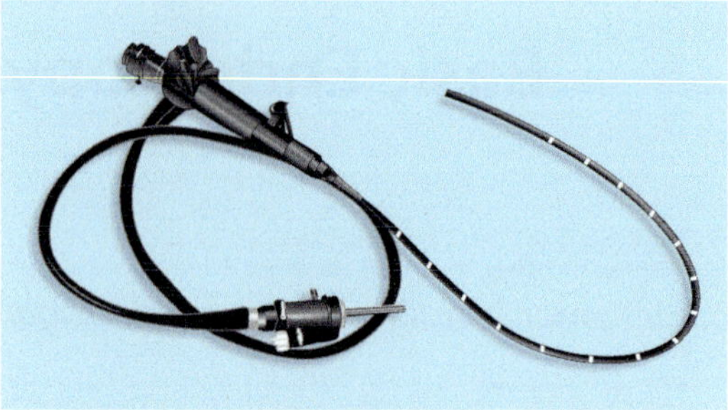

Fig. 2: Upper gastrointestinal (GI) endoscope.

Esophagus

- *Location:* Posterior to the trachea
- *Starts:* Distal to the cricoid cartilage
- *Ends:* Cardiac orifice of the stomach
- *Dimensions:*
  - *Diameter:* 4–6 mm
  - *Length:*
    - *Term infant:* 9–10 cm
    - *Adult:* Approximately 25 cm
- *Mucosa transition:* From pale to reddish pink at the Z line (esophagus to gastric epithelium).

Stomach

- *Location:* Beneath the diaphragm
- *Distance from incisors:* Approximately 40 cm in adults
- *Structural parts:*
  - *Gastric cardia:* Where esophagus enters the stomach
  - *Fundus:* Upper portion, visible in retroflexed endoscopic view
  - *Stomach body:* Main portion
  - *Incisura:* Along lesser curvature, separates body from antrum
  - *Antrum:* Lower part of stomach
- *Endoscopic features:*
  - *Transition from body to antrum:* Rugae to flat mucosa
- *Pylorus:* Muscular opening to duodenum bulb

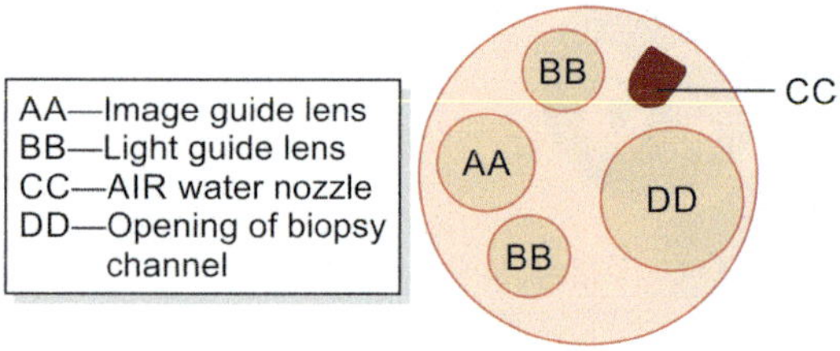

Fig. 3: Scope anatomy.

Duodenum

- *Extent:* From pylorus to duodenojejunal angle
- *Duodenum bulb:* Expanded region immediately after pylorus
- *Course:*
  - *C-shaped loop:*
    - *Posterior and right:* 2.5 cm
    - *Descending portion:* 7.5–10 cm
    - *Anterior and left:* Approximately 2.5 cm
- *Connection:* Joins jejunum at ligament of Treitz

INDICATIONS FOR UPPER GASTROINTESTINAL ENDOSCOPY

Diagnostic Indications

- Persistent upper abdominal pain or pain with alarming symptoms (e.g., weight loss and anorexia)
- Dysphagia, odynophagia, or feeding problems
- Intractable or chronic symptoms of gastroesophageal reflux disease (GERD)
- Unexplained irritability in a child
- Persistent vomiting of unknown cause or hematemesis (vomiting blood)
- Iron deficiency anemia with suspected chronic GI bleeding when upper GI source is suspected after normal colonoscopy
- Chronic diarrhea or malabsorption
- Assessment of acute injury after caustic ingestion

- Surveillance for malignancy in high-risk patients (e.g., polyposis syndromes, previous caustic ingestion, and Barrett esophagus).

Therapeutic Indications

- Foreign body removal
- Dilation or stenting of strictures
- Esophageal variceal ligation
- Control of upper GI bleeding
- Placement of feeding or draining tubes
- Management of achalasia (e.g., botulinum toxin injection and balloon dilation).

CONTRAINDICATIONS FOR UPPER GASTROINTESTINAL ENDOSCOPY

Absolute Contraindications

- Perforated bowel
- Peritonitis
- Toxic megacolon in an unstable patient.

Relative Contraindications

- Severe neutropenia
- Coagulopathy
- Severe thrombocytopenia or impaired platelet function
- Increased risk of perforation (e.g., connective tissue disorders, recent bowel surgery, and bowel obstruction)
- Aneurysm of the abdominal or iliac aorta.

ESOPHAGOGASTRODUODENOSCOPY PROCEDURE STEPS

- *Positioning the patient:*
    - Place the patient in the left lateral position.
    - Apply buccopharyngeal and hypopharyngeal topical anesthesia.
    - Insert a mouthpiece between the teeth or gums.
- *Inserting the endoscope:*
    - Advance the flexible tip of the endoscope carefully, staying in the midline and at the interface between the tongue and hypopharyngeal mucosa.
    - Visualize structures such as the tongue, uvula, epiglottis, and cricoarytenoid cartilages.
    - Guide the endoscope past the cricoarytenoid cartilages to the cricopharyngeus muscle, which closes off the esophagus.
    - Apply gentle local pressure and ask the patient to swallow to help pass the endoscope into the cervical esophagus.
- *Maintaining visualization:* Use insufflation and suction intermittently to keep the esophagus distended and ensure the endoscope remains centered in the esophageal lumen.
- *Navigating the esophagus:* Note the first extrinsic compression from the left main bronchus and the subsequent pulsations of the heart.
- *Identifying the gastroesophageal junction:*
    - Identify the gastroesophageal junction by the distinct change in mucosal color and texture.
    - Gently advance the endoscope beyond the upper gastroesophageal junction.
- *Examining the stomach:*
    - Aspirate the gastric fluid completely once inside the stomach.
    - Rotate the tip of the endoscope to examine the anterior and posterior walls of the stomach.
    - Advance the scope along the greater curvature of the stomach, examining all structures.
- *Visualizing the duodenum:*
    - Gently advance the scope beyond the pylorus to visualize the first part of the

    - duodenum, including the superior duodenal angle.
    - If necessary, further advance the scope to view the second part of the duodenum.
- *Performing the J maneuver:* Pull the scope back and perform a J maneuver by angling the scope 180° upward to visualize the proximal curvatures and fundus of the stomach.
- *Completing the examination:* Gently withdraw the scope to complete the examination.

CLINICAL PRACTICE UPDATE ON ESOPHAGOGASTRODUODENOSCOPY QUALITY

- *Optimization of endoscopic detection:*
    - Enhance mucosal cleansing.
    - Improve visualization time.
- *Evaluation of suspected premalignancy:*
    - Utilize image-enhanced endoscopy.
    - Follow standardized biopsy protocols and document findings.
- *Postprocedure follow-up:*
    - Test for *Helicobacter pylori* and manage treatment.
    - Determine the need and timing for subsequent endoscopic surveillance.
    - Manage medications, including the timing for resuming antithrombotics.

Patient and instrument preparation:

- Overnight fasting is mandatory.
- The patient is adequately counseled regarding the procedure in the outpatient as well as in the endoscopy suite.
- Lignocaine gargle or spray can be used for topical anesthesia of the pharynx and hypopharynx and sedation must be used for anxious patients.
- A mouthpiece is placed between teeth or gums.

Position

The patient lies down in a lateral decubitus position.

Steps

- The patient lies in the left lateral position after buccopharyngeal, and hypopharyngeal topical anesthesia has been applied. A mouthpiece is installed between the teeth or gums, and the flexible tip of the endoscope is advanced, taking care to stay in the midline and at the interface between the tongue and hypopharyngeal mucosa **(Fig. 4A)**. Tongue, uvula, epiglottis, and cricoarytenoid cartilages are seen. Passing beside the midline, the cricoarytenoid cartilages are passed and the tip of the endoscope stops on the cricopharyngeus which closes the entry to the esophagus **(Fig. 4B)**. Gentle local pressure while asking the patient to swallow allows the tip of the endoscope to pass into the cervical esophagus **(Figs. 4A to E)**.
- Insufflation and suction are intermittently used to keep the esophagus distended while the endoscope is kept in the center of the esophageal lumen.
- First extrinsic compression encountered is compression by the left main bronchus, and subsequently the pulsations of the heart are appreciated.
- The gastroesophageal junction is then identified by the distinct change in color and texture of the mucosa, and the scope is gently negotiated beyond the upper gastroesophageal junction.
- Once inside the stomach, the gastric fluid is aspirated completely.
- Tip of the scope is rotated to examine the anterior and posterior walls of the stomach.

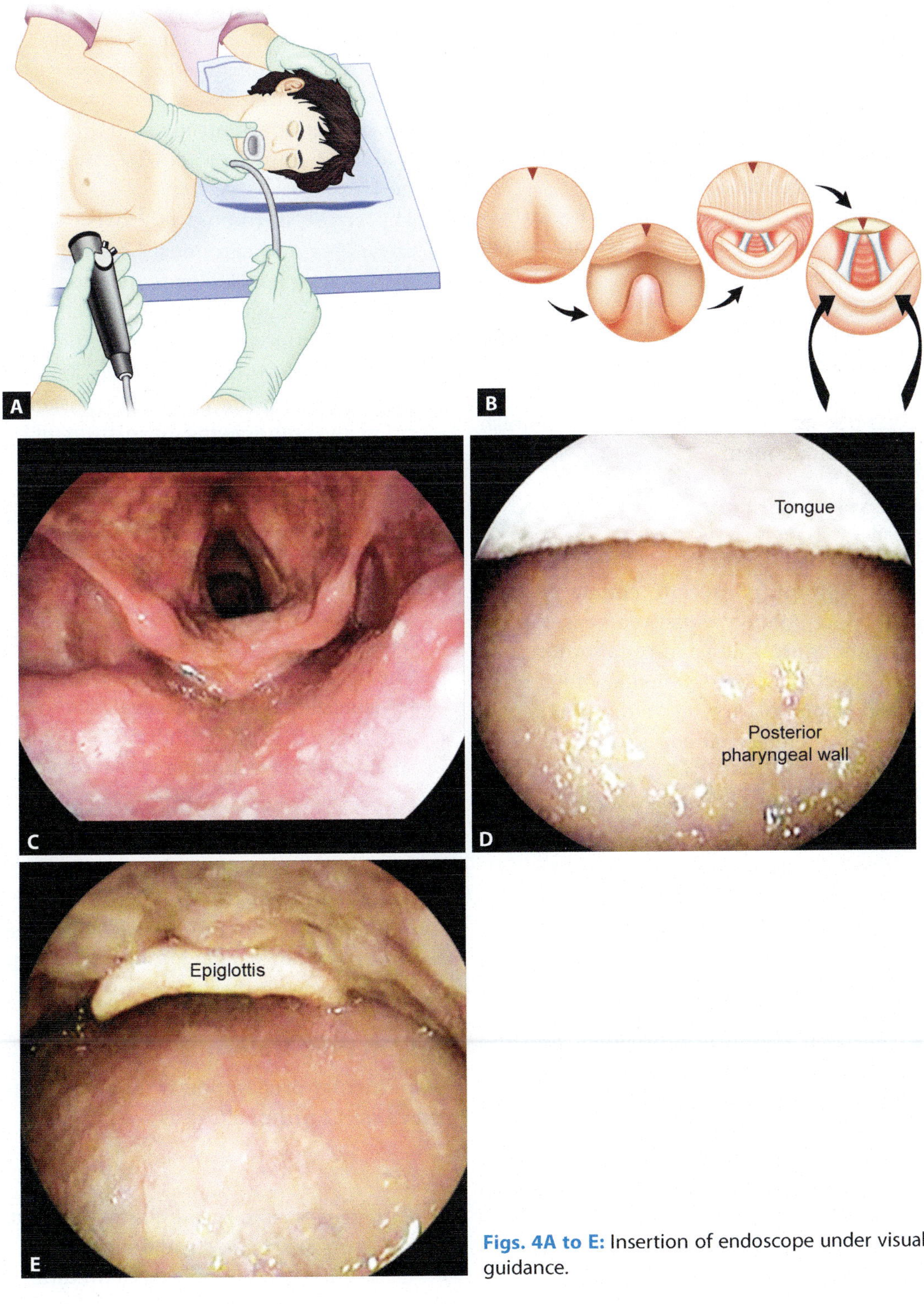

Figs. 4A to E: Insertion of endoscope under visual guidance.

- Scope is advanced along the greater curvature of the stomach while examining all structures.
- Scope is gently negotiated beyond the pylorus to visualize the first part of duodenum including the superior duodenal angle.
- If indicated the scope may be further advanced to visualize the second part of the duodenum
- Scope is pulled back, and the J maneuver is performed by complete 180° upward angulation to visualize the proximal curvatures and fundus.
- The scope is gently pulled back to finish the examination.

COLONOSCOPY

Preparation

About 100 mL phosphate enema without dietary preparation usually suffices in most patients. More extensive preparation may be needed in selected patients with chronic constipation or stricture. Mild sedation may be administered in patients to allay anxiety.

Position

Left lateral position. If there is a difficulty in negotiation, one can change to other positions such as supine or prone.

Steps

- Digital examination of the rectum is performed.
- Perianal region is lubricated, and the scope is gently inserted **(Fig. 5)**.
- Air is insufflated to obtain a view of the intestinal mucosa.
- Scope is pushed keeping the lumen in view at all times, and instrument should be pulled back repeatedly after passing any major bend in order to straighten the scope.
- *N Loop management:* N Loop is formed on reaching the junction of sigmoid and descending colon. The scope is passed into the descending colon and hooked retroperitoneally, and the scope is moved out 20–30 cm to straighten the loop.
- The scope is rotated clockwise while advancing and care must be taken that the distance traveled by scope should be equal to the length of scope inserted.
- Entry into the ascending colon beyond the hepatic flexure again requires looping the scope into the proximal transverse colon and withdrawing the instrument by 30–50 cm.
- Pressure may be applied in the left iliac fossa to prevent the formation of a loop in the sigmoid colon.
- The hepatic flexure is a 180% turn and as soon as the ascending colon is visualized, it is shortened by aspiration and deflated. The scope is subsequently inserted further to visualize the ileocecal valve.
- The scope is gently withdrawn using the single-handed technique.

CYSTOSCOPY (FIG. 6)

Cystoscopy is an important but invasive tool available to the urologist. It offers a diagnostic and therapeutic tool and is performed as a day care procedure under local anesthesia or regional spinal anesthesia.

Patient Preparation

No particular preparation is required apart from a sterile urine culture.

Steps

- Patient is placed in lithotomy position, and parts are cleaned and draped.
- Lignocaine jelly is instilled per urethra.

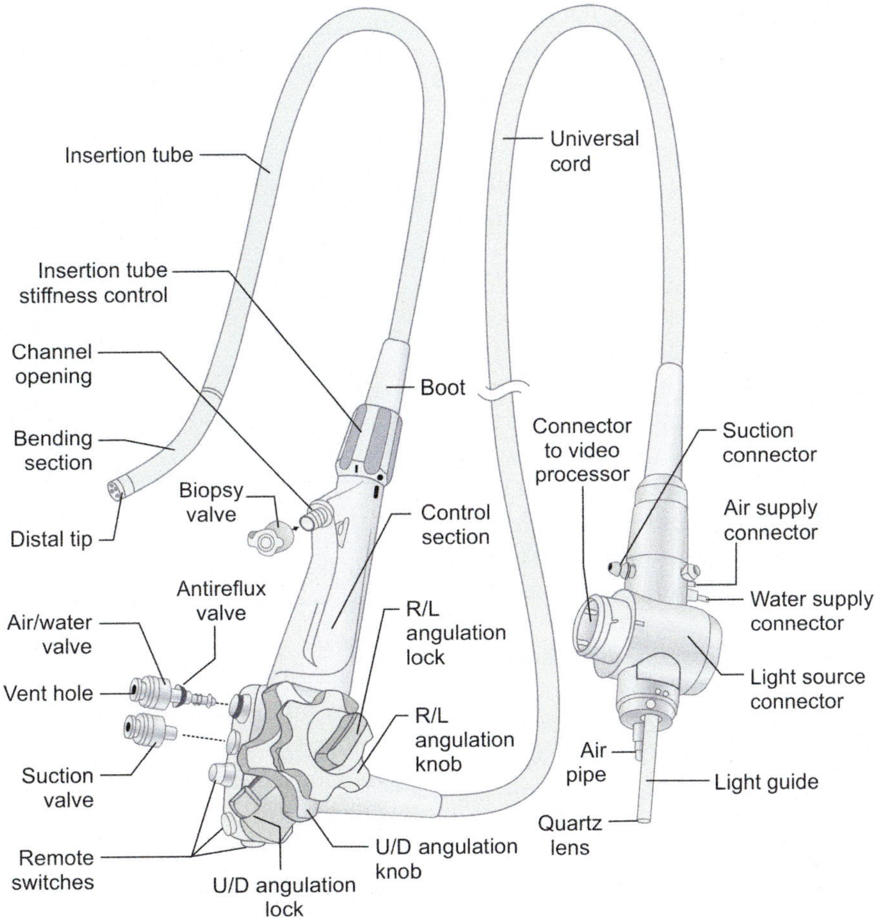

Fig. 5: Colonoscope. (R/L: right/left; U/D: up/down)

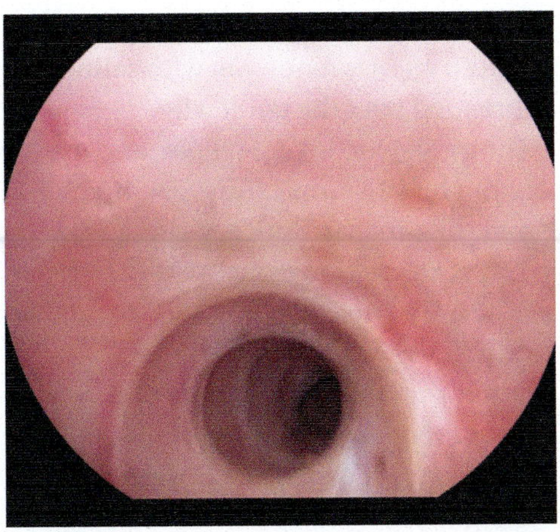

Fig. 6: Urethroscopy showing urethral stricture.

- The cystoscope, bridge, and sheath are assembled and connected to a light source and camera.
- Irrigation is connected to the inlet.
- Cystoscope is introduced into the urethra while keeping the penis stretched.
- The cystoscope is advanced while making a note of the caliber, condition of urethral mucosa, and any associated anomalies
- Cystoscope is advanced till the membranous narrowing is reached and the patient is asked to relax, and flow of irrigation may be increased to gently negotiate beyond the membranous

urethra. At this conjuncture, the operator has to dip the entire scope to negotiate the bulbomembranous angle. (in the male patient follow steps 7–9).

- The scope now enters the prostatic urethra, and the grade of prostatic enlargement and length of the prostatic urethra are noted.
- Scope is negotiated beyond the bladder neck into the bladder by further depressing the scope.
- Within the bladder, the entire cavity is examined in a sectoral fashion starting from the trigone area and subsequently tracing the ureteric orifices on each side. The condition of the mucosa and back pressure changes if any must be assessed.
- Efflux of urine and peristalsis is appreciated on each side.
- Lateral walls are subsequently visualized from the neck to the dome.
- The scope may be rotated 180% to visualize the dome of the bladder, which is identified by the bubbles of air occupying the region.
- Anterior wall of the bladder, especially the region proximal to the neck, is difficult to visualize without exerting some pressure using the other hand over the abdomen.
- The bladder is then emptied partially, and the scope is removed gently under vision while measuring the prostatic urethra using the finger as a guide to mark the initial point.

DOUBLE-J STENTING (FIG. 7)

Common indications for double-J (DJ) stenting are:

- To relieve ureteric obstruction due to any pathology.
- To prevent steinstrasse after extracorporeal shock wave lithotripsy (ESWL) of the stone is more than 2 cm.

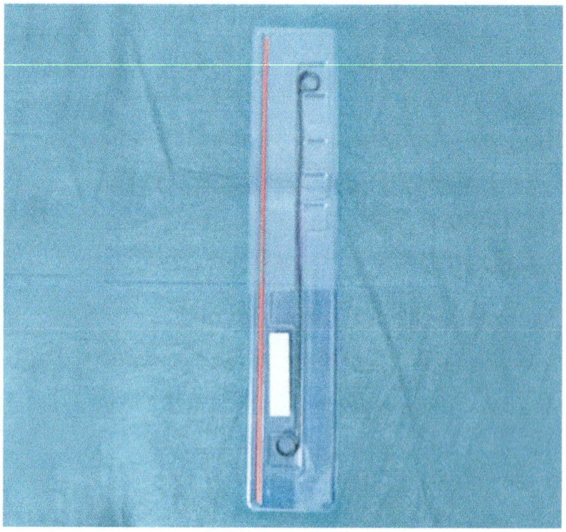

Fig. 7: Double-J stent.

- During complex pelvic surgery, ureters can be stented with self-illuminating stents, which makes identification of ureter easy.
- After any endoscopic urological procedures, e.g., ureteroscopy (URS), percutaneous nephrolithotomy (PCNL), then a DJ stent is inserted.

Steps for Double-J Stenting

- The desired orifice to be stented is visualized, and guidewire is negotiated through the working channel into the orifice till about 20–25 cm.
- The DJ stent is made wet with saline and is threaded over the guidewire.
- The guidewire is kept taught, and the stent is pushed through the working channel and the ureteric orifice.
- The various graduations on the stent are noted as the stent passes through the orifice.
- Once the entire length of the stent has traversed the working channel of the cystoscope, a pusher is threaded over the guidewire, and the remaining length of the stent is pushed such that the last

graduated mark also crosses the ureteric orifice.

- The scope is now brought back to the bladder. neck and if the stent has been adequately pushed the junction of the stent and the pusher will be visible.
- At this conjuncture, the guidewire is pulled keeping the junction in vision.
- Once the entire guidewire has been pulled, the vesical end of the stent will coil upon itself, leaving the pusher free which can be subsequently withdrawn.

KEY POINTS

- With the advances in design of endoscopy it has become very easy to learn endoscopic techniques.
- Endoscopy can diagnose many unsuspecting conditions and many of then can be treated endoscopicallt.

Index

Page number followed by *f* refer to figure, and *t* refer to table.

T

U

V

W

X

Y

Z